MW00844924

# Laser Systems Engineering

# Laser Systems Engineering

**Keith J. Kasunic**

**SPIE PRESS**
Bellingham, Washington USA

Library of Congress Cataloging-in-Publication Data

Names: Kasunic, Keith J., author.
Title: Laser systems engineering / Keith J. Kasunic.
Description: Bellingham, Washington : SPIE Press, [2016]
Identifiers: LCCN 2016025819 | ISBN 9781510604261 (hard cover) | ISBN 151060426X (hard cover) | ISBN 9781510604278 (pdf) | ISBN 1510604278 (pdf) | ISBN 9781510604285 (epub) | ISBN 1510604286 (epub) | ISBN 9781510604292 (kindle/mobi) | ISBN 1510604294 (kindle/mobi)
Subjects: LCSH: Lasers. | Optical engineering.
Classification: LCC TA1675 .K37 2016 | DDC 621.36/6–dc23 LC record available at https://lccn.loc.gov/2016025819

Published by

SPIE
P.O. Box 10
Bellingham, Washington 98227-0010 USA
Phone: +1 360.676.3290
Fax: +1 360.647.1445
Email: books@spie.org
Web: http://spie.org



Cover photograph courtesy of Shutterstock, Inc.

Printed in the United States of America.
First Printing.
For updates to this book, visit http://spie.org and type "PM271" in the search field.

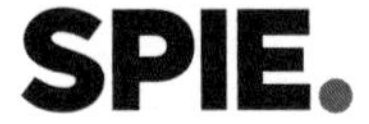

# Contents

# Preface

How did it happen that more than 50 years after the invention of the laser, almost all of the books that have the word "laser" in their title emphasize the design of the lasers themselves, rather than the development of optical systems that incorporate these unique sources of light? A quick web search reveals thousands of books that focus on laser design; very few books, however—*Building Electro-Optical Systems* by Hobbs, *Laser Communications in Space* by Lambert and Casey, *Field Guide to Lidar* by McManamon, and *Electro-Optical Instrumentation* by Donati, for example—address aspects of the design and engineering of laser systems.

As a result, and aside from the many books available for fiber-optic communication systems, the design of laser systems that use free-space optics—manufacturing, biomedical systems, laser radar, laser displays, and so on—is still a hit-or-miss proposition, with little systematic guidance available. The purpose of this book is to take an initial step in addressing this gap.

The perspective taken to do this—that of the laser systems engineer—is sometimes thought of as "designing the right laser" versus "designing the laser right." Unfortunately, this approach is both incomplete and overly centered on the laser designer's goal of designing the laser right. Designing (or selecting) the right laser—i.e., one that meets system-level requirements—is certainly key, but designing the right optical, scanning, and detector subsystems is equally important.

Starting with a description of what the "right" laser might look like, this book addresses all of these topics. Laser selection will depend on the application, with Chapter 2 reviewing the available laser types (semiconductor, solid-state, fiber, and gas) in the context of what makes them uniquely suited to meet specific requirements such as average power, peak power, linewidth, power consumption, cost, size, and so on.

Chapter 3 then looks at Gaussian beam propagation and associated non-idealities for aberrated and higher-order beams; Chapter 4 uses these concepts to develop the details of the optical subsystem, including the unique properties of Gaussian-beam focusing, as well as truncation, aberrations, surface figure, surface ripple, surface roughness, surface quality, material absorption, back-reflections, optical coatings, and laser damage threshold.

In addition to the laser and optical subsystems, scanning and beam control are required for directing photons onto a biomedical specimen, manufacturing workpiece, projection screen, or target. The scanning technologies, optical components, and system trades for these subsystems are covered in Chapter 5.

Finally, many laser systems require the use of a detector—single-pixel or focal plane array—to collect an image or otherwise obtain information about the beam. Before we can measure photons, however, we first need to understand how many are expected, their wavelengths, and their spatial distribution. This is reviewed in Chapter 6, where we examine the notion of laser brightness, and then use the concept to estimate the power collected by the optical and detector subsystems. Chapter 7 then ties everything together from the point of view of photon detection, including detector types, geometries, sensitivities, and selection.

The emphasis in all chapters is on real-world design problems and the first-order equations and commercial off-the-shelf components used to solve them. As with any book, not every topic can be included; however, readers may also find my previous books useful for understanding the many differences between lasers and incoherent sources [*Optical Systems Engineering* (McGraw-Hill, 2011)] or obtaining additional details on the optomechanical aspects of building laser systems [*Optomechanical Systems Engineering* (John Wiley & Sons, 2015)].

**Keith J. Kasunic**
*August 2016*
*Palo Alto, California, USA*

# Chapter 1
# Introduction

For many years, lasers had been considered by engineers to be a problem in search of a solution—not the other way 'round, as is often repeated in the scientific literature. The problem was getting the laser to work properly, reliably, cost-effectively, etc.—and then getting it to "play" well with the other components in the system. This historical difficulty in obtaining working hardware with these unique sources of photons led to the many Immutable Laws of Lasers:

- The optimum number of lasers in any system is zero.
- The only likely result of a laser development program is that all available funds will be expended.
- The performance of any given laser cannot be predicted based on the measurements of the performance of any other laser.
- Lasers are the wave of the future—and always will be!

Fortunately, these laws have mutated over the years to the point where they are now mostly obsolete, and lasers are used in a number of difficult environments ranging from the manufacturing floor to the ceiling of outer space. Examples vary from the obvious to the obscure, including:

- Driverless cars and autonomous vehicles[1]
- Biomedical microscopes with sub-diffraction-limited resolving power, resulting in a Nobel prize for its inventors[2]
- The Internet and laser communications[3]
- Manufacturing applications requiring material heating, removal, or addition[4]
- Laser projection systems and displays[5]
- Directed energy (aka "Star Wars") for planetary defense against asteroids[6]

Despite their many applications—and the prominence of lasers in popular culture as well[7]—there is still a surprising lack of information available on how to design and engineer a laser *system*. The development of lasers themselves has for years dominated academic research, yet the money has not flowed to the broader issues and intricacies involved in using these high-tech "flashlights" in industrial, commercial, biomedical, or defense applications. The purpose of this book is to take an initial step in filling this gap.

A laser is a source of both light and heat. Light is an electromagnetic wave with a wavelength $\lambda$ and frequency $\nu$ with energy propagating at the speed of light $c$ in vacuum:

$$\nu = \frac{c}{\lambda} \qquad [\mathrm{Hz}] \tag{1.1}$$

The wavelengths that correspond specifically to "light" are shown in Fig. 1.1 as ultraviolet (UV), visible (VIS), and infrared (IR). The different types of lasers reviewed in this book can emit in any or all of these wavelength bands. Table 1.1 divides these bands into smaller units such as vacuum UV (VUV), midwave IR (MWIR), and so on.

In this chapter, we give an overview of the book by first looking in more detail at some laser systems that illustrate important laser properties (Section 1.1). As these properties depend on the design of the lasers themselves,

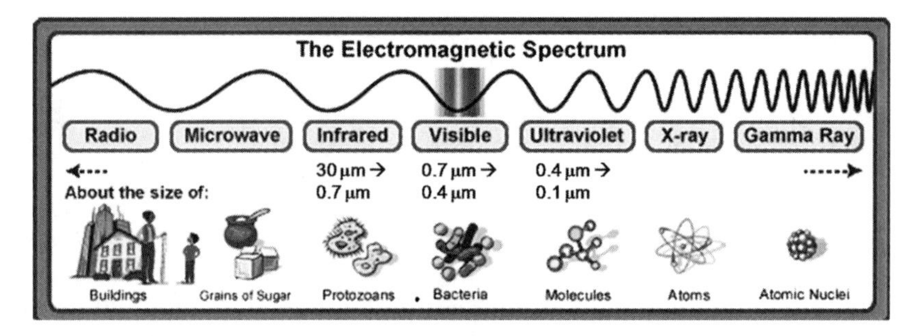


**Figure 1.1** Optical electromagnetic wavelengths ("light") can be divided into infrared, visible, and ultraviolet bands. [Credit: NASA (www.nasa.gov)]. (See color plate.)

**Table 1.1** Laser wavelength bands from Fig. 1.1 can be subdivided into near ultraviolet (NUV), near infrared (NIR), and so on.

| Wavelength Band | Abbreviation | Wavelength (μm) |
|---|---|---|
| Vacuum ultraviolet | VUV | 0.1–0.18 |
| Deep ultraviolet | DUV | 0.18–0.32 |
| Near ultraviolet | NUV | 0.32–0.40 |
| Visible | VIS | 0.4–0.7 |
| Near infrared | NIR | 0.7–1.0 |
| Shortwave infrared | SWIR | 1–3 |
| Midwave infrared | MWIR | 3–5 |
| Longwave infrared | LWIR | 8–12 |
| Very longwave infrared | VLWIR | 12–30 |

we then review in Section 1.2 the principles of laser engineering. Finally, we preview the book contents in Section 1.3 with an overview of the components used in typical laser systems, and some of the design trades required for optimizing overall laser system performance.

## 1.1 Laser Systems

As illustrated in Fig. 1.2, a generic laser system consists of lasers, optics, scanners, detectors, and a propagation medium such as air. As a result, the required tasks for laser system development may include laser selection, beam propagation, optical design, beam scanning, radiometry, detector selection, and possibly atmospheric compensation.

The heart of the laser system is, of course, the laser—of which there are nearly an infinite number of types and wavelengths (Fig. 1.3). One of the goals of this book is to narrow down the number of options to those that will cover 90% or so of the possible systems, with the more-obscure 10% not included. Some common laser systems—and the critical laser properties that make them useful—are reviewed in the rest of this section.

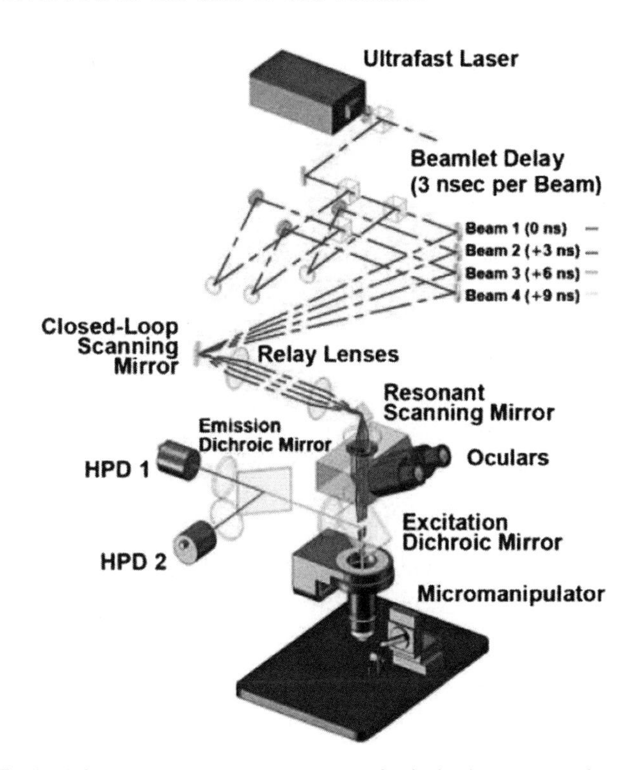


**Figure 1.2** Typical laser system components include lasers, optics, scanners, and detectors. [Reprinted with permission from: A. Cheng et al., "Simultaneous two-photon calcium imaging at different depths with spatiotemporal multiplexing," *Nature Methods* **8**, 139–142 (2011).] (See color plate.)

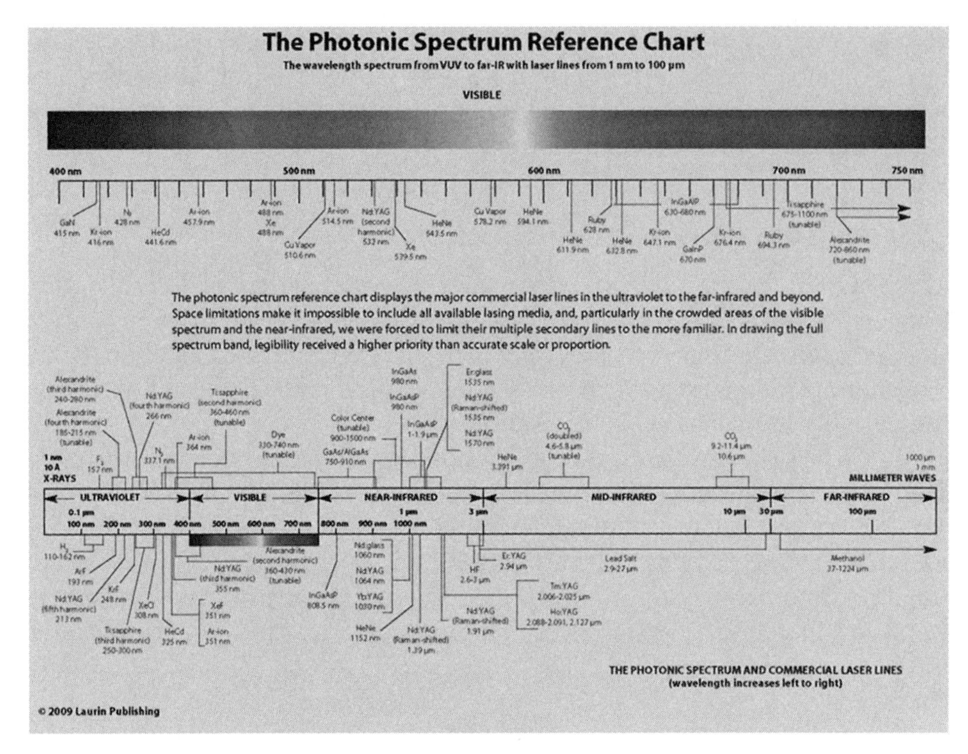


**Figure 1.3** The large number of laser types and wavelengths makes laser selection for system development a complex task. (© 2009 Laurin Publishing; reprinted with permission.) (See color plate.)

The first system is that of optical data storage (Fig. 1.4) such as CD, DVD, and HD-DVD players, and holographic data storage. In this case, low-power semiconductor diode lasers are commonly used because a property known as *beam quality* (Chapter 3) allows focusing to the smallest possible, diffraction-limited spot size ($\sim \lambda/D$ for an objective lens with an aperture diameter $D$). This ensures the highest possible storage capacity on the limited surface area of a disk; a shorter wavelength also increases capacity, with wavelengths evolving from $\lambda = 780$ nm for CD systems down to 405 nm for HD-DVDs such as Blu-ray™. Additional benefits of diode lasers—critical for the consumer market—include their low cost, size, and electrical power consumption.

Another common laser application is that of testing the irregularity of optical surfaces.[8] Such testing requires a laser with a large coherence length, i.e., the distance over which its phase is approximately unchanged (Section 1.2.1). For example, the laser's coherence length must exceed twice the distance between the reference surface and the test surface in Fig. 1.5, as any difference in phase will interfere and appear incorrectly as an error in the surface of the test mirror. Helium-neon (HeNe) gas lasers are often used for interferometers because they have both a long coherence length and good

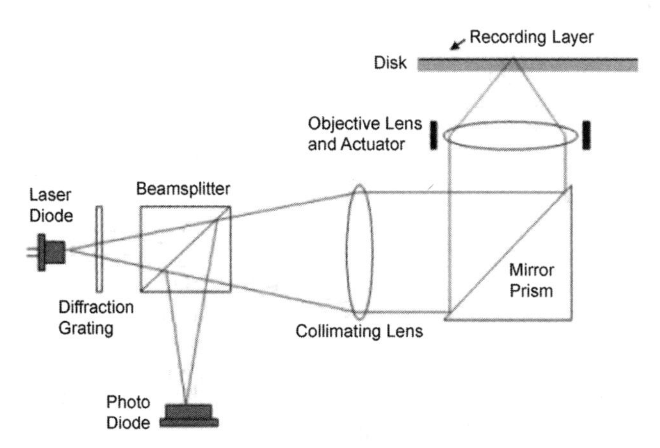


**Figure 1.4** Optical data storage requires lasers with beams that can be focused to the smallest possible spot size. [Reprinted from W.-S. Sun et al., "Compact HD-DVD pickup head with a lens-prism," *Proc. SPIE* **5174**, 128–135 (2003).] (See color plate.)

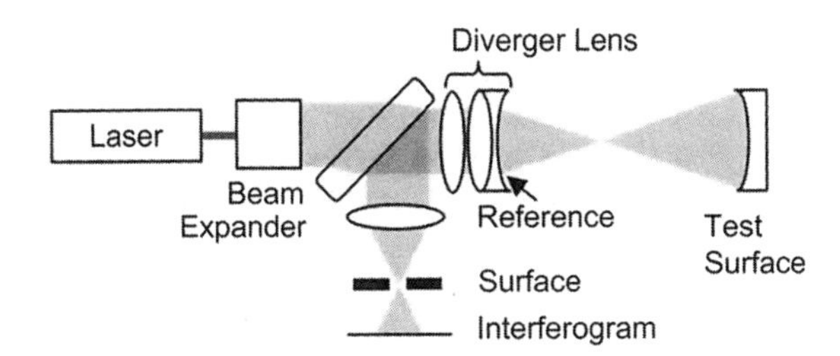


**Figure 1.5** A Fizeau interferometer used for testing optical surfaces requires the long coherence length of a laser. (Reprinted with permission from Ref. 8, p. 59.)

spatial coherence across the wavefront. Helium-neon wavelengths of 633 nm (VIS) and 3.39 μm (MWIR) are common, as are carbon dioxide ($CO_2$) gas lasers with a wavelength of 10.6 μm for testing LWIR optics.

A third laser application is that of directed energy (DE), where it is necessary to deposit the highest amount of power in the smallest area at a large distance. This places a requirement on the laser brightness; distinct from simply output power, laser brightness is a measure of how spatially efficient a source is at emitting power. For example, if the output power of two lasers is the same, the laser emitting with fewer atoms (a smaller area) into a smaller divergence angle has a higher brightness (Chapter 6). Solid-state and fiber lasers can deliver more than 10 kW of average power from a small, near-diffraction-limited beam and are thus an option for DE applications requiring high irradiance ($W/cm^2$) or fluence ($J/cm^2$) on a target.

Finally, a fourth common laser application is that of confocal microscopy. As illustrated in Fig. 1.6, these microscopes obtain high-resolution 3D images

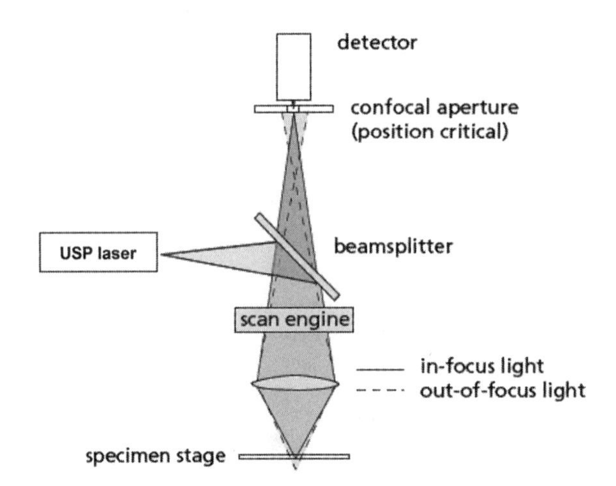


**Figure 1.6** MPE confocal microscopy relies on ultrashort-pulse (USP) lasers with high peak power and low average power. (Credit: CVI Laser, LLC.)

by blocking out-of-focus photons with a detector pinhole (confocal aperture). Using a technique known as multiphoton excitation (MPE), image contrast can be improved by using a low-average-power laser that creates one short-λ photon from two (or more) longer-λ photons. The key laser properties that allow MPE are a high peak power (to efficiently generate long-λ photons) and low average power (to minimize heat absorption by the specimen). This requires ultrashort-pulse (USP) lasers that can release energy in a short pulse or "shot" on the order of 1–10 psec (Section 2.1.5). Fiber lasers allow the generation of such pulses in a product size appropriate for clinical use.

Summarizing, we see that various laser properties—beam quality, coherence length, brightness, pulse width, and so on—may or may not be important depending on the application. There are, of course, many other laser systems besides the four discussed in this section (see Table 1.2), and we will look at a number of these throughout the course of the book. As well, the different types of lasers—semiconductor, gas, solid-state, and fiber—and their properties will be reviewed in more detail in Chapter 2.

## 1.2 Laser Engineering

While the intent of this book is to go into detail on the development of laser systems, a brief introduction to the design of lasers themselves makes their use in a system a more-intelligent endeavor. Many references are available for details on laser design; Ref. 9 is recommended.

One of the primary goals of laser engineering is to meet system requirements by controlling the unique features of lasers that determine the properties of coherence length and beam quality, namely, the degree of

**Table 1.2** Critical system properties (or key performance parameters) required for various laser applications. The laser types and properties will be reviewed in detail in Chapter 2.

| Laser Application | Wavelength and Laser Type | Key Performance Parameters (KPPs) |
|---|---|---|
| HD-DVD Players | 405 nm; diode | Spot size, size, cost |
| Bar-Code Scanners | 670 nm; diode | Size, cost |
| Laser Communications | 1550 nm; diode | Modulation rate, noise |
| Fluorescence Microscopy | 400–1100 nm; multiple | Spot size, peak power |
| Eye Surgery ("LASIK") | 193 nm; excimer | Spot size, power stability |
| Precision Manufacturing | 0.3–10.6 μm; multiple | Spot size, peak power, PRF |
| Interferometry | 633 nm, 3.39 μm; gas | Coherence |
| Semiconductor Lithography | 193 nm; excimer | Spot size, energy stability |
| Laser Pumping | 808, 980 nm; diode | Wavelength, power |
| Laser Rangefinder | 1.55 μm; solid-state | Peak power, beam quality |
| Laser Radar | 1.064 μm; solid-state | Peak power, beam quality |
| Directed Energy | 1 μm; solid-state, fiber | Brightness, efficiency |
| IR Countermeasures | 3-5 μm; QCL | Wavelength, brightness |

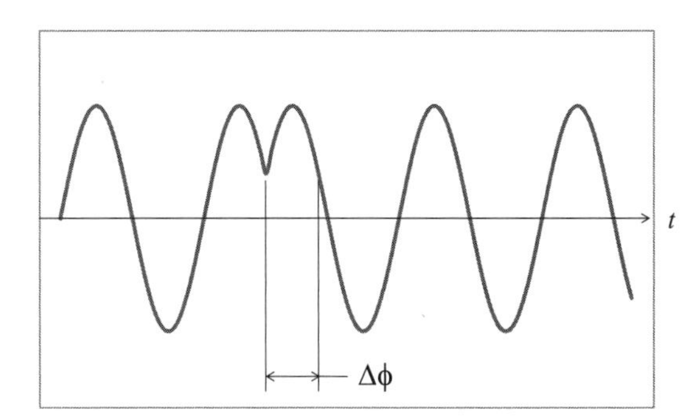


**Figure 1.7** Collisions between gas molecules create temporal phase jumps $\Delta\phi$ in their emitted wavefronts, affecting the propagating frequencies and the laser's temporal coherence.

phase coherence. That is, the wavefronts must be in phase along the propagation direction (temporal coherence, Fig. 1.7); in addition, the wavefronts must also be in phase across the beam diameter (spatial coherence, Fig. 1.8). There are also variations on these themes, where specialized lasers have low temporal coherence but good spatial coherence (white-light or super-continuum lasers), or high temporal coherence but poor spatial coherence ("random" lasers).

As shown in Fig. 1.9, what's needed for a laser's temporal and spatial coherence is:

- A gain medium (and associated pump energy $h\nu_p$) to create a population inversion (or gain) of the medium's electron energy states [Fig. 1.9(a)], allowing photon amplification.

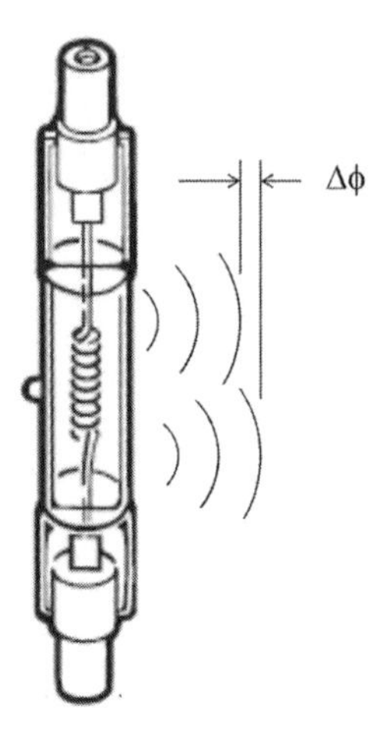


**Figure 1.8** Atoms emitting independently across an incoherent source such as a tungsten-filament lamp results in a phase difference $\Delta\phi$ and poor spatial coherence of the wavefronts. (Permission to reprint granted by Newport Corporation; all rights reserved.)

- A resonant cavity—two mirrors, for example—to control the number, direction, and phase coherence of the amplified photons [Fig. 1.9(b)].

The amplification of photons is in phase with the incident wavefront and is known as stimulated emission, while atoms that spontaneously emit photons before they interact with the laser beam have a random phase relationship (i.e., are not coherent) with the wavefront (Fig. 1.10). As a result, higher gain has a larger fraction of amplified in-phase photons in comparison with the incoherent photons.

If the energy of the incident electromagnetic field more-or-less matches that of the electron's excited state energy $E_2$ compared with some lower-energy state

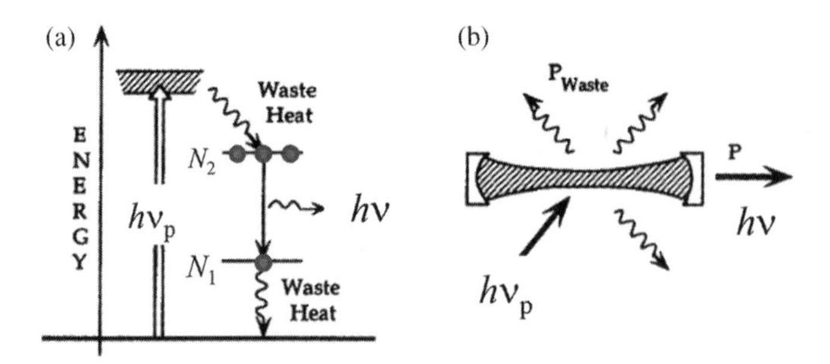


**Figure 1.9** (a) Changes in the gain medium's electron energy states result in the emission of a photon with energy $h\nu$. (b) The back-and-forth reflections in a two-mirror resonant cavity increase the number of stimulated photons. (Reprinted from Ref. 10.)

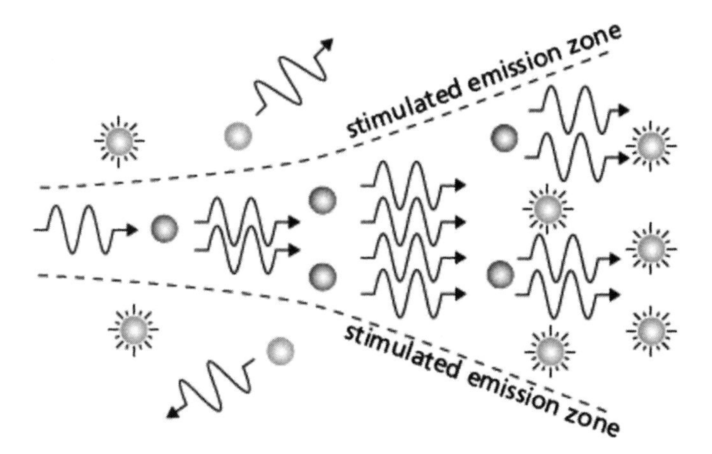


**Figure 1.10** The wavefronts of stimulated photons are emitted in phase with the incident photons. (Credit: CVI Laser, LLC.)

$E_1$, then there is a high probability the electron will give up its energy in the form of a stimulated photon whose energy $E_p$ in Fig. 1.9(a) is

$$E_p = E_2 - E_1 = h\nu = \frac{hc}{\lambda} \qquad [\mathrm{J}] \tag{1.2}$$

where $h = 6.626 \times 10^{-34}$ J-sec is Planck's constant. Physically, a higher-frequency, shorter-wavelength photon has more energy, as would be expected for an electromagnetic wave that changes at a faster rate.

The population inversion—defined as $N_2 - N_1$ in Fig. 1.9(a), with more electrons in the gain medium in an excited energy state $E_2$ than a lower state $E_1$—has a distribution of excited-state energies and thus amplifies more than a single wavelength. In its simplest form, this distribution is a result of the inevitable Heisenberg uncertainty fluctuations of the excited-state lifetime, resulting in a spread of photon energy $\Delta E_p = h\Delta\nu$ that is known as the *gain bandwidth* (in units of energy).

Building on these principles, laser engineering entails a large number of complexities, some of which are reviewed in the next subsections under the categories of temporal coherence, spatial coherence, pulse generation, and wavelength conversion.

### 1.2.1 Temporal coherence

We have seen in Section 1.1 how the coherence length affects the performance of an interferometer; in this section, we take another look at this idea from the laser designer's perspective.

Even though it is common to talk of a pure "red" or 633-nm wavelength, no laser emits at a single (monochromatic) wavelength. Instead, there are unavoidable gain medium, quantum-mechanical, and optomechanical

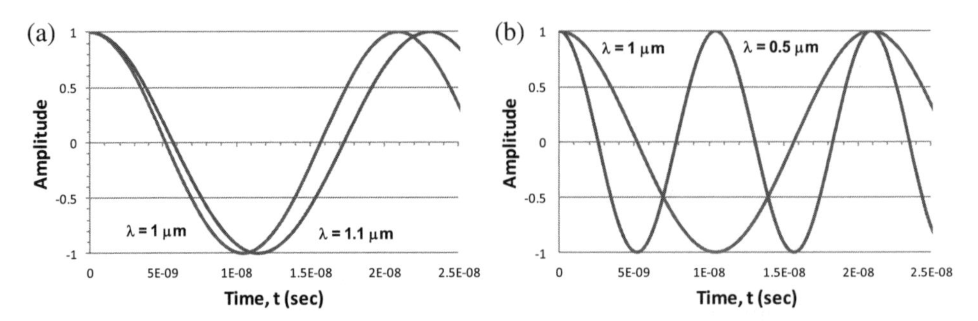


**Figure 1.11** Coherence length $d_c = c\tau_c$ is the distance over which different wavelengths become out of phase, with (a) a smaller $\Delta\lambda$ giving a longer coherence length, and (b) a larger $\Delta\lambda$ giving a shorter coherence length.

broadenings of any laser's wavelength, and the degree of broadening—or *linewidth* $\Delta\lambda$—determines the laser's temporal coherence and coherence length.

Temporal coherence can be understood by using a physical picture of two wavelengths propagating along the laser's longitudinal axis. Even if the speed of light is the same for both wavelengths, Fig. 1.11 shows that they will eventually get completely out of phase. The distance over which this occurs is known as the coherence length $d_c$.

The coherence time $\tau_c$ over which the emitted wavelengths are considered to be in phase—that is, are temporally coherent—thus depends inversely on the absolute value of the wavelength difference $|\Delta\lambda|$ or frequency difference $\Delta\nu = c|\Delta\lambda|/\lambda^2$ [from differentiating Eq. (1.1)]:

$$\tau_c \approx \frac{1}{2|\Delta\nu|} = \frac{1}{2c}\frac{\lambda_o^2}{|\Delta\lambda|} \qquad \text{[sec]} \tag{1.3}$$

clearly showing that a narrow-spectrum laser with small $\Delta\nu$ has a longer time over which different frequencies propagate before they are no longer considered to be in phase. Typical numbers for a HeNe laser used for interferometeric optical testing are a coherence time $\tau_c = 0.33$ nsec and a coherence length $d_c = c\tau_c = 100$ mm for a linewidth $\Delta\lambda = 2$ pm (see Table 1.3). Note that the results shown in Fig. 1.11(b)—where the different wavelengths

**Table 1.3** Coherence length $d_c = c\tau_c$ of commonly used lasers; see Chapter 2 for more detail on each of these laser types.

| Laser Type | Center Wavelength, $\lambda_o$ | Linewidth, $\Delta\lambda$ or $\Delta\nu$ | Coherence Length, $d_c$ |
|---|---|---|---|
| High-Power Diode | 808 nm | 3 nm | 100 μm |
| Nd:YAG | 1064 nm | 50 pm | 10 mm |
| He-Ne | 633 nm | 2 pm | 100 mm |
| Low-Power Fiber | 1070 nm | 10 kHz | 15 km |

are out of phase at a time $t \approx 10^{-8}$ sec—are not consistent with the estimates from Eq. (1.3), as the equation assumes that $\Delta\lambda$ is small in comparison with the center wavelength $\lambda_o$.

What determines the lasing wavelength $\lambda_o$ and linewidth $\Delta\lambda$? Ideally, three factors: the axial modes based on the length of the laser cavity, the bandwidth of the gain medium, and the type of gain medium (homogeneous versus inhomogeneous).

Axial (or longitudinal) modes are determined by the geometrical fit (or *resonance*) of a given wavelength in the laser cavity. That is, if the two mirrors that define a laser cavity are nearly planar and perfectly reflecting—an ideal assumption, given that one mirror will be designed *not* to be so that light can escape the cavity as output power—then Fig. 1.12 shows that an integer number $m = 1, 2, 3$, etc., of half-wavelengths of the electric field fit in the cavity length $L$:

$$m\frac{\lambda}{2n} = L \qquad [\mathrm{m}] \tag{1.4}$$

where the refractive index $n$ of the gain medium is included to account for the reduction in wavelength in comparison with its free-space ($n = 1$) value. With the exception of a specific type of semiconductor laser known as a vertical-cavity surface-emitting laser (VCSEL) with a cavity length $L \approx \lambda$, the number of half-wavelengths is large in practice. For example, for a HeNe laser emitting at $\lambda = 633$ nm with $L = 100$ mm and $n \approx 1$, $m = 2L/\lambda = 2 \times 0.1$ m/633 nm $= 315{,}955$ half-wavelengths.

Unless they are specifically "locked" together in phase (as in Section 1.2.3), these axial modes are emitting independently of one another, and are thus all potential wavelengths at which the laser can oscillate. Solid-state lasers using titanium-doped sapphire as a gain medium, for example, may emit hundreds of thousands of axial-mode wavelengths (Section 2.2.2). These lasers are commonly specified by the frequency difference between each axial mode,

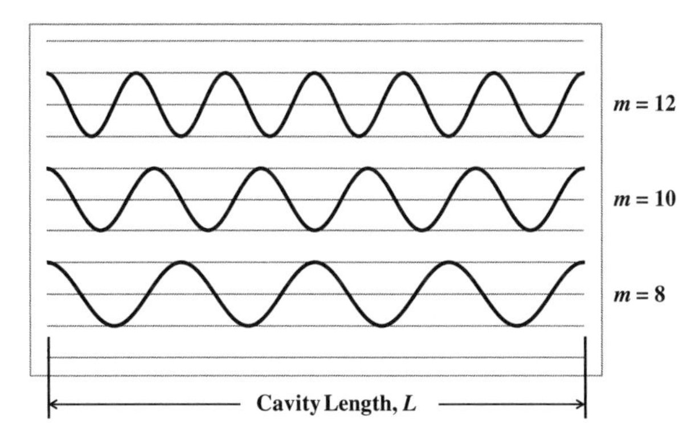


**Figure 1.12** An integer number $m$ of half-wavelengths ($m\lambda/2n$) of the electric field fit inside a perfectly reflecting resonant cavity, a simplifying assumption used to describe axial modes.

where each frequency $\nu_m$ for a planar cavity is obtained by combining Eqs. (1.1) and (1.4),

$$\nu_m = \frac{c}{\lambda_m} = \frac{mc}{2nL} \qquad [\text{Hz}] \tag{1.5}$$

and the frequency difference $\Delta\nu_a$ between adjacent axial modes—also known as the free spectral range (FSR) of the laser cavity—is given by

$$\Delta\nu_a = \nu_{m+1} - \nu_m = \frac{c}{2nL} \qquad [\text{Hz}] \tag{1.6}$$

For example, a HeNe laser with $L = 100$ mm has an axial mode spacing $\Delta\nu_a = (3 \times 10^8$ m/sec)/(2 × 1 × 0.1 m) = 1.5 GHz, while a short-cavity semiconductor laser with $L = 100$ μm and $n = 3$ gives $\Delta\nu_a = (3 \times 10^8$ m/sec)/ $(2 \times 3 \times 100 \times 10^{-6}$ m) = 500 GHz.

Whether or not multiple axial modes will lase depends, in part, on the cavity-mode spacing $\Delta\nu_a$ in comparison with the frequency spectrum (or gain bandwidth) $\Delta\nu_g$ of the gain medium. This is shown in Fig. 1.13, where the gain curve is superimposed over the longitudinal modes of an ion laser. The gain bandwidth is determined by a number of possible gain-medium mechanisms: natural broadening due to spontaneous decay of excited-state energies, Doppler broadening due to atomic or molecular motion, collision broadening due to intermolecular impacts of gas molecules that change the phase of the emitted wavefront (Fig. 1.7), or phonon broadening due to imperfections and variations in lattice spacings in semiconductor, solid-state and fiber lasers. Independent of mechanism, a gain bandwidth wider than the axial mode spacing—as shown in Fig. 1.13—has the potential to lase at more than one axial-mode wavelength.

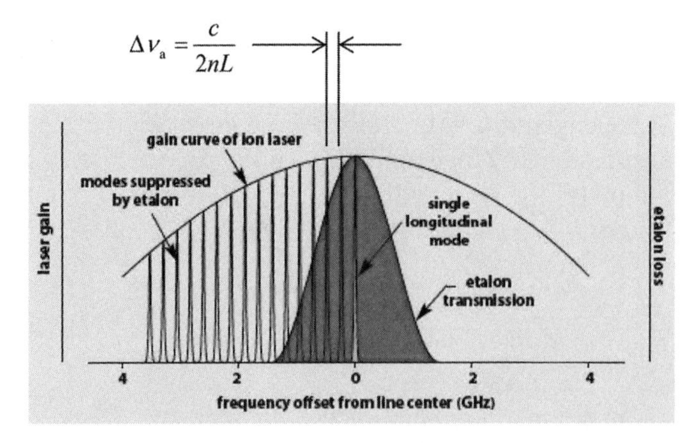


**Figure 1.13** The gain bandwidth $\Delta\nu_g$ of many lasers exceeds the longitudinal-mode spacing $\Delta\nu_a$. (Permission to reprint granted by Newport Corporation; all rights reserved.)

Whether or not this occurs depends on the third contributor to the emission wavelength and linewidth, namely, how the gain medium responds (saturates) to power levels inside the cavity. There are two possibilities: (1) the gain decreases equally across the entire gain bandwidth as excited-state population levels are used up to increase the output power (homogeneous saturation), or (2) the gain decreases only at specific wavelengths depending on the gain-broadening mechanism (inhomogeneous saturation).

For homogeneous gain saturation—as is found with natural, collision, and homogeneous phonon broadening—the peak of the gain at steady state will drop to equal the cavity losses, and this will occur at or near one axial mode. This mode will thus lase, and homogeneous saturation typically leads to single-longitudinal-mode (SLM) lasing at one axial mode (aka single-frequency), rather than over the entire gain curve.[11] Stimulated emission thus results in a narrowing of the output spectrum from its spontaneous width $\Delta\nu_g$, a principal reason for the narrow linewidth of a laser; as a result, semiconductor lasers have a smaller $\Delta\lambda$ than spontaneously emitting LEDs made from the same material.

For inhomogeneous saturation, on the other hand, the gain saturates only at those axial-mode wavelengths preferred by the gain medium—with Doppler and inhomogeneous (strained lattice) phonon broadening being typical examples. This can lead to lasing at more than one axial mode, and such multi-longitudinal-mode lasers emit at discrete frequency spacings given by Eq. (1.6).

For a long coherence length, then, the first option for the laser systems engineer is a frequency-stable SLM laser, as is required for interferometry, coherent sensing, and holography. Because the drop-off of the gain curve might not be sufficient to prevent small cavity and refractive-index fluctuations from causing the axial mode to "hop" to an adjacent wavelength, laser designers might also use an additional frequency-stabilization component in the cavity.

The most commonly used component is a Fabry–Pérot (FP) etalon. In its simplest form, this is a flat piece of glass whose thickness $d_{FP}$ is much smaller than the laser cavity's, and its axial mode spacing is thus much larger [Eq. (1.6)]. As seen in Fig. 1.13—where only one axial mode of the etalon is shown—the wavelengths that can lase are now based on the superposition of the etalon transmission and the longitudinal modes of the laser. The full-width at half-maximum (FWHM) bandwidth $\Delta\nu_R$ of the etalon transmission is based on its finesse $F_R$ and axial mode spacing $\Delta\nu_{FP} = c/2nd_{FP}$:

$$\Delta\nu_R = \frac{\Delta\nu_{FP}}{F_R} \approx \frac{c}{2nd_{FP}} \cdot \frac{1-\sqrt{R_{p1}R_{p2}}}{\pi(R_{p1}R_{p2})^{1/4}} = \frac{c}{2nd_{FP}} \cdot \frac{1-R}{\pi\sqrt{R}} \quad \text{[Hz]} \tag{1.7}$$

for surface power reflectivities $R_{p1}$ and $R_{p2}$, valid for $R \equiv (R_{p1}R_{p2})^{1/2} \geq 0.4$ or so. The etalon's transmission bandwidth is usually much smaller than its mode spacing; e.g., using an etalon with $R = 0.9$ gives $F_R = \pi R^{1/2}/(1 - R) \approx 30$.

Because the mode spacing of the etalon is so much larger than that of the laser, however, even a relatively wide $\Delta\nu_R$ may drop off faster with laser frequency than the gain curve (Fig. 1.13); as a result, the laser is less sensitive to small fluctuations in power, cavity length, or refractive index, and mode hops are less likely to occur. In practice, the etalon bandwidth also depends on the parallelism and flatness of its surfaces—effects that can be controlled to such a degree with the fabrication of the etalon as to still make the etalon a useful frequency-stabilization component.

Even a frequency-stabilized SLM laser has a linewidth—an unavoidable consequence of random spontaneous-emission phase variations resulting from quantum fluctuations in excited-state energy levels. For such lasers, the ideal single-mode (Schawlow–Townes) linewidth $\Delta\nu_{ST}$ for a laser cavity $\Delta\nu_R$ (not its etalon) is given by Refs 9 and 12 as

$$\Delta\nu_{ST} = \frac{\pi h\nu \cdot (2\pi\Delta\nu_R)^2}{P} \quad [\text{Hz}] \tag{1.8}$$

where $P$ is the output power of the given axial mode. Physically, the higher power has a larger fraction of amplified in-phase photons in comparison with the incoherent, out-of-phase photons from spontaneous emission, reducing $\Delta\nu_{ST}$ to something smaller than the cold-cavity FWHM bandwidth $\Delta\nu_R$ of the *laser's* axial modes [also Eq. (1.7)] given the laser-cavity reflectivity $R$.

Equation (1.8) represents the ultimate lower limit on linewidth, with no commercial products able to achieve this level of frequency stability ($< 1$ Hz). In practice, some SLM fiber lasers have a linewidth smaller than 10 kHz—limited by "technical noise" (fluctuations in optical and optomechanical parameters, e.g.), and resulting in a coherence length $d_c \geq 15$ km.

There are, of course, many applications where coherence length is either unimportant or a hindrance to system performance. One example is that of speckle, where the reflections from a rough surface coherently interfere to produce a spotted image—a huge disadvantage for laser-based displays. In such cases, the system might still be limited by a different property of importance to both laser designers and systems engineers, namely, spatial coherence.

### 1.2.2 Spatial coherence

We have mentioned in Section 1.1 how the concept of beam quality affects focused spot size for optical data storage; in this section, we take a closer look at this idea from the laser designer's perspective. We have also seen in Section 1.2.1 how the laser wavelength is determined by three factors, but in practice additional factors such as mode hopping play a role. In this section we will see that yet another factor—the spatial coherence—also affects the lasing wavelength.

As discussed by Siegman (Ref. 9, pp. 55–58), the concepts of spatial coherence and beam quality arise because there may be phase variations $\geq \lambda/4$ across the diameter of each mirror in any laser cavity. These variations can result from manufacturing imperfections in each mirror, refractive-index non-uniformities of the gain medium, or misalignments of the mirrors.[13]

A typical laser cavity for solid-state and gas lasers[14,15] is shown in Fig. 1.14. Known as a confocal resonator, this particular type of cavity is designed with the radius of curvature of each mirror ($R_1$ and $R_2$) centered on the surface of the opposing mirror one cavity length $L$ away. In the absence of manufacturing imperfections and index non-uniformities, this cavity is relatively stable against misalignments and produces a beam with a Gaussian irradiance profile and has no phase variations across it. In addition, the electric and magnetic fields are transverse to the longitudinal axis, and the combined irradiance and phase profiles are known as a Gaussian beam, i.e., a spatially coherent transverse electro-magnetic ($TEM_{00}$) mode of order (0, 0).

In practice, unavoidable misalignments between mirrors are one of the most common causes of excessive phase variations across the beam (Fig. 1.15)—and resulting loss of beam quality. For a small misalignment angle $\Delta\theta$, which keeps the on-axis length $L$ the same by pivoting around the mirror surface at the longitudinal (or $z$) axis, there is still an optical axis determined by the line connecting the center of curvature of each mirror. However, there is also the potential for an asymmetry in the phase of the wavefront if the optical axis propagates through a solid-state crystal or Brewster window at an angle (see Section 2.1.12). Such asymmetries—astigmatism and coma, for example—can also result from manufacturing imperfections in each mirror or refractive-index non-uniformities in the gain medium.

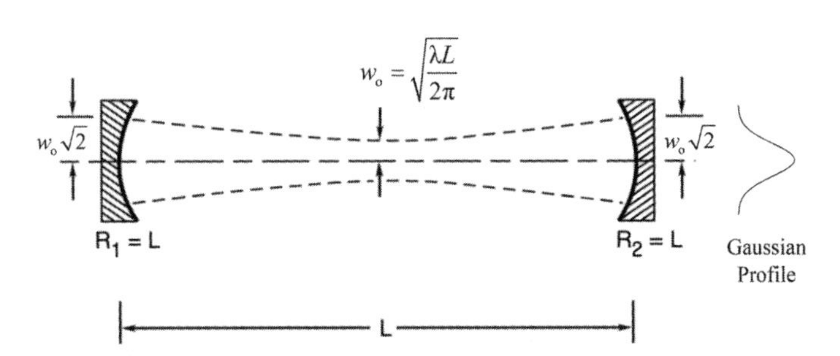


**Figure 1.14** A symmetric confocal laser cavity with the radius of curvature of each mirror ($R_1$ and $R_2$) equal to the cavity length $L$. The minimum beam radius (or *waist*) $w_o$ is at the center of the cavity where the focal length $f = R_i/2 = L/2$ of each mirror coincides. [Adapted from R. Scheps, *Introduction to Laser Diode-Pumped Solid State Lasers*, SPIE Press, Bellingham, Washington (2002).]

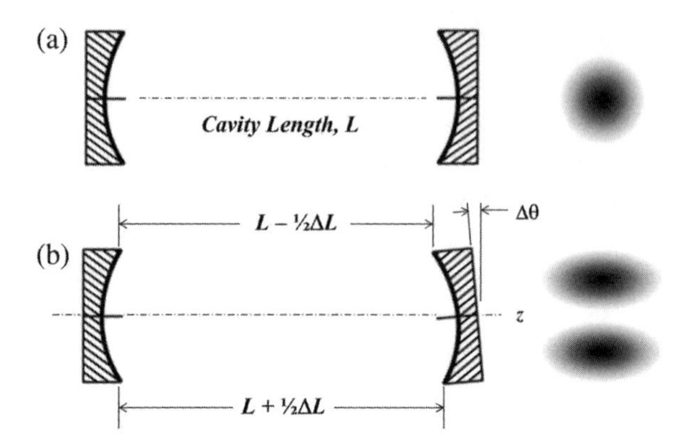


**Figure 1.15** An angular misalignment $\Delta\theta$ can distort the Gaussian $TEM_{00}$ profile in part (a), creating a phase difference across the beam and a lobed, circularly asymmetric irradiance profile in part (b) known as a $TEM_{01}$ spatial mode. Higher- and multi-order spatial modes are also possible.

To first order, the asymmetries result in an approximate phase difference $\Delta\phi$ across the beam proportional to the change in cavity length $\Delta L$ at the edges of the mirrors:

$$\Delta\phi \propto \frac{2\pi n}{\lambda}\Delta L \qquad [\text{rad}] \tag{1.9}$$

where the type of mirror determines the actual phase difference. Two flat mirrors, for example, give $\Delta L = D\Delta\theta$, while curved mirrors will modify the phase with an additional quadratic term ($\Delta L = D^2/2R_i$) that depends on the diameter $D$ and radius of curvature $R_i$ of the mirrors.

As a Gaussian beam starts to develop from spontaneous emission within the cavity, there are additional phase terms—Gaussian wavefront propagation (see Chapter 3), Guoy phase shift, and so on—that become important with misaligned mirrors. Independent of these details, the phase variations across the mirrors modify the Gaussian beam in three ways: (1) an increase in the divergence angle at which the beam exits the laser; (2) an increase in spot size if the beam is focused with a lens; and (3) a small shift in the emission wavelength, and a possible linewidth broadening as well.

The beams that result can be either aberrated Gaussians (for small misalignments) or are no longer circularly symmetric, with the asymmetric profile of the misalignment direction [Fig. 1.15(b)] and one (or more) zero-irradiance lines (or *nodes*). The mode shown in Fig. 1.15(b), for example, is a $TEM_{01}$ mode because there are no nodes in the horizontal direction and one node in the vertical. Depending on the degree of phase shift across the mirror, there might be higher-order modes as well, specified as $TEM_{pq}$ for the integers $p > 0$ and $q > 0$ defining the number of nodes in the profile.

It sometimes happens that the transverse irradiance profile from a misaligned cavity is circularly symmetric, even though the profile shown in Fig. 1.15(b) is not. This occurs when the misalignments in both directions combine to produce a symmetric beam. A common example is the "donut" mode—a combination of $TEM_{01}$ and $TEM_{10}$ profiles—which is circularly symmetric. This is perhaps the most common multi-transverse-mode profile, as it is likely that there will be a slight angular misalignment of the cavity mirrors about both the $x$ and $y$ axes. In practice, it is unusual to obtain a pure higher-order mode such as $TEM_{31}$, as other contributors such as contamination or manufacturing imperfections of each mirror and refractive-index nonuniformities contribute to the phase profile, leading to combinations of modes.

Whether single- or multiple-spatial mode, the paraxial transverse irradiance distribution in free-space lasers is described mathematically by the product of the circularly symmetric Gaussian distribution and the Cartesian-coordinate Hermite polynomials.[9] Experimentally, the spatial-mode "content" is determined by a quantity known as $M^2$ which, as we will see in detail in Chapter 3, can be used to determine the increase in divergence angle and/or focused spot size. An ideal, diffraction-limited beam has an $M^2 = 1$; lasers with $M^2 \leq 1.5$ or so are said to have good beam quality.[16]

The third modification of a Gaussian beam that results from transverse spatial modes is a small shift in the emission wavelength, in addition to a possible linewidth broadening. This is shown in Fig. 1.16, where each longitudinal-mode frequency $\nu_m$ has transverse-mode frequencies associated with it. That is, the transverse modes—$TEM_{01}$, $TEM_{11}$, $TEM_{12}$, $TEM_{22}$, and so on—each have a slightly different frequency, given by

$$\nu_{pqm} = \frac{c}{2nL}\left[m + \frac{1}{\pi}(1 + p + q)\cos^{-1}\sqrt{(1 - L/R_1)(1 - L/R_2)}\right] \quad [\text{Hz}] \quad (1.10)$$

where the $1 - L/R_i$ term is also referred to in the literature as a cavity stability parameter $g_i$.[9] In addition, the terms inside the square brackets in Eq. (1.10)

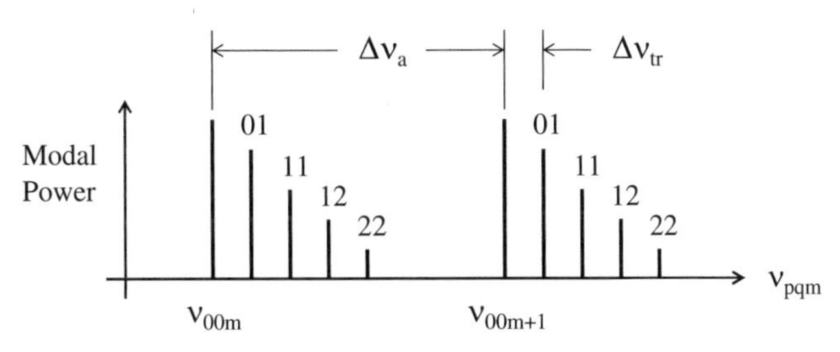


**Figure 1.16** Transverse modes associated with a $TEM_{00}$ axial mode have a frequency that differs from that of the axial, potentially leading to a broadening of the linewidth (and decrease in coherence length) for multi-spatial-mode lasers.

show that each Gaussian $TEM_{00}$ mode may or may not have the same optical frequency as that given in Eq. (1.5) for a planar cavity.

As an example of the transverse-mode frequencies for a confocal cavity with $L = R_i$, we have $\cos^{-1}(0) = \pi/2$, giving $\nu_{00m} = (c/2nL) \times (m + ½)$ and $\nu_{01m} = (c/2nL) \times (m + 1)$. The transverse mode spacing $\Delta\nu_{tr}$ is then $\nu_{01m} - \nu_{00m} = c/4nL$, or one-half of the axial mode spacing $\Delta\nu_a$. Also note that the absolute value of the axial-mode frequency $\nu_{00m}$ has shifted to a higher frequency by the same amount, given the factor of $m + ½$ in comparison with the factor of $m$ in Eq. (1.5) for a near-planar cavity [for which the $\cos^{-1}(1)$ term for $R_i \approx \infty$ is zero, reducing Eq. (1.10) to Eq. (1.5) for $TEM_{00}$ modes].

There are other cavity designs—semi-confocal, spherical, hemispherical, etc.—where the transverse mode spacing is much smaller than that for the confocal cavity.[9] For designs that are relatively insensitive to misalignments—confocal and the widely used near-hemispherical (or half-concentric)—it is feasible to control the misalignments, fabrication errors, index non-uniformities, and mirror cleanliness to such a degree that single-spatial-mode lasers with near-$TEM_{00}$ beam quality are common and inexpensive. These lasers will be reviewed in detail in Chapter 2.

In summary, beam quality is a measure of the phase variations across a beam.[16] The resulting transverse spatial mode properties—the systems-level consequences of which will be reviewed in Chapters 2 and 3—are an increase in beam divergence angle and focused spot size, as well as the possibility of a shift in wavelength in comparison with an ideal near-planar cavity. Also note that the term "multimode laser" can be ambiguous, as we have seen in this section that in addition to multi-longitudinal-mode lasers, there are also multi-transverse-modes that must be considered in system design. More typically, "multimode" refers to spatial modes, while "multifrequency" refers to axial modes.

### 1.2.3 Pulse generation

The lasers considered up to this point have been continuous wave (CW), with no obvious change in power level over time. In many applications, however, there is a need to concentrate the lasing energy into a shorter period of time—a pulse of width $\Delta t_p$—to increase the *peak* output power $P_{peak} = Q_p/\Delta t_p$ for a pulse energy $Q_p$ (Section 2.1.4). As we will see, applications for which this is important include nonlinear wavelength conversion (Section 1.2.4), "cold" laser machining (Section 2.1.5), multiphoton microscopy, as well as laser ranging and active imaging where the detector responds to reflected peak power (Chapter 7).

The first and most obvious approach to generating pulses is to switch the pump (and thus the gain) on-and-off—resulting in pulse widths shorter than the pump pulse, but with low peak power.[9] This is a result of the dynamic interaction between excited-state electrons and photons leading to relaxation oscillations as the excited-state energies "relax" (and are stimulated) to a lower-energy state; reducing these oscillations limits the degree of above-threshold pumping and thus the peak powers obtained. Despite its limitations, such gain switching is necessary for some types of $CO_2$ and excimer lasers for which other types of switching are not practical.

To avoid the relaxation oscillations and generate much higher peak power than is possible with gain switching, two methods are used for pulse generation: Q-switching and mode locking.

The concept of Q-switching refers to changing the quality $Q_c$ of the laser cavity. "Quality" in this case is not the transverse beam quality, but the cavity's ability to store laser energy:

$$Q_c = 2\pi\nu_{pqm}\frac{Q_{store}}{P_{loss}} = \frac{\nu_{pqm}}{\Delta\nu_{pqm}} \tag{1.11}$$

where the stored photon energy $Q_{store} = n_p h\nu$ for $n_p$ photons, each with energy $h\nu$, and the power loss $P_{loss} = Q_{store}/\tau_p$ for a photon lifetime $\tau_p$ in the cavity. This gives a cavity quality $Q_c = 2\pi\nu\tau_p$ with a photon lifetime that depends on the internal cavity losses $\alpha_{int}$ (due to internal absorption and diffraction) and coupling losses $\alpha_m$ (i.e., output power through the cavity mirrors). The photon lifetime is given as

$$\tau_p = \frac{1}{v_g}\cdot\frac{1}{\alpha_{int}+\alpha_m} \qquad [\text{sec}] \tag{1.12}$$

for a pulse traveling with a group velocity $v_g$. If the power reflectivity of each mirror is $R_{pi}$ and the internal losses are small, then the round-trip power-conservation condition [i.e., $R_{p1}R_{p2}\exp(2gL) = 1$] shows that the mirror loss that must be compensated by the gain $g$ at threshold is

$$\alpha_m = -\frac{1}{2L}\ln(R_{p1}R_{p2}) \qquad [1/\text{cm}] \tag{1.13}$$

For example, if the laser cavity length $L = 100$ mm and the power reflectivity $R_{p1} = R_{p2} = 0.98$ for each mirror, then $\alpha_m \approx 0.002$/cm. Increasing the cavity length allows photons more time to travel around the cavity before being "expelled" by the mirror as output power, thus decreasing the mirror loss on a per-centimeter basis.

Physically, a low-loss cavity with high-reflectivity mirrors has a long photon lifetime and thus efficiently stores energy (i.e., has a large $Q_c$), while a high-loss cavity with low-reflectivity mirrors has a short photon lifetime and thus dissipates (or damps) energy (i.e., has a small $Q_c$). A typical gas-laser cavity has a $Q_c$ value of $\approx 10^8$–$10^9$, indicating an extremely long photon lifetime: $\tau_p = Q_c/2\pi\nu \approx 0.025$–$0.250$ μsec for visible-wavelength light.

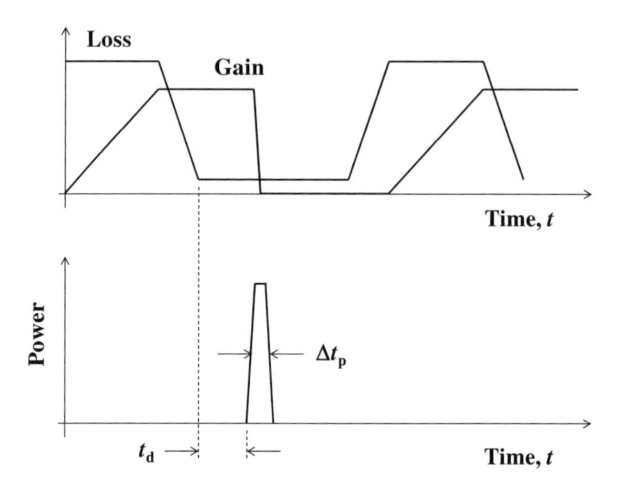


**Figure 1.17** Q-switching is based on a buildup of gain when the cavity loss is high and a quick release of this energy in the form of a short pulse with $\Delta t_p \approx$ 1–10 nsec when the loss is removed.

Q-switching, then, changes the laser cavity's losses to create shorter pulses than can be obtained with gain switching. By initially keeping the loss high (low $Q_c$) while the pump is activated, the population inversion and gain build up (Fig. 1.17); lasing is not possible, however, as the cavity loss from the switch is kept too high for the gain to overcome.

When the switch is turned off, the losses decrease (high $Q_c$) and the gain is then much higher than the total cavity loss; after a slight delay $t_d$, this gain is quickly utilized to create photons in the form of a short pulse with a FWHM width $\Delta t_p$. The Q-switch is then turned back on to increase the cavity loss again; if this did not happen, no additional pulses would be generated, and lasing would start at a steady-state power where gain balances losses.

Both active and passive technologies are available for Q-switching. Active switching typically uses an acousto-optic (AO) modulator to reduce the laser's internal losses in synchronization with the pulse's round-trip through the laser cavity, producing pulse widths on the order of 1–10 nsec.[17,18] Unfortunately, the AO modulator, while allowing large pulse energies and a variable switching rate, has a number of size, weight, and speed disadvantages in comparison with passive Q-switching.

Passive Q-switching with a *saturable absorber* generally produces lower-energy pulses but at a higher rate than an AO modulator. That is, just as the population inversion $N_2 - N_1$ in Fig. 1.9 can saturate to zero at a sufficiently high power, so can the absorption that is proportional to its negative (or $N_1 - N_2$). A saturable absorber thus has *less* loss—i.e., is "bleached"—as the incident power increases; the absorption at high power decreases as the number of atoms in a higher energy state approaches that in the lower, and the absorption (low-to-high energy transitions) approaches the emission (high-to-low energy transitions). In this way, even a slight increase in peak pulse power reduces the loss of a saturable absorber, with the pulse Q-switching itself into narrower pulses in a self-reinforcing feedback loop with multiple round-trips through the laser cavity.

Typical materials with large saturable absorption include $Cr^{4+}$:YAG crystals for use at $\lambda \approx 1064$ nm,[19] semiconductor saturable-absorber mirrors (SESAMs) such as GaAs-InGaAs multilayers for $\lambda = 1064$ nm, and the recent development of low-loss graphene for broadband Q-switching.[20] Passive Q-switching—with its lower size, weight, complexity, and cost—is preferred over active switching unless large pulse energies are required. For either type of switching, peak power on the order of $10^4 \times$ larger than the average power ($P_{peak} \approx$ 10–100 MW) is common—though only for 1–10 nsec, so not nearly enough kilowatt hours to bring down the power grid (in most cases).

In practice, a number of non-ideal characteristics limit the laser systems engineer's use of Q-switching. For example, the fast change in gain can lead to multi-axial-mode lasing; the time between pulses (or *timing jitter*) for saturable absorbers changing due to the high spontaneous emission rate from the large gain; and the lifetime of the saturable absorber being limited due to the high power densities.

For shorter pulses than are possible with Q-switching, a method known as *mode locking* is widely used.[21] That is, the axial modes determined by the combination of cavity length and gain bandwidth (Fig. 1.13)—which normally lase independently of each other—are coherently added in time (in phase, or *constructively interfere*) to produce short pulses on the order of 10 psec or less. This can occur for both inhomogeneous and homogeneous broadening of the gain, as an inhomogeneous gain medium normally supports multiple axial modes, and the homogeneous medium does so as well under non-steady-state (i.e., pulsed) conditions.

The modes must be shifted in phase by exactly the right amount to ensure that they all have the same phase at the same time somewhere in the cavity [for example, at the output mirror where the mode peaks line up on the right-hand side (RHS) of Fig. 1.12]. Even though the relative phase of any mode with respect to another is not initially known, we can modulate the beam—either actively or passively—so that the relative phase "locks" into a fixed value.

To understand how this can be achieved, an oscillating sinewave that is amplitude-modulated (AM) has frequency sidebands—a well-known result from Fourier analysis.[22] The frequency shift from the sinewave frequency $\omega = 2\pi\nu$ (in units of radians/sec) is simply the modulation frequency $\Omega$, giving AM frequencies of $\omega - \Omega$, $\omega$, and $\omega + \Omega$.

If the sinewave frequency corresponds to a laser mode frequency $\omega_m = 2\pi\nu_m$, and the modulation frequency $\Omega = 2\pi\Delta\nu = \pi c/nL$ equals the axial mode spacing $\Delta\omega_a$, then the AM sideband frequencies of $\omega - \Omega$ and $\omega + \Omega$ are superimposed on the neighboring axial modes $\omega_{m-1}$ and $\omega_{m+1}$. If all of the axial modes that are lasing are modulated at $\Omega$, then all modes will be coupled to their neighbors, to their neighbor's neighbors, and so on. To the degree that $\Omega$ is constant, the modes are thus locked together—in frequency difference and in phase.[23]

Once locked, the modes coherently add together to produce pulses that are much shorter than implied by the amplitude-modulation frequency $\Omega$ (Fig. 1.18). With the peaks of $N$ modes coinciding, for example, the sum from all modes increases the peak power by a factor of $N$ if the power from each mode is the same, which is not the case given the dropoff in the gain curve, but is useful for understanding the concept of axial-mode addition.

In addition, Fig. 1.18 shows that the sum of in-phase axial modes also narrows the FWHM pulse width by a factor of $N$. This is analogous to a diffraction grating, where the beam reflected from the grating lines constructively interfere at a particular direction in space, with the width of the interference pattern decreasing as more lines are illuminated. The net effect of more modes, then, is to increase the peak power by a factor of $N^2$—one factor of $N$ from power addition and one factor of $N$ from pulse narrowing.

Given that the locking of more modes decreases the pulse width $\Delta t_p$, and a wider gain bandwidth $\Delta\nu_g$ allows more modes to have enough gain to lase, the pulse width is approximately

$$\Delta t_p = \frac{1}{N} \cdot \frac{2nL}{c} \approx \frac{1}{\Delta\nu_g} \qquad \text{[sec]} \tag{1.14}$$

for $N \approx \Delta\nu_g/\Delta\nu_a$ and $\Delta\nu_a = c/2nL$. Titanium-doped sapphire (or $Ti{:}Al_2O_3$) lasers, for example, have an extremely large gain bandwidth ($\Delta\lambda_g \approx 300$ nm) and are thus commonly used for generating pulses as short as 10 fsec.

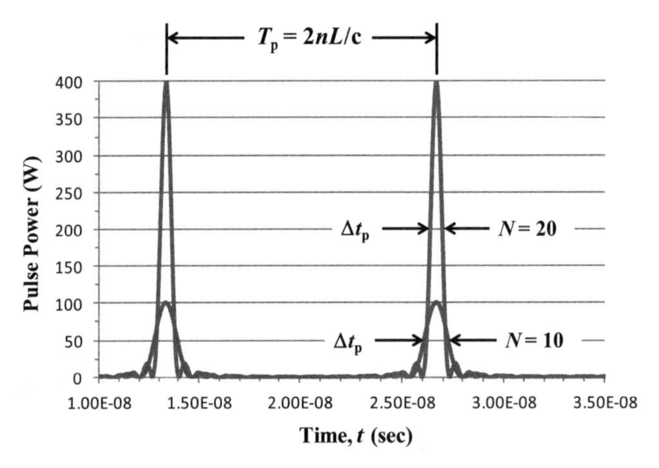


**Figure 1.18** Mode-locked period $T_p$ and FWHM pulse width $\Delta t_p$ for $N = 10$ and $N = 20$ axial modes with equal power in each mode.

Finally, the pulse period $T_p = 2nL/c$ equals the round-trip time of a pulse as it circulates around the laser cavity. While the axial-mode picture in Fig. 1.12 appears to be static, the dynamic picture is that each mode reflects from the output mirror and coherently combines as an in-phase pulse after each round-trip transit $2L$ through the cavity, after which it is partially transmitted through the output mirror. Long fiber lasers, for example, have a long pulse period and relatively low pulse repetition frequency PRF $= 1/T_p$, while much-shorter semiconductor lasers can in principle produce pulses at gigahertz rates.

As with Q-switching, both active and passive technologies are available for mode locking. Active mode locking typically uses a Pockels-cell electro-optic (EO) modulator[24] to create AM (or possibly frequency-modulated) sideband frequencies such that all of the axial modes that are lasing are modulated at $\Omega$. Alternatively, we can think of the modulator as reducing the laser's internal losses in synchronization with the pulse's round-trip through the laser cavity, producing pulse widths on the order of 10 psec.[17]

Passive mode locking with a saturable absorber—using materials such as SESAMs—produces even shorter pulses. The power-dependent absorption modulates the beam power, creating frequency sidebands for each mode that are locked to the other modes. Alternatively, by transmitting the peak power while absorbing the leading and trailing edges of the pulse, saturable absorption narrows the pulse width; the process is ultimately limited by the gain bandwidth and, with much more hardware complexity than is described here, leads to pulses on the order of 10 fsec to 10 psec. As with Q-switching, passive mode locking is generally preferred to active mode locking with its increase in size, weight, complexity, and cost.

Typical examples of mode-locked USP applications include Ti:$Al_2O_3$ (also known as Ti:sapphire) lasers for research into molecular dynamics, and fiber lasers for "cold" laser machining to reduce thermal damage. This is an active area of product development and there are, of course, many engineering details required to implement mode locking. Practical limitations include variations in EO modulation frequency $\Omega$, refractive-index variations across the gain bandwidth that modify the mode spacing, thermal expansion causing changes in cavity length and mode spacing, etc. For more details, see Paschotta[18] and Chapter 2.

### 1.2.4 Wavelength conversion

It sometimes happens that the inherent laser wavelength—1064 nm for a neodymium (Nd)-doped yttrium-orthovanadate ($YVO_4$) crystal as a gain medium, for example—is not useful for the task. In these cases, the laser designer must provide some mechanism of wavelength conversion, where the laser wavelength based on the gain medium is converted to some other wavelength of interest to meet the system requirements.

A common example is the conversion of 1064-nm light to 532 nm—a wavelength that the human eye can detect. Such conversion has been used for many years in low-cost laser pointers (Fig. 1.19), where the green (532-nm) light is easily obtained using a potassium titanium-oxide phosphate (KTP) crystal.[25] Another example is the conversion of 1064-nm light to 1570 nm; this conversion is useful because the 1570-nm photons are not as damaging to the eye as the 1064-nm photons, allowing the development of eye-"safer" laser rangefinders.

Figure 1.19 illustrates the wavelength-conversion hardware for second-harmonic generation (SHG). That is, by sending 1064-nm light of a sufficiently high peak power density (W/m$^2$) through a KTP crystal, second-harmonic wavelengths (one-half of 1064-nm) are generated. This occurs because the crystal's electrons cannot respond linearly to the large EM field; instead, an incident sinusoidal wave is re-emitted as a distorted waveform, which Fourier analysis tells us requires wavelengths shorter than the fundamental sinusoid—i.e., "harmonics"—to create. These harmonic wavelengths are in fact generated by the crystal, and the nonlinear conversion process of SHG is also known as *frequency doubling*.[26]

Another example of wavelength conversion is the use of an optical parametric oscillator (OPO) to create eye-"safer" photons at $\lambda = 1570$ nm

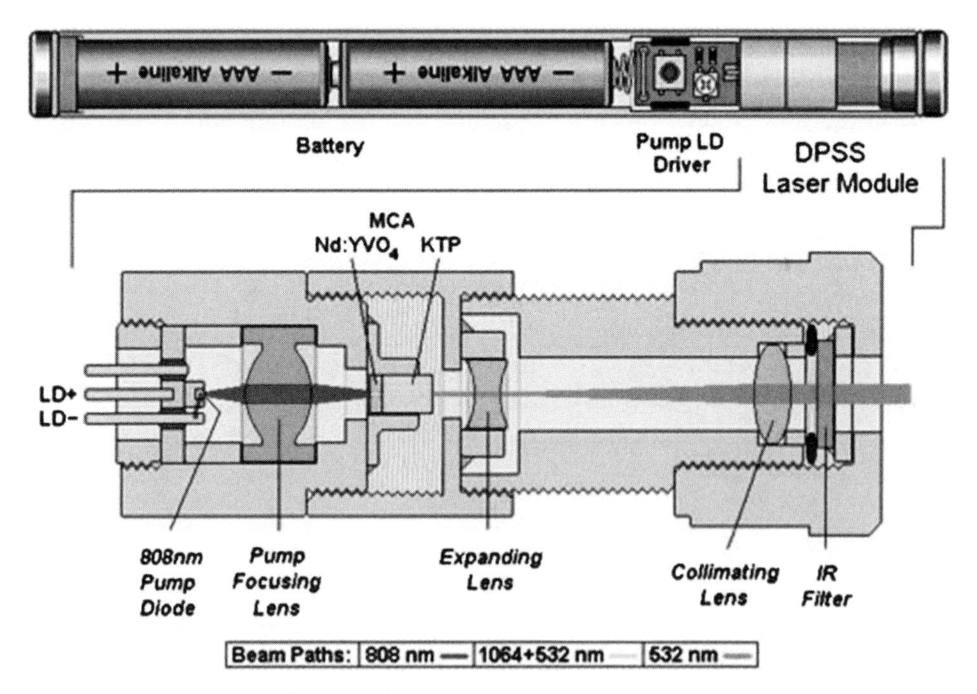


**Figure 1.19** Second-harmonic generation (SHG) of 1064-nm photons from a Nd:YVO$_4$ laser into 532-nm photons uses a nonlinear crystal such as KTP. (Credit: Chris Chen, Wikimedia Commons.) (See color plate.)

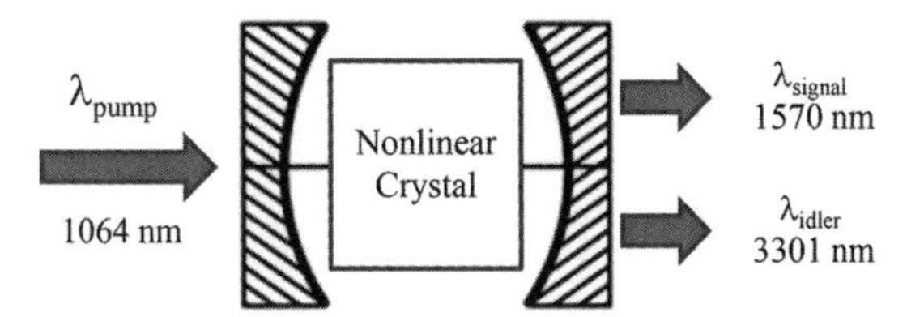


**Figure 1.20** A high-energy photon at $\lambda_{pump}$ = 1064 nm is converted to two lower-energy (longer-wavelength) photons by a nonlinear crystal such as KTP in a resonant cavity.

(Fig. 1.20). In this case, KTP (or some other nonlinear crystal) is used in a resonant cavity, thus assuring high-power density—for a nonlinear wavelength-conversion mechanism known as sum-frequency generation (SFG).

This nonlinear wavelength-conversion process relies on the conservation of photon energy to convert one short-wavelength (higher-energy) photon into two longer-wavelength (lower-energy) photons. With $E_{pump} = E_{signal} + E_{idler} = h\nu_{pump} = hc/\lambda_{pump}$ [from Eq. (1.1)], we have

$$\frac{1}{\lambda_{pump}} = \frac{1}{\lambda_{signal}} + \frac{1}{\lambda_{idler}} \qquad [1/\text{nm}] \tag{1.15}$$

where the sum of photon energies [or the sum of frequencies using Eq. (1.2)] gives this nonlinear mechanism its name. The labeling of a photon as a "signal" or "idler" is a bit arbitrary, as there are also applications where the MWIR 3301-nm wavelength shown in Fig. 1.20 is the desired output and is therefore the signal in that case.

In addition to SHG and SFG, there are a number of other nonlinear mechanisms used for wavelength conversion: frequency tripling or third-harmonic generation (THG), frequency quadrupling or fourth-harmonic generation (FHG), difference-frequency generation (DFG), etc.[26] To implement these technologies, the laser designer must consider wavelength range, nonlinear response, phase matching, temperature sensitivity, angular sensitivity, walk-off angle, and laser damage threshold, among other parameters.

In practice, two requirements play a key role for the laser systems engineer in the use of wavelength-conversion technologies:

- Conversion efficiency: Energy is lost in the conversion of wavelengths, and the conversion efficiency is the transmitted energy in comparison with the incident energy. The large peak power from pulsed lasers is more efficient at generating nonlinear effects than CW lasers. Up to 80% efficiency has been obtained for SHG using a KTP crystal at $\lambda = 1064$ nm, and >65% efficiency has been obtained for SHG with a lithium triborate (LBO) nonlinear crystal at $\lambda = 1064$ nm and $\Delta t_p \sim 2$ nsec.[27]
- Temperature tuning: The requirements on the laser pointer in Fig. 1.19 are not difficult to meet, while the power stability (Section 2.1.8) and

frequency stability (Section 2.1.9) requirements for a complex laser radar system that uses both 1064-nm and 532-nm photons to obtain information on the Earth's atmosphere from a low-Earth orbit may be extremely challenging. In such cases, temperature tuning of the nonlinear crystal—i.e., controlling the refractive indices $n(\nu)$ and $n(2\nu)$ to maintain phase matching—may be required; see Ref. 27 for more details.

Summarizing Section 1.2, laser designers must control a number of important parameters, including: (1) axial modes for "color" purity and temporal coherence, (2) transverse modes for directionality and spatial coherence, (3) pulse width and period, and (4) wavelength conversion. Many more engineering specifications of importance to the user of lasers—i.e., the laser systems engineer—will be reviewed in Chapter 2. A brief overview of the laser systems engineering process and the remainder of the book are first given in Section 1.3.

## 1.3 Laser Systems Engineering

An awareness of the laser designer's options will only simplify the laser systems engineer's job, as many of the tasks are similar. But even with this understanding, an obvious first question to ask for any system architecture is: why—or under what conditions—is a laser even necessary? While we have reviewed some of the properties of lasers, answering a question such as this requires a follow-on question: What are the properties of the alternatives?

The alternatives to lasers are incoherent sources—solar energy, arc lamps, tungsten-halogen bulbs, and so on[28]—and the first comparison (or design trade) to make is how much power is available from each type of source. This may seem like a strange design trade; after all, if the laser and the incoherent source both emit 100 mW of power, then isn't 100 mW available from both for material ablation, biomedical sample fluorescence, or any other application?

Figure 1.21 illustrates why this is not the case. In Fig. 1.21(a), we see that an incoherent source on the left of the lens is imaged to something resembling the source with a magnification $m_{\text{lens}} = -s_i/s_o$ for an object distance $s_o$ and an image distance $s_i$. In Fig. 1.21(b), on the other hand, a laser of the same size and placed at the same object distance $s_o$ is imaged to a focused spot whose size depends on the laser wavelength $\lambda$, the lens diameter $D$, and the beam quality $M^2$.

The reason for the difference in Fig. 1.21 is that the wavefronts from the incoherent source are emitted by each point on the source independently of the other (Fig. 1.8), and thus recombine to an image independently of each other as well. Each point on the source is in fact focused to a small spot, but

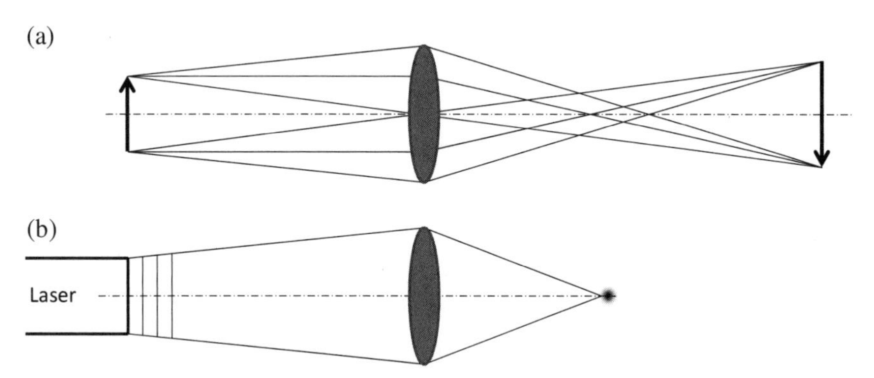


**Figure 1.21** (a) A lens reproduces a nearby incoherent source into an image resembling the source. (b) A lens images a nearby laser beam of the same size into a small focused spot.

because each point emits independently of the others—i.e., incoherently—they recombine as shown on the RHS of Fig. 1.21(a).

For the laser, however, the points are to a large degree emitting in phase, and thus coherently recombine into a small, focused spot. The degree to which they are in phase depends on the spatial coherence, which as we will see in Chapter 3 determines in part the size of the spot.

In addition, essentially all of the power emitted by the laser is collected by the lens, while a large fraction of the power emitted by the incoherent source is not. That is, the laser's full-divergence angle (or directionality) $2\theta_o \approx \lambda/D$, while an incoherent source typically emits at least some power into a sphere encompassing the source. Sizing a lens to capture the laser's divergence angle is thus relatively straightforward (see Chapter 6), while specialized reflectors are required to capture even a decent fraction of an incoherent source's power.

Finally, the incoherent source emits an extremely large wavelength band, while the laser typically does not (exceptions such as super-continuum lasers will be reviewed in Section 2.2.3).

It turns out that it is possible to use an incoherent source in such a way that it has many of the properties of lasers—but at a cost. Figure 1.22 illustrates how this is possible using a small aperture size $s$ (such as a pinhole after the source itself) and a narrow bandpass filter (BPF) to transmit only a small fraction of the wavelengths emitted. In addition, if the pinhole is placed

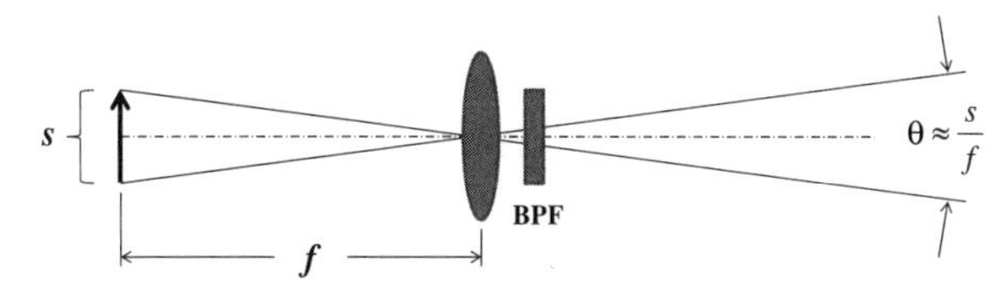


**Figure 1.22** An incoherent source can be designed with a small aperture size $s$ to increase spatial coherence, and a bandpass filter (BPF) to control temporal coherence.

at the focal length of the lens, the lens collimates the incoherent source with a divergence angle $\theta \approx s/f$.[28] As the pinhole is made smaller—and the wavefront across it is thus more coherent—the divergence angle will approach the full divergence angle $2\theta_o$ of a laser, after which $\theta$ is limited by wavefront diffraction and cannot be made any smaller (see Problem 1.10).

So with some additional optics, it is possible to design an incoherent source with a spatial and temporal coherence similar to a laser's—but at the cost of a huge loss of power. The pinhole, for example, allows only a small fraction of the incoherent source's light through it, as does the BPF. One of the unique features of a typical laser, then, is not the directionality and narrow wavelength band, but these properties *combined with* almost all of its output power available for useful tasks such as material ablation, fluorescence microscopy, or directed energy.

For a laser *system*, however, laser output power is not the whole story, and there are other requirements, components, and subsystems that must be considered as well. The perspective taken to do this—that of the laser systems engineer—is sometimes thought of as "designing the right laser" versus "designing the laser right." Unfortunately, this is both incomplete and overly centered on the laser designer's goal of designing the laser right. Designing the right laser—i.e., one that meets system-level requirements such as output power—is certainly key, but designing the right optical, scanning, and detector subsystems is equally critical.

Table 1.4 is a common systems-engineering tool that illustrates one way in which these other subsystems are taken into account. Known as a trade table, it compares three different design options for a laser radar system. The options evaluated in this case—and there are many other criteria that must also be used—are based on a power budget, i.e., is there enough power reflected from the target to be "useful" to the detector?

In this simple example, system performance depends on three components: the laser output power, the size of the telescope aperture collecting the reflected power, and the detector's sensitivity (i.e., the smallest power it can detect). In Design 1, it was assumed by the laser-system architect that a laser with 1 W of output power was available, as well as a telescope aperture of 100 mm and a minimum power for the detector (or *sensitivity*) of 1 nW.

**Table 1.4** A trade table summarizing component specifications for laser radar system design options.

| Component | Design 1 | Design 2 | Design 3 |
|---|---|---|---|
| Laser Power | 1 W | 0.1 W | 0.1 W |
| Telescope Aperture | 100 mm | 316 mm | 100 mm |
| Detector Sensitivity | 1 nW | 1 nW | 0.1 nW |

In reviewing the architecture with the laser designer, however, it was found that the 1-W laser would not be ready for product development for quite a while, and that a 100-mW laser was the only reliable option for now.

So with a factor of $10\times$ less power available from the laser, a factor of $10\times$ increase in telescope area (Design 2)—or a $10^{1/2} = 3.16\times$ increase in aperture size—was considered to compensate. At this point, the optical engineer on the project mentioned that such an aperture was much larger in terms of size and weight than the customer would consider, thus removing Design 2 as one of the options.

Fortunately, in reviewing the architecture with the detector specialist, it was found that detectors with $1/10^{th}$ the sensitivity were available as commercial off-the-shelf (COTS) parts, thus allowing Design 3 to proceed as the baseline architecture.

As we will see in Chapter 6, there are a number of additional details such as beam quality to consider when developing power budgets, and this simple example illustrates only one of the many design trades between the subsystems—laser, optics, scanning, and detector—to be reviewed in this book. Included are chapters on laser types and selection (Chapter 2), the unique requirements on using optical components in laser systems (Chapter 4), scanning technologies and system trades (Chapter 5), and detector types and selection (Chapter 7). Interspersed between these chapters are the concepts needed to understand beam propagation (Chapter 3) and radiometry (Chapter 6). The book does not include software or electrical[29] subsystems.

The emphasis in all chapters is on real-world design problems and the first-order equations and COTS components used to solve them. As with any book, not every topic can be included; however, readers may also find my previous books useful for understanding the many differences between laser systems and conventional optical systems using incoherent sources [*Optical Systems Engineering*, McGraw-Hill (2011)], or obtaining additional details on the optomechanical aspects of building laser systems [*Optomechanical Systems Engineering*, John Wiley (2015)].

## 1.4 Problems

**1.1** Analyze the 1950s Laser-Eyed Monster from the perspective of the laser systems engineer. For example, is there a possible eye-safety issue associated with launching a high-power beam through one's eyes? In addition, how would such a laser be powered, how would the heat be removed, and how would the wavelength be controlled? Hint: See Chapter 2 for additional considerations.

**1.2** What is the linewidth $\Delta\lambda$ for an inhomogeneously broadened laser that lases at five axial-mode frequencies based on Eq. (1.6)?

**1.3** Does the transmission of an etalon drop off faster or slower with laser frequency as the etalon reflectivity $R$ is increased? Are there disadvantages to using a higher reflectivity?

**1.4** What is the cold-cavity (zero gain) FWHM bandwidth $\Delta\nu_{SLM}$ of the individual longitudinal modes of a laser resonator based on the mirror reflectivities? (Hint: What is the finesse of the laser cavity?) And is this result consistent with that obtained from Eqs. (1.11), (1.12), and (1.13)?

**1.5** What is the axial mode spacing $\Delta\nu_a$ for the confocal cavity? How does it compare with that of the planar-mirror cavity?

**1.6** Are there any laser cavity designs that have the same absolute value of the axial-mode frequency as the planar-mirror cavity? Hint: See Ref. 9.

**1.7** What is the approximate cavity length $L$ needed to obtain the mode-locked pulse period $T_p$ shown In Fig. 1.18? The gain medium's refractive index $n \approx 1$.

**1.8** In a mode-locked laser, what is the relation between the coherence length $d_c$ and the pulse width $\Delta t_p$?

**1.9** If a SFG oscillator creates one 2128-nm photon from 1064-nm photons, what is the wavelength of the second long-wavelength photon that an OPO must produce to conserve energy?

**1.10** Referring to Fig. 1.22, what pinhole size is required to give the same collimated-beam full-divergence angle as a laser with $2\theta_o = 4\lambda/\pi D$? Assume that the wavelength $\lambda = 1$ μm and the smallest relative aperture available for the lens is $f/D \equiv f/\# = 1$.

## Notes and References

1. See, for example, A. Samman, L. Rimau, J. R. McBride, R. O. Carter, W. H. Weber, C. Gmachl, F. Capasso, A. L. Hutchinson, D. L. Sivco, and A. Y. Cho, "Potential use of near, mid, and far infrared laser diodes in automotive LIDAR applications," *IEEE Vehicular Technology Conference*, pp. 2084–2089 (2000); or R. Halterman and M. Bruch, "Velodyne HDL-64E lidar for unmanned surface vehicle obstacle detection," *Proc. SPIE* **7692**, 76920D (2010) [doi: 10.1117/12.850611].
2. S. W. Hell, "Nanoscopy with focused light," *Proc. SPIE* **8882**, 888203 (2013) [doi: 10.1117/2032261].
3. G. P. Agrawal, *Fiber-Optic Communication Systems*, Fourth Edition, John Wiley & Sons (2010).

4. J. König and T. Bauer, "Fundamentals and industrial applications of ultrashort pulsed lasers at Bosch," *Proc. SPIE* **7925**, 792510 (2011) [doi: 10.1117/12.878593].

5. K. V. Chellappan, E. Erden, and H. Urey, "Laser-based displays: A review," *Applied Optics* **49**(25), F79–F98 (2010).

6. P. Lubin, G. B. Hughes, J. Bible, J. Bublitz, J. Arriola, C. Motto, J. Suen, I. Johansson, J. Riley, N. Sarvian, D. Clayton-Warwick, J. Wu, A. Milich, M. Oleson, M. Pryor, P. Krogen, M. Kangas, and H. O'Neill, "Toward directed energy planetary defense," *Optical Engineering* **53**(2), 025103 (2014).

7. See, for example, Salvador Dali, "The Laser Unicorn Disintegrates the Horns of the Cosmic Rhinoceros," 1974.

8. E. P. Goodwin and J. C. Wyant, *Field Guide to Interferometric Optical Testing*, SPIE Press, Bellingham, Washington (2006) [doi: 10.1117/3.702897].

9. A. E. Siegman, *Lasers*, University Science Books, Sausalito, California (1986).

10. H. Weichel, "Lasers" in *The Infrared & Electro-Optical Systems Handbook* Vol. **3**, W. D. Rogatto, Editor, ERIM, Ann Arbor, Michigan and SPIE Press, Bellingham, Washington, Chapter 10 (1993).

11. In practice, small time-varying fluctuations in cavity spacing, lattice strain, and the refractive index of the gain medium lead to *mode hops*; see Section 2.1.9 for more details.

12. A. Mooradian, "Laser linewidth," *Physics Today* **38**(5), 42–50 (1985).

13. See, for example, R. Hauck, H. P. Kortz, and H. Weber, "Misalignment sensitivity of optical resonators," *Applied Optics* **19**(4), 598–601 (1980); or Ref. 9, Section 19.4.

14. This section does not apply to lasers that rely on total-internal-reflection (TIR) waveguiding between the mirrors, with semiconductor and fiber lasers being the most common. For those lasers that do not rely on waveguides, i.e., solid-state and gas lasers, the free-space modes in this section are applicable; see Ref. 15 for more information on waveguide modes.

15. C. R. Pollock, *Fundamentals of Optoelectronics*, Richard D. Irwin Publishing, Homewood, Illinois (1994).

16. Spatial coherence is defined by correlations across the wavefront (stationary phase). Unfortunately, this leaves open the possibility that

a wavefront with phase errors (a single $TEM_{01}$ mode, for example) is spatially coherent. As we will see in detail in Chapter 3, the concept of beam quality avoids this limitation by using a comparison of a wavefront not with itself, but with an ideal (uniphase), diffraction-limited ($M^2 = 1$) $TEM_{00}$ mode with zero phase errors across it, and which can be focused to the smallest-possible spot size.

17. R. Paschotta, *Field Guide to Lasers*, SPIE Press, Bellingham, Washington (2008) [doi: 10.1117/3.767474].

18. R. Paschotta, *Field Guide to Laser Pulse Generation*, SPIE Press, Bellingham, Washington (2008) [doi: 10.1117/3.800629].

19. J. Zheng, S. Zhao, and L. Chen, "Laser-diode end-pumped passively Q-switched intracavity doubling Nd:$YVO_4$KTP laser with $Cr^{4+}$:YAG saturable absorber," *Opt. Eng.* **41**(8), 1970–1975 (2002) [doi: 10.1117/1.1486245].

20. Z. Zheng, C. Zhao, S. Lu, Y. Chen, Y. Li, H. Zhang, and S. Wen, "Microwave and optical saturable absorption in graphene," *Optics Express* **20**(21), 23201–23214 (2012).

21. H. A. Haus, "Mode-locking of lasers," *IEEE Journal on Selected Topics in Quantum Electronics* **6**(6), 1173–1185 (2000).

22. J. F. James, *A Student's Guide to Fourier Transforms*, Cambridge University Press, Cambridge (1995).

23. C. C. Cutler, "Why does linear phase shift cause mode locking?" *IEEE Journal of Quantum Electronics* **28**(1), 282–288 (1992).

24. V. V. Matylitsky, F. Hendricks, and J. Aus der Au, "Femtosecond laser ablation properties of transparent materials: Impact of the laser process parameters on the machining throughput," *Proc. SPIE* **8611**, 861112 (2013) [doi: 10.1117/12.2003691].

25. Such lasers can also present a hazard to the eye due to leakage of 1064-nm light. For more details, see J. Galang, A. Restelli, E. W. Hagley, and C. W. Clark, "A red light for green laser pointers," *Optics and Photonics News*, pp. 11–13, Oct. 2010.

26. R. W. Boyd, *Nonlinear Optics*, Third Edition, Academic Press, San Diego (2008).

27. N. W. Sawruk, P. M. Burns, R. E. Edwards, T. Wysocki, A. Van Tujil, V. Litvinocitch, E. Sullivan, and F. E. Hovis, "ICESat-2 laser technology readiness level evolution," *Proc. SPIE* **9342**, 93420L (2015) [doi: 10.1117/12.2080531].

28. K. J. Kasunic, *Optical Systems Engineering*, McGraw-Hill, New York (2011).

29. P. C. D. Hobbs, *Building Electro-Optical Systems*, Second Edition, John Wiley & Sons, Hoboken, New Jersey (2009).

# Chapter 2
# Laser Selection

Of the many emerging applications of laser systems, one of the most intriguing is three-dimensional (3D) printing. That is, rather than manufacturing a component by starting with a bar or rod and removing material, 3D printing starts with fine grains of material and builds up layers by using the heat from absorbed laser light to thermally fuse the grains together (Fig. 2.1). Such laser additive manufacturing (LAM) allows complexity not readily available using material removal—lattice structures in the axles of high-performance racecars requiring low weight and high strength, for example.[1] While there are still a number of details being worked out—design rules, material strength, process reliability, manufacturing throughput, etc.—indications at this point are that the benefits of LAM exceed the costs for some low-volume applications.[2]

Another approach to manufacturing parts of increasing complexity and precision is to improve on the "material removal" model by using USP lasers for micromachining of very fine features that are otherwise obtainable only at high cost or insufficient quality. An example is the use of USPs for the cost-effective manufacture of flow injectors for regulating fuel consumption in

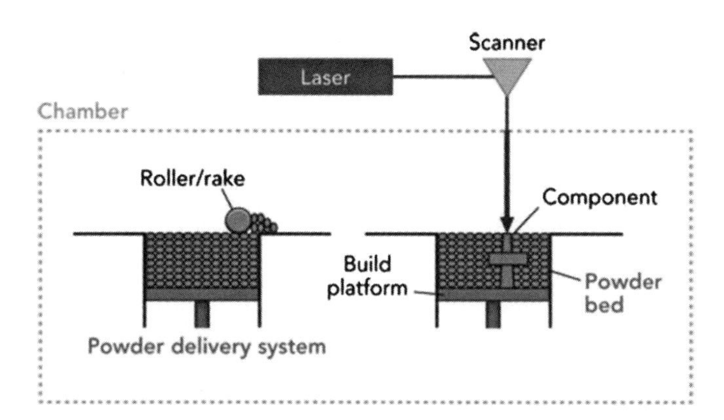


**Figure 2.1** 3D printing uses lasers to melt powders together to manufacture complex components. [Reprinted with permission from C. Dunsky, "Process monitoring in laser additive manufacturing," *Industrial Laser Solutions* **29**(5) (Sept. 12, 2014). © PennWell Corp. 2014.]

diesel engines—thus improving fuel efficiency and reducing carbon emissions.[3] The type of laser that allows this type of manufacturing is also used for a number of other applications, ranging from laser eye surgery—which is not yet additive—to the trade show demonstration of scribing a customer's name in the interior of a block of plastic.

The purpose of this chapter is to review the various types of lasers that might be useful for given system requirements such as LAM or material removal. As part of this, we first identify in Section 2.1 laser specifications such as average power, peak power, linewidth, pulse repetition frequency, etc., that are unique to specific applications such as manufacturing, biomedical systems, laser radar, laser communications, laser displays, directed energy, and so on. We then review in Section 2.2 the various types of lasers, classified as semiconductor, solid-state, fiber, and gas. Finally, Section 2.3 pulls everything together from the perspective of laser selection to meet overall system requirements. The emphasis is on commercially available lasers that can be used for most applications; we do not include "hero" experiments or rarely used lasers such as dye, chemical, free-electron, or x-ray.

## 2.1 Laser Specifications

We have seen in Chapter 1 how four key laser properties—also known as specifications, or "specs"—can occupy the laser designer's time: temporal coherence (coherence length), spatial coherence (focusing and directionality), pulse generation, and wavelength conversion. In this section, we dig a little deeper into the uses, consequences, and non-idealities of these specs, as well as review a number of additional properties of importance to the laser systems engineer.

### 2.1.1 Wavelength

Driven by requirements, wavelength is often the most important spec in developing laser systems. Table 2.1 lists the most-common wavelengths, the laser type (see Section 2.2), and some typical applications. In practice, these wavelengths have non-idealities associated with their use, including tolerances—i.e., plus-or-minus variations from the nominal wavelengths listed in Table 2.1—as well as drift with temperature and the potential need for tuning.

Tolerances from the nominal wavelength can be critical for many applications. As one example, the pump diode shown in Fig. 1.19—a type of semiconductor laser (see Section 2.2.1)—has a nominal wavelength of 808 nm; the reason is that the absorption required for the population inversion of the $Nd:YVO_4$ solid-state gain medium is particularly strong at this wavelength, and different wavelengths result in less absorption, thus lowering the efficiency of the laser.

**Table 2.1** Laser wavelengths as emitted by commonly used laser types, and typical applications; the different laser types will be reviewed in Section 2.2.

| Wavelength | Laser Type | Typical Applications |
|---|---|---|
| 157 nm | Excimer ($F_2$) | Semiconductor lithography |
| 193 nm | Excimer (ArF) | Eye surgery; semiconductor lithography |
| 248 nm | Excimer (KrF) | Semiconductor lithography |
| 266 nm | Nd:YAG (4×) | Manufacturing |
| 325 nm | HeCd | Stereolithography |
| 355 nm | Nd:YAG (3×), VECSEL | Manufacturing; biomedical |
| 405 nm | Diode (InGaN) | HD-DVD data storage |
| 455 nm | VECSEL | Laser-based displays |
| 532 nm | Nd:YAG (2×), VECSEL | Manufacturing; laser-based displays |
| 577 nm | VECSEL | Biomedical |
| 620–680 nm | Diode (AlGaInP) | Laser-based displays; bar-code scanners; laser pointers |
| 633 nm | HeNe | Interferometry; optical testing |
| 670–1100 nm | Ti:sapphire | Research |
| 808 nm | Diode (AlGaAs) | Laser pumping; manufacturing |
| 980 nm | Diode (InGaAs) | Laser pumping; manufacturing |
| 1030 nm | Disk (Yb:YAG) | Manufacturing |
| 1030–1070 nm | Fiber (Yb:Glass) | Manufacturing; laser radar |
| 1064 nm | Nd:YAG | Manufacturing; biomedical; directed energy |
| 1540 nm | Er:Glass | Rangefinders |
| 1550 nm | Diode (InGaAsP), fiber | Fiber-optic communications |
| 3.30 μm | Nd:YAG (+OPO) | Infrared countermeasures |
| 3.39 μm | HeNe | Interferometry; optical testing |
| 4.60 μm | QCL | Infrared countermeasures; spectroscopy |
| 10.6 μm | $CO_2$ | Manufacturing; optical testing; lithography |

Unfortunately, the pump diode is typically specified by the manufacturer as having a ±3 nm tolerance, so unless told otherwise they will supply pump diodes with a wavelength ranging anywhere from 805 nm to 811 nm—diodes that will be unacceptable for many applications. A wavelength screening process (and associated cost increase) is usually sufficient to narrow the wavelength range received from the diode vendor.

For the same reason, drift of the diode's wavelength with temperature $T$ may also need to be controlled. A typical edge-emitting diode has a wavelength sensitivity $d\lambda/dT \approx 0.3$ nm/K—a result of a shift in the peak wavelength of the gain curve with temperature—in which case a 10-K temperature increase results in a 3-nm wavelength shift—more than enough to exceed some wavelength-drift requirements. The consumer-market Nd:$YVO_4$ laser pointer shown in Fig. 1.19 is not overly sensitive to such wavelength shifts, while a Nd:YAG laser used for manufacturing or displays will be to within ±0.5 nm. As a result, thermoelectric coolers (TECs) are often used for diode-laser temperature stabilization[4] and wavelength control, thus allowing a looser requirement on wavelength screening.

Note that while it is easier to heat something up than it is to cool it down, diode lifetime decreases exponentially as it gets hotter, so it is

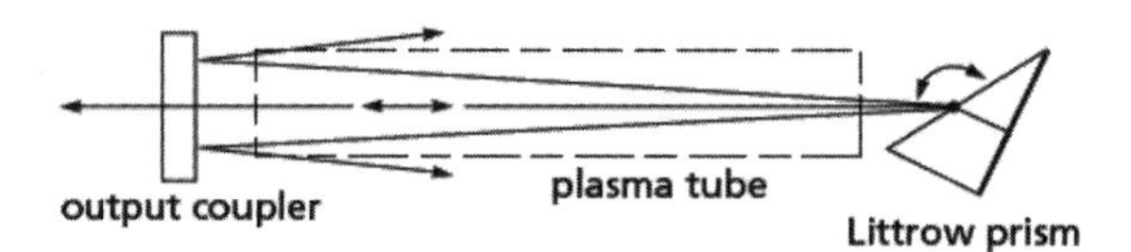


**Figure 2.2** Wavelength tuning of a gas (plasma) laser using angular adjustments of a prism in a Littrow configuration. (Credit: CVI Laser, LLC.)

better for temperature-critical applications to start with diodes specified as 808 nm +3/–0 nm (for example), ensuring that any temperature changes for wavelength control will cool the laser and not decrease the lifetime by doing so.

Solid-state lasers themselves are also susceptible to wavelength drift from temperature changes; see Section 2.1.9 for more details.

Finally, temperature control is also used not for shifting a laser's peak wavelength to a specific value such as 808 nm, but for obtaining a range of wavelengths. Such tuning might be necessary, for example, to determine the reflectivity or absorption of a material sample over a waveband, or spectroscopic sensing of gas components. Alternatives to low-speed thermal tuning include piezoelectric transducer (PZT) "stretchers" to change the length $L$ of a solid-state or fiber laser at high frequency, as well as prisms or gratings used as an external-cavity mirror to change the reflected wavelength when the prism is rotated (Fig. 2.2). Because of the longer cavity length, these lasers also have a high cavity quality $Q_c$ [see Eq. (1.11)].

A common example of a tunable laser is a Ti:sapphire solid-state laser. The wide bandwidth that is effective for producing short pulses also has a peak wavelength that can be varied by tuning. In the case of Ti:sapphire, the tuning is obtained using a polarization component known as a birefringent filter that controls the wavelength of the linearly polarized light created by the laser cavity.[5]

Independent of the method of tuning—temperature, cavity length, angle, or polarization—critical specs for tunable lasers include:

- Range – The Ti:sapphire laser has the largest tuning range ($\approx$400 nm), while PZT cavity-length tuning of fiber and solid-state lasers can be limited to ranges of <30 MHz. The disadvantage of a large tuning range is the change in output power as the wavelength is tuned away from the peak of the gain curve. OPOs also have a wide tuning range, using either thermal or angle tuning of the OPO crystal.
- Resolution – Ideally, tuning is continuous, allowing an infinitesimal resolution (or difference between tuned wavelengths). In practice, a number of non-idealities and competing effects prevent this from happening. For example, thermal tuning of a semiconductor laser changes its refractive index, cavity length, and peak wavelength of the gain curve. The balance of the change in these three parameters results

in discontinuous changes in wavelength (mode hops) that make it difficult to obtain a particular wavelength without using additional stabilizing hardware such as an on-chip (distributed feedback) grating or an external cavity. For an external cavity, the resolution is then determined by the resolution of the angular-positioning mechanism, with discrete changes $\delta\lambda_t \approx 0.5$–1 nm for semiconductor quantum-cascade lasers (QCLs).

- Speed – How quickly the wavelength can be changed to a different value depends primarily on the tuning method. For example, PZT stretchers can have a tuning rate on the order of 30 kHz, while thermal tuning of semiconductor lasers has a much-slower response time of 100 msec or more, depending on tuning range.
- Stability – Instabilities such as wavelength drift and/or jitter during or after tuning can occur for a number of reasons. For example, the angular pointing stability of an external prism or grating determines the variations in reflected wavelength, possibly requiring vibration isolation to avoid.[4] We will look in more detail at wavelength stability and its effect on laser system performance in Section 2.1.9.

### 2.1.2 Temporal coherence

As we have seen in Chapter 1, the laser bandwidth—either single mode or multimode—determines the temporal coherence and coherence length. In this section, we take a closer look at some of the reasons for a wide bandwidth—mode hopping, spatial hole burning, and so on—as well as the use of fiber dispersion and nonlinearities to create an ultrawide-bandwidth "white light" source known as a supercontinuum laser.

Before getting to these topics, one point that needs clarification is that the coherence length $d_c$ given in Section 1.2.1 is measured in air. If the beam is propagating in a window, lens, or other component with index $n > 1$, however, then the coherence length $d_{c,n}$ is smaller by $n$:

$$d_{c,n} = \frac{d_c}{n} \qquad [\mathrm{m}] \tag{2.1}$$

This is illustrated in Fig. 2.3, where the wavelength is shorter in the higher-index material,[6] and with more waves that can fit in the length of the optic, the shorter the coherence length before neighboring wavelengths separated by $\Delta\lambda$ becoming out of phase. This is also characterized using the concept of optical path length (OPL) = $nd$, with OPL/$\lambda_o$ equal to the number of free-space wavelengths in a distance $d$, and increases with either physical path length $d$ or refractive index $n$. The OPL can be the same in a distance $d$ of air or $d/n$ of high-index material, and the number of wavelengths and coherence length is the same in such cases as well.

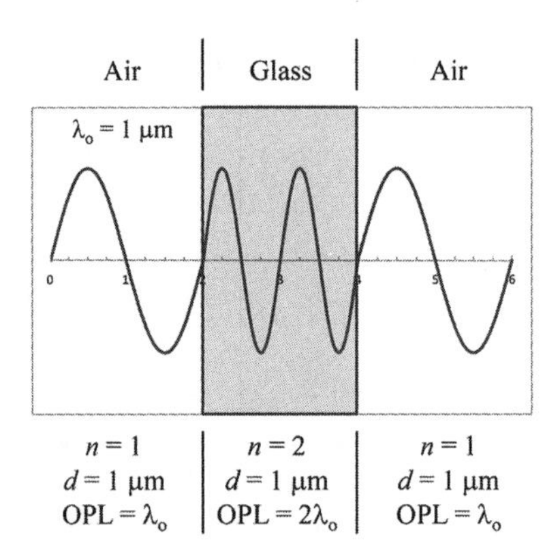


**Figure 2.3** The optical path length (OPL) = $nd$, with OPL/$\lambda_o$ equal to the number of wavelengths in a physical path length $d$ with index $n$.

Recalling from Chapter 1 that the coherence length ideally depends on the longitudinal modes based on the length of the laser cavity, the bandwidth of the gain medium, and the type of gain medium (homogeneous versus inhomogeneous), we expand on these concepts in this section to include additional linewidth broadening due to spatial hole burning and mode hops.

Spatial hole burning occurs because the power distribution of a longitudinal mode has the peaks and valleys associated with a standing wave, and only the peaks utilize gain to create stimulated emission; i.e., the peaks "burn holes" in the spatial gain distribution along the length of the laser cavity. This allows an additional longitudinal mode to utilize the gain, with one peak located at one valley of the shifted mode. The wavelengths of these two modes are slightly different,[7] and the laser linewidth $\Delta\lambda$ of even homogeneously broadened lasers is wider as a result; Eq. (1.3) shows that the coherence length is also reduced.

Small perturbations of the laser cavity—due to optical feedback from downstream components reflected back into the cavity through the output mirror, for example—may cause the laser to switch ("hop") its output wavelength between these longitudinal modes. Diode lasers are particularly susceptible to such hops, as the low reflectivity of the output mirror (the diode facet) allows a relatively large amount of feedback back into the cavity. Mode hops can also change the output power or energy (Section 2.1.8), as the different modes will have slightly different gain.

The consequences of spatial hole burning and associated mode hops for the laser systems engineer are that: (1) reflections from downstream optical components back into the laser cavity should be minimized using antireflection coatings, tilted windows, and other methods described in Chapter 4; and (2) as laser pumping is increased to increase output power, spatial hole burning can result in multiple longitudinal modes and therefore a linewidth that gets broader at higher power—not smaller as expected for the single-mode linewidth given in Eq. (1.8). We will see more on these topics in Sections 2.1.8 and 2.1.9.

Finally, ultrawide-bandwidth sources known as supercontinuum "white light" lasers with ultrashort coherence lengths have recently been developed. Some years ago it was commonly thought that the idea of a white-light laser was contradictory—that a laser had an inherently narrow optical linewidth, incompatible with a broad-band spectrum. Linewidth, however, is only one of many unique laser characteristics; others include spatial coherence (Section 2.1.3) and stimulated emission resulting in second-order photon statistics that are different from those of conventional sources[8]—characteristics that are maintained by supercontinuum lasers.

A supercontinuum is not created with broadening non-idealities such as spatial hole burning or mode hopping; instead, fiber nonlinearities generated by the peak power from USPs (Section 2.1.5) create a continuous band of wavelengths encompassing a huge number of longitudinal modes. Coherence length is thus usually not a requirement for the use of these lasers; more details on the use and selection of supercontinuum lasers are given in Section 2.2.3.

### 2.1.3 Spatial coherence

We have also seen in Chapter 1 how phase errors across a beam can determine its spatial coherence and beam quality. A beam with "poor" quality, for example, has a large divergence angle and focused spot size. Also associated with these phase errors are variations in the irradiance profiles (Fig. 2.4) that can reduce the usefulness of the laser in applications where a uniform or Gaussian profile is required.

There are many reasons that divergence angles and focused spot sizes are important to the laser systems engineer. As we have seen in Chapter 1, for

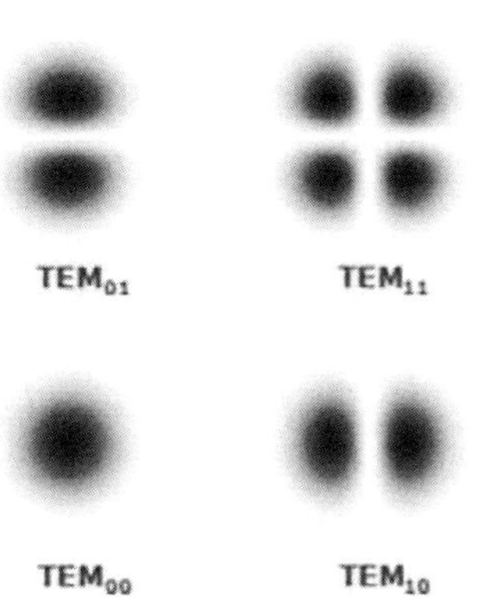


**Figure 2.4** Irradiance profiles for $TEM_{00}$ (Gaussian), $TEM_{01}$, $TEM_{10}$, and $TEM_{11}$ transverse modes. [Reprinted from R. Paschotta, *Field Guide to Lasers*, SPIE Press, Bellingham, Washington (2008).]

example, a smaller spot size increases the number of bits of information that can fit on a CD or DVD. As we will see in Chapter 6, in other cases it is the power density (power per unit area) that determines a laser's ability to heat a target, also putting an emphasis on controlling spatial coherence and spot sizes. In addition, it is easier to collect light with a lens from a low-divergence beam. In contrast, there are applications such as laser-based projectors where poor spatial coherence is an advantage, as it reduces the speckle of the image (see Chapter 7).

The degree of "poorness"—that is, how much the divergence angle or spot size increases—is usually measured with respect to the Gaussian ($TEM_{00}$) mode shown in Fig. 2.4. For example, a higher-order $TEM_{11}$ mode has a divergence angle and spot size that is 3× larger than the $TEM_{00}$ mode (see Chapter 3). Such situations are not common, and more often the laser emits an aberrated Gaussian or multimode beam consisting of a combination of higher-order modes such as $TEM_{01}$ and $TEM_{10}$. In addition, there are also non-idealities in spot size and shape that make it difficult to measure the mode quality; more details are given in Chapter 3.

### 2.1.4 Output power: CW, QCW, and pulsed

Independent of the degree of temporal and spatial coherence, the output power of the beam can be measured as a single number. Typical continuous wave (CW) values range from 1 μW for low-power semiconductor lasers to 100 kW for high-power fiber lasers. The term CW refers to the fact that there is no obvious attempt such as quasi-CW (QCW) or pulsing to change the output power; instead, any changes in power are considered to be errors in stability (see Section 2.1.8).

Output power first increases with pumping, i.e., an increase in either optical pumping or electrical current, depending on the type of laser. Figure 2.5 shows that the increase in output power $P$ for an edge-emitting semiconductor laser depends on drive current $i$. Characteristics of these curves include the threshold current $i_{th}$ (the current at which the laser first emits coherent light) and the slope efficiency $\eta_s = \Delta P/\Delta i$ (units of W/A) above threshold. This measures how much the output power changes as the current changes, with large slope efficiencies requiring less current (and electrical power) to increase the optical power emitted.

As the current increases, the wall-plug efficiency can decrease because the fraction of the electrical power that does not go towards increasing the laser output power instead increases the semiconductor temperature and internal losses; for the same reason, there may also be a "roll-over" of the output power at even higher current.

Mathematically, we can express the linear slope efficiency in terms of laser design parameters:

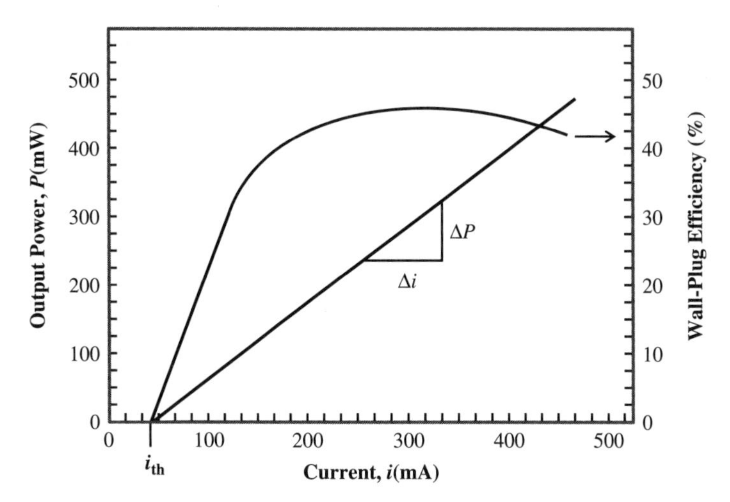


**Figure 2.5** Output power $P$ and wall-plug efficiency for an edge-emitting semiconductor laser depends on the laser drive current $i$ in comparison with the threshold current $i_{th}$.

$$P = \frac{h\nu}{2q} \frac{\alpha_m}{\alpha_{int} + \alpha_m} (i - i_{th}) \qquad [W] \tag{2.2}$$

for an internal loss $\alpha_{int}$ and mirror loss $\alpha_m$, with the laser designer's goal to minimize the internal loss in comparison with the mirror loss. Physically, the increase in pump current does not increase the laser gain; instead, the gain is clamped by the total loss $\alpha_{int} + \alpha_m$ at a fixed value, and the increase in current beyond threshold goes directly into increasing the output power.

A variation on the CW theme is the use of QCW changes in drive current, typically used for semiconductor lasers. A common example is the use of a semiconductor laser as an optical pump for a Q-switched solid-state laser; in this case, it is not necessary to continuously drive the semiconductor laser, and there is a thermal advantage as well to interrupting the current. That is, by reducing the drive-current duty cycle—equal to $t_{on}/(t_{on} + t_{off})$ for an on-time $t_{on}$ and an off-time $t_{off}$ (Fig. 2.6)—the average power dissipation and thermal load on the semiconductor pump laser are reduced for a given QCW power level; alternatively, the QCW power can be increased if the average power is kept the same.

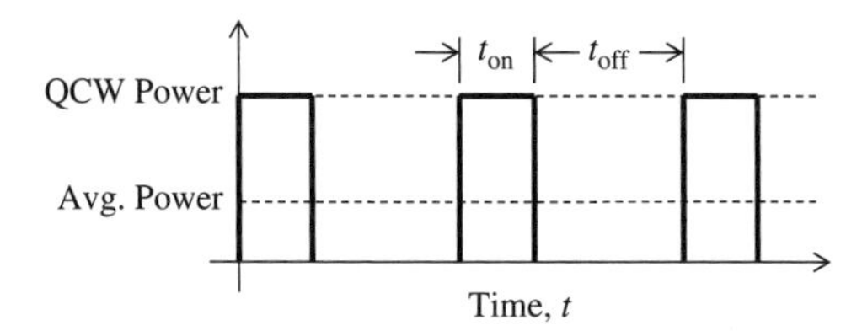


**Figure 2.6** A duty cycle of less than 100% can be used to either increase the QCW power or reduce the average power dissipation.

As internal losses for semiconductor lasers generally increase with temperature, reducing the thermal load with a QCW pump increases the wall-plug efficiency and reduces the power consumption of the pump laser. Pulsed QCW pumping with the same average power is also commonly used and allows the highest-possible Q-switch energy, with the limitation of a lower pulse repetition frequency (PRF) given the allowable on-off times for a semiconductor laser. For example, a rectangular on-time of 0.1 msec and a duty cycle of 10% have a QCW output power that is 10× that of the CW power but is limited to a PRF of 1/(0.1 msec × 10) = 1 kHz.

The concepts of pulse width and PRF are needed for understanding two high-PRF modes of characterizing output power, namely, those of Q-switching and mode locking. Seen previously in Section 1.2.3, the peak power can now be much larger than that obtained using low-PRF QCW pulsing of the pump power. As shown in Fig. 2.7, the peak power $P_{\text{peak}}$ depends on how quickly the pulse energy $Q_{\text{p}}$ is changed:[9]

$$P_{\text{peak}} = \frac{\Delta Q_{\text{p}}}{\Delta t_{\text{p}}} \qquad [\text{W}] \tag{2.3}$$

The peak power of a diode-pumped solid-state (DPSS) laser can be as much as $10^6\times$ larger than the average power. Applications for which a large peak power is important include nonlinear wavelength conversion (Section 1.2.4), "cold" laser machining (Section 2.1.5), multiphoton microscopy, and laser ranging and active imaging where the detector responds to the peak power reflected off of a target (Chapter 7).

If the pulse width and period are known, the peak power can be related to the average power as

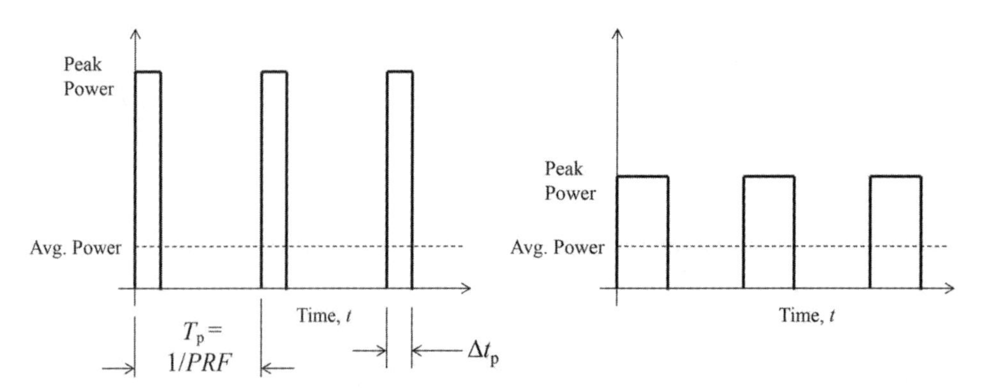


**Figure 2.7** With the same average power, a shorter pulse width $\Delta t_{\text{p}}$ in comparison with the pulse period $T_{\text{p}} = 1/PRF$ increases the peak power for Q-switched and mode-locked pulses.

$$P_{\mathrm{peak}} = P_{\mathrm{avg}} \frac{T_{\mathrm{p}}}{\Delta t_{\mathrm{p}}} = \frac{P_{\mathrm{avg}}}{\Delta t_{\mathrm{p}} \cdot PRF} \qquad [\mathrm{W}] \tag{2.4}$$

illustrating that if the average power is not changed, shorter pulses result in higher peak power. The PRF also plays a role, as $T_{\mathrm{p}} = 1/PRF$ is the pulse period (or time between pulses), and Eq. (2.4) and Fig. 2.7 show that reducing the pulse width in comparison with the period increases the peak power—physically a result of concentrating more average energy into a shorter period of time. As a result, even though the average power of a Q-switched solid-state laser may only be 10 W, the peak power is 100 kW for 10-nsec pulses switching on and off at a PRF of 10 kHz.

The distinction between average and peak power is clearly illustrated in a current application of pulsed lasers, namely, laser machining of glass and sapphire covers for smart phones, watches, and the like. Specifically, materials that look transparent to our eye transmit low-power light based on a linear mechanism of electron oscillation—so how can we use VIS-wavelength lasers for machining and material removal when the output of these lasers is typically transmitted by such materials?

The key is that a high peak power induces nonlinear electron oscillations that result in absorption and, in extreme cases, electron ionization. Such nonlinear absorption and multiphoton ionization processes no longer allow laser power to be transmitted; instead, the material is ablated, resulting in efficient laser machining. The degree to which a transparent material can be machined, then, depends on the peak power (which may or may not be dominated by pulse width). As we will see in the next section, laser machining of materials such as metals that are inherently absorptive at low power depends more directly on the pulse width.

### 2.1.5 Pulse width

A key parameter for estimating peak power, then, is the pulse width $\Delta t_{\mathrm{p}}$. Typical numbers run from 1–10 nsec for Nd:YAG solid-state lasers, to 10 psec or less for fiber and disk lasers, to 100 fsec or less for Ti:sapphire lasers. This is currently an important area of laser development, as short pulses have a number of advantages beyond that implied by peak power alone. Specifically, if the pulse width is shorter than the thermal diffusion time of the absorbed energy, then there will be no *thermal* damage (vaporization) to the work piece or biomedical sample (Fig. 2.8). Instead, material removal (ablation) is based purely on electron ionization, and with minimal heat-affected zone (HAZ) surrounding the machined area, manufacturing quality improves to the point where new applications requiring higher precision of mechanical dimensions are possible.

USPs, then—typically defined as $\Delta t_{\mathrm{p}} \leq 10$ psec, although this depends on the thermal diffusivity of the machined material—allow both a high peak

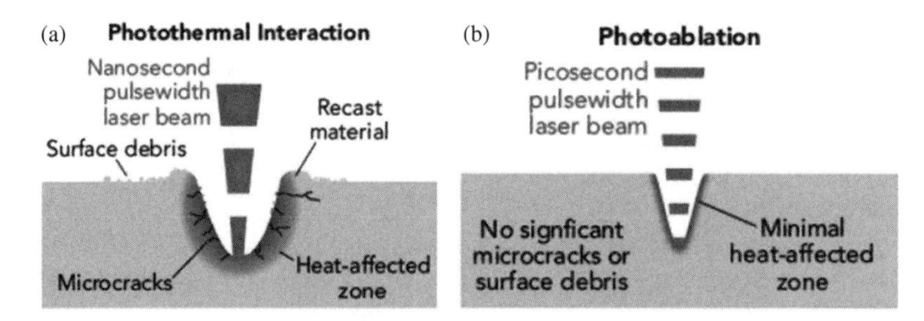


**Figure 2.8** Picosecond pulses shorter than the thermal diffusion time of the material minimize photothermal damage, allowing "cold" photoablation. (Reprinted with permission from Coherent, Inc.)

power and "cold machining" of absorbing materials with minimum photothermal effects. If the average power is large enough, however, the relatively slower thermal processes can still cause heating and damage if energy is accumulated over a number of pulses near the same location. A key goal of some USP laser applications is thus a large peak power with low average power; Eq. (2.4) shows that this requires control of both the pulse width and PRF (also see Section 2.1.7).

Another application for which pulse width has a large effect on laser-system performance is laser radar for self-driving vehicles, where pulses are directed at objects such as nearby automobiles or pedestrians to determine their distance (or range $R$). A key requirement for such systems is the minimum measurable distance $\Delta R$ between objects; known as the range resolution, it depends on the pulse width such that $2\Delta R = c\Delta t_p$. To date, such systems have typically relied on non-USP systems such as semiconductor or Nd:YAG solid-state lasers capable of reliably producing 1- to 10-nsec pulses with sufficiently high peak power.

From Section 1.2.3 we know that USP lasers—also known as ultrafast lasers—require mode locking to generate pulses. It is only recently that laser developers have introduced mode-locked products that have the flexibility, reliability, low maintenance, and low cost sufficient for a manufacturing or commercial environment. We will see these types of lasers in more detail in Section 2.2.

Independent of laser type, it is often the case that laser pulses are not approximately rectangular, and it is useful to estimate the pulse width in these cases. Table 2.2 lists the FWHM pulse width in comparison with the rectangular pulse. A value >1 indicates that the peak power obtained using Eq. (2.3) is smaller by the same factor, as expected when the pulse energy does not change as quickly for a pulse with a slower rise and fall time. For example, a Gaussian pulse shape has a FWHM width that is 1.4× larger than the ideal rectangular pulse and a peak power that is 1.4× smaller for the same pulse energy.

**Table 2.2** Normalized FWHM pulse widths for commonly used pulse shapes.[10]

| Pulse Shape | FWHM $\Delta t_p$ |
|---|---|
| Rectangular | 1.00 |
| Gaussian | 1.41 |
| $Sech^2$ | 1.54 |
| Lorentzian | 2.00 |

### 2.1.6 Pulse energy

Pulse energy, then, is the second component of peak power; it may also be useful as an alternative to specifying peak power, as there are physical processes that depend on energy and not power. That is, pulse energy $Q_p$ is the power integrated over the time of the pulse,

$$Q_p = \int P(t)dt = P_{peak} \cdot \Delta t_p \qquad [J] \qquad (2.5)$$

for a rectangular pulse. Pulse energy is also known as *dose*, with laser systems such as semiconductor photolithographic manufacturing depending on the energy a photoresist is exposed to, rather than the peak power. Damage to optical components may also be specified in terms of energy density or *fluence* (units of $J/cm^2$), as we will see in Chapter 4.

Typical pulse energies supported by current laser designs are on the order of 1 mJ, with 1 μJ being small, 1 J being relatively large, and 1 MJ being researched at Livermore's National Ignition Facility (NIF) for nuclear fusion. In general, Q-switching has higher pulse energies in comparison with mode locking.[11]

Pulse energy (and therefore peak power) depends on:

- How long the laser can store energy before releasing it; i.e., the rate at which the inverted population loses its excited-state energy must be slow for a large $Q_p$
- The number of atoms that are emitting (i.e., the mode volume)
- Loss of energy due to absorption by harmonic generation or OPO components
- Wavelength—shorter-λ UV photons have more energy than longer-λ VIS photons, given that photon energy $E_p = hc/\lambda$

The first three items are parameters controlled by the laser designer, but the last item may be a factor for the systems engineer to consider in laser selection (see Section 2.3).

Differences in pulse energy do not necessarily imply a smaller peak power. For example, a solid-state Nd:YAG laser with $Q_p = 1$ mJ and $\Delta t_p = 10$ nsec has $P_{peak} = 0.001$ J/($10 \times 10^{-9}$ sec) = 0.1 MW; a disk laser with a typical

$Q_p = 0.1$ mJ and $\Delta t_p = 10$ psec, on the other hand, has $P_{peak} = 0.0001$ J/$(10 \times 10^{-12}$ sec$) = 10$ MW. The 100× larger peak power of the USP disk laser—even with its 10× lower pulse energy—is a key factor in the selection of these lasers for manufacturing and biomedical applications.

### 2.1.7 Pulse repetition frequency

Yet another spec of importance for Q-switched and mode-locked lasers is the PRF (also known as pulse repetition rate, or PRR). The combination of pulse energy and PRF determines the average optical power,

$$P_{avg} = Q_p \cdot PRF \qquad [\text{W}] \tag{2.6}$$

where the pulse energy times the number of pulses per second (the PRF) is the average output power of the laser.

Typical PRFs range from 1–10 Hz for Q-switched laser rangefinders to 200 MHz for high-throughput manufacturing and biomedical imaging using mode-locked lasers. As shown in Fig. 2.9, however, an excessively high PRF can reduce the pulse energy—and therefore the peak and average power. The figure shows that at low PRF (0.1–1 kHz), the pulse energy of a solid-state laser stays more-or-less constant, initially increasing the average power with PRF [Eq. (2.6)]. At the same time, the pulse width is also constant, so the peak power does not increase [Eq. (2.3)].

When the PRF approaches 2 kHz, however, the pulse energy starts to drop, as the extraction of energy from the excited-state atoms exceeds the rate at which they can supply it. Simultaneously, the pulse width increases because the excited-state dynamics do not allow pulsing at the higher PRF. The combination of these two effects decreases the peak power and keeps the average power approximately constant—a combination that can result in excess heating of the target or sample, without the benefits of high peak

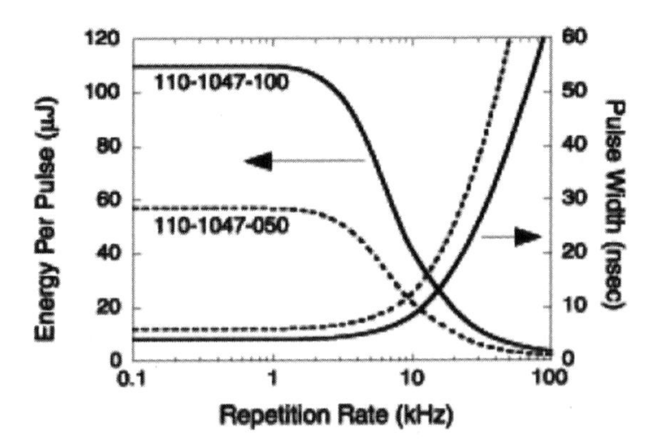


**Figure 2.9** Pulse energy and width from a solid-state laser are approximately constant until the PRF is excessively high. [Data for the M110 Series nonplanar ring oscillator (NPRO) laser courtesy of JDSU.]

power. A key goal of some USP laser applications is thus a large peak power with low average power, which Eq. (2.4) shows us requires control of both the pulse width and PRF.

Nonetheless, there are applications where a larger PRF is useful. The first is when the higher average power density ($W/m^2$) allows larger areas to be simultaneously processed and increases manufacturing throughput for those non-USP applications—lithography, for example—that do not rely on peak power. In addition, using more pulses with a lower energy per pulse allows less variation in total dose—i.e., one big pulse with all of the required energy has a large $\Delta Q_p$.

In practice, a non-ideality that arises with pulsed lasers is that of timing jitter.[12] That is, the pulse period $T_p = 1/\mathrm{PRF}$ is not exactly the same from pulse to pulse, and relying on it to be so results in system errors. For example, direct-detection laser radar systems use the change in distance $\Delta R$ over the time $T_p$ between pulses to determine an object's velocity; any errors in the time will therefore result in errors in the calculated velocity. Timing jitter's dominant contributor is often optomechanical noise, usually seen as vibration-induced variations in cavity spacing that result in changes in round-trip time and thus PRF.

### 2.1.8 Power and energy stability

Given the dependence of peak power on pulse energy, the energy repeatability (or stability) is a critical spec for a number of applications. For example, cold micromachining of the human cornea using LASIK or similar techniques depends on the peak power, and variations in this power can have disastrous consequences for the eyesight of the patient. A less critical application—that of laser-based projection systems—requires a certain degree of power stability to maintain color fidelity with only one calibration, thus saving field-service expenses.[13]

Power and energy stability can be divided into short-term (pulse-to-pulse) and long-term (drift) changes. Figure 2.10 shows the long-term power output of a semiconductor laser, where the power is seen to drift to a slightly smaller value over a period of 2500 hours of CW operation. Depending on the application, such drift can render the laser useless, thus requiring the vendor to specify the power drop over a given time period—a condition known as "end of life" (EOL), which must be clearly specified by the laser systems engineer.[14]

For pulsed lasers, Fig. 2.11 shows the variation in pulse-to-pulse energy with PRF (or repetition rate) for an excimer laser used for semiconductor lithography, with very tight requirements on energy stability to ensure high-volume production yield of computer chips.[15] The figure shows a higher PRF having a larger standard deviation in pulse energy, with the shorter cavity required for a faster PRF having less time for the pulse energy to stabilize. For

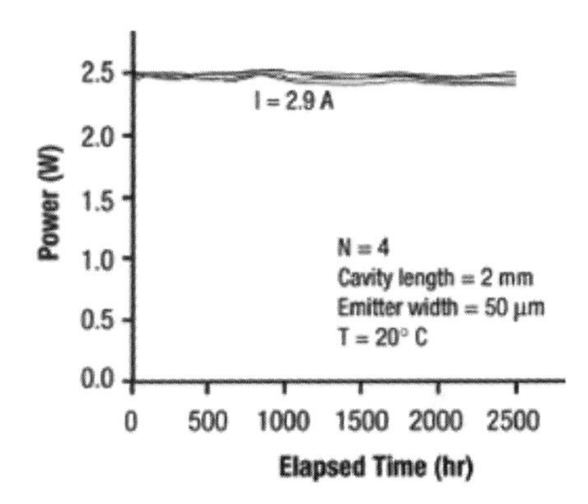


**Figure 2.10** Power drift over a specified number of operating hours determines the EOL performance. (Reprinted with permission from Newport Spectra-Physics; all rights reserved.)

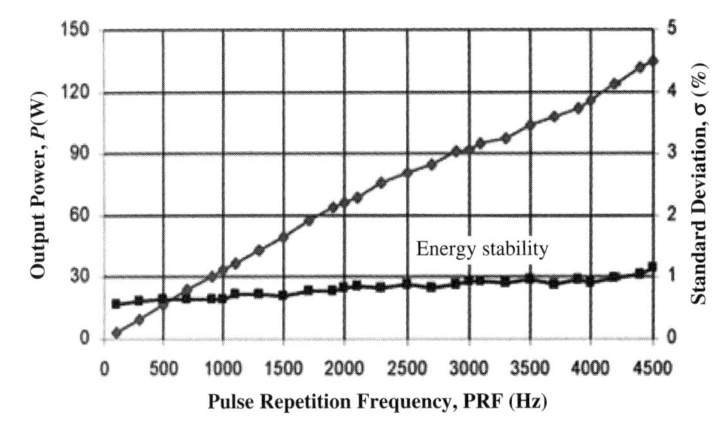


**Figure 2.11** Pulse-to-pulse energy instability—measured as a standard deviation $\sigma$ of the pulse energy—increases with PRF for an excimer laser. (Data courtesy of Coherent, Inc.)

the same reason, other types of lasers will have better or worse stability than the 1% shown in Fig. 2.11—short-cavity quantum-cascade lasers, for example, are specified with <4% pulse-to-pulse energy stability based on variations in pulse power and width.[16]

If EOL power or pulse-to-pulse stability is not specified, then some other time scale must be supplied by the vendor. For example, to avoid down-time for the re-calibration of pulse energy, long-term pulse stability for excimer lasers used in lithography must be known. The definition of "long term" can depend on either the application or the lifetime of the laser itself, with the application being preferred, but such data is not always available from the vendors. A common spec is the use of a root-mean-square (RMS) power change over a 1- to 12-hour period, with longer periods having a larger power variation.

Power and energy stability are also known as amplitude stability; *intensity noise* is also used, although the term *noise* often implies frequency dependence.

For example, a power drift over an 8-hour period implies a measurement frequency of once per 8 hours, equal to 1/(8 hours × 3600 sec/hour) = 34.7 μHz. If the measurement frequency is higher, however—as it clearly is for laser-communication systems operating at data rates of 10 GHz or higher—then the intensity noise must be specified at these frequencies.

The concept of relative intensity noise (RIN) is most common, where the laser's optical power variance $\sigma_P^2(f)$ is measured relative to the mean optical power $P$ at a specific electrical frequency $f$ and over a small electrical bandwidth $\Delta f$:

$$RIN(f) = \frac{1}{\Delta f}\left[\frac{\sigma_P(f)}{P}\right]^2 \qquad [1/\text{Hz}] \tag{2.7}$$

where $1/\Delta f$ gives units of 1/Hz, and the unitless power ratio $[\sigma_P(f)/P]^2$ is often expressed in terms of decibels (dB), giving equivalent units of dB/Hz. As shown in Fig. 2.12, RIN is then measured over the frequency range needed for the particular system—0.1 to 10 GHz for high-data-rate laser communications systems, for example—with features specific to the laser being used (such as high-frequency relaxation oscillations for semiconductor lasers). Laser RIN can be one factor of many determining pump noise or the system signal-to-noise ratio (SNR)—see Chapter 7 for more details.

Design options available to the laser systems engineer for improving power and energy stability include:

- High PRF – More pulses at lower energy per pulse generally allows less variation in total dose, even though the energy variance of each pulse may be a bit larger.

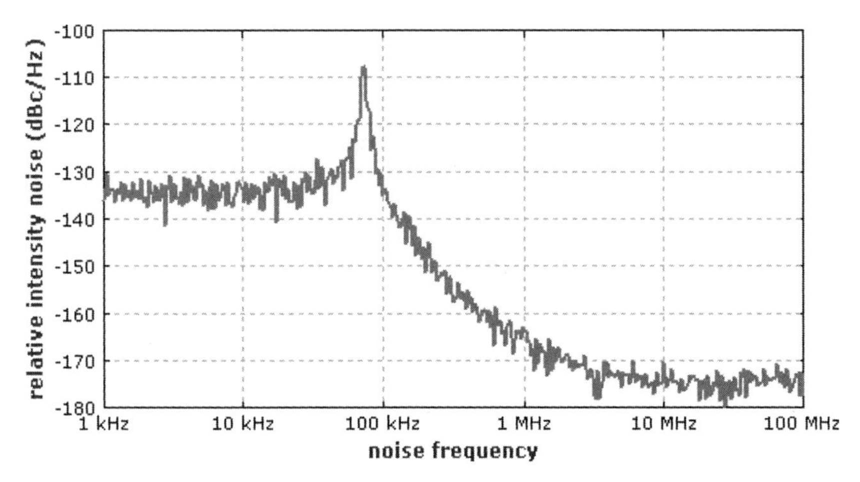


**Figure 2.12** Relative intensity noise peaks at a relaxation-oscillation frequency specific to the laser type. [Reprinted from R. Paschotta, *Field Guide to Lasers*, SPIE Press, Bellingham, Washington (2008).]

- Temperature control – As we have seen, temperature drift results in changes in cavity length $L$ and refractive index $n$; such changes also change the peak laser wavelength, and thus the output power as the different wavelengths have slightly different gain. This affects both semiconductor and solid-state lasers, placing an emphasis on temperature control. For example, a high-stability solid-state laser specifies a 5% peak-to-peak power drift over 8 hours if the temperature is kept constant to less than 5 °C, and after a 30-minute warm-up to stabilize the temperature.[17]
- High power – RIN is reduced at higher power, as the proportion of spontaneous emission noise is smaller in comparison with the stimulated output power.[18]
- Laser selection – RIN peaks at a relaxation-oscillation frequency $f_{RO}$ that depends on the laser type, and drops quickly at higher frequencies (see Fig. 2.12). As a result, solid-state or gas lasers—with a peak RIN at $f_{RO} < 1$ MHz—can have a lower RIN than a semiconductor laser with a peak RIN at $f_{RO} \approx 1$ GHz.
- Longitudinal modes – The output power of a multiple-longitudinal-mode (MLM) laser is averaged over many modes (e.g., Nd:YLF solid-state lasers). However, while the total power might remain relatively constant, the power of each mode can change dramatically, thus increasing the RIN of the main mode by factors of as much as 100× at frequencies up to $f_{RO}$.[18] Such mode-partition noise (MPN) can be avoided by the use of a single-longitudinal-mode (SLM) laser as the quietest option; alternatively, a highly MLM laser will have more noise than an SLM, but less noise than a few-mode laser, as the change in power of each highly MLM laser mode is a smaller fraction of the overall power.
- Optical feedback – Optical feedback from downstream components reflected back into the cavity can result in power and energy changes. Diode lasers are particularly susceptible to such switching, as the low reflectivity of the output mirror (the diode facet) allows a relatively large amount of feedback back into the cavity, changing the refractive index and increasing laser noise.[18] As we will see in Chapter 4, solutions to feedback-induced power instabilities include antireflection coatings, changes in lens surface curvature, and tilted components.
- Pump stabilization – Low-level variations in gain pumping result in output instabilities, including RIN power changes and relaxation oscillations; one common "noise eating" solution is to feedback-stabilize the pump drive circuit.
- Electrical noise reduction – See Hobbs for an excellent discussion.[19]

While power and energy stability are common requirements for laser systems, these fluctuations can also result in frequency and phase instabilities, with consequences discussed in the next section.

### 2.1.9 Frequency stability

In certain types of systems—interferometry, coherent laser communications, or coherent laser radar—the phase relationship between signals must be maintained. For example, we saw in Section 1.2.1 that two signals of a different frequency (or wavelength) become out of phase after a propagation distance known as the coherence length $d_c$. As a result, any frequency instabilities that increase the range of frequencies emitted by a laser also decrease the coherence length.

Equation (2.8) allows us to estimate the frequency shift $\Delta\nu_L$ for a common cause of frequency instabilities, namely, changes in mirror spacing or cavity length $\Delta L$:

$$\Delta\nu_L = -\frac{mc}{2n}\frac{\Delta L}{L^2} \Rightarrow \frac{\Delta\nu_L}{\nu} = -\frac{\Delta L}{L} \tag{2.8}$$

where the negative sign indicates a shift to lower frequencies as the cavity length $L$ increases. Depending on the system requirements, frequency stability may require extremely robust optomechanical stabilization of the laser cavity. For example, for a HeNe laser emitting at a wavelength $\lambda = 632.8$ nm (or $\nu = c/\lambda = 4.74 \times 10^{14}$ Hz) with a cavity length $L = 250$ mm, we find from Eq. (2.8) that $\Delta\nu_L \approx 190$ MHz ($\Delta\lambda_L = 0.00025$ nm) for $\Delta L = 100$ nm. In general, it can be shown that a cavity change $\Delta L = \lambda/2n$ shifts the laser frequency by one mode spacing (Problem 2.8), or $\Delta\nu_L = c/2nL$—an extremely sensitive change given the small dimensions of optical wavelengths. Physically, this is a result of changing the round-trip distance $2L$ such that a different longitudinal mode is resonant with the cavity length.

Two of the largest contributors to frequency instabilities are vibration-induced jitter and temperature-induced drift. If the jitter occurs during the measurement time, then the frequency is broadened approximately as given by Eq. (2.8) for $\Delta\nu << \Delta\nu_L$. To minimize vibration jitter of the cavity, lasers must be mounted on a stiff, stable structure with a high mechanical-resonance frequency and energy dissipation (damping) to reduce the changes in cavity length (as well as mirror angular misalignments, which cause changes in transverse-mode frequency). Vibration isolation from floor motion, air flow, cooling fans, laser water pumps, etc., may also be required at frequencies ranging from 0.1–100 Hz—typically difficult for frequencies <10 Hz or so using instrument-size commercial isolators.[4]

On a longer time scale—minutes and hours—changes in cavity length due to changes in operating temperature result in a drift of the emission frequency, rather than a broadening; this drift is also given by Eq. (2.8). To minimize such thermal drift, lasers might need to be mounted on low-thermal-expansion materials such as Invar, graphite epoxy (GrE), ceramic, or titanium using low-strain kinematic or semi-kinematic mounts.[4] For example, given a thermal expansion $\Delta L_t = \alpha_t \times L \times \Delta T$ of the mount that is entirely transferred to the laser cavity—this can usually be avoided in practice—for a linear coefficient of thermal expansion (CTE) $\alpha_t$ and a change in mount temperature by $\Delta T$, the fractional frequency shift $\Delta \nu_L/\nu = \Delta L_t/L = \alpha_t \Delta T$, emphasizing the need for a small CTE and control of environmental temperature changes.

In addition to vibration and temperature control, different laser types will have varying levels of frequency stability. For example, diode lasers—which are more susceptible to feedback because of the low reflectivity of their cavity mirrors—will generally have more frequency noise as the reflected power affects the number of free electrons and thus the diode's refractive index.

For solid-state and semiconductor lasers with refractive index $n > 1$, temperature changes will also change the index via the thermo-optic ($dn/dT$) effect, resulting in an additional contribution to thermal drift. Such index changes are minimized with a low thermal resistance from the laser to the heat sink to minimize the $\Delta T$ based on heat generated internally to the laser—an approach useful for minimizing changes in laser cavity length as well.[4]

The combined effect of changes in length, index, and peak of the gain curve is summarized by the laser vendor's specs. For example, a highly stable NPRO solid-state laser has a specified frequency drift of less than 50 MHz per hour if the system is designed to meet certain specs, including a 30-minute warm-up time and base temperature change $\Delta T \leq 2$ °C.[20] Other vendors offer frequency-stabilized HeNe lasers with a frequency drift of ±1 MHz over a 1 minute period or ±2 MHz over 8 hours, obtained with temperature control of $\Delta L$.[21]

Pushing the technological limits of laser frequency stability has resulted in the award of the Nobel Prize in Physics in 2005. Figure 2.13 illustrates the experimental method named after Pound, Drever, and Hall (PDH), which has proven to be the most successful. The method allows the stabilization of laser frequency to less than 1 Hz, although only for a second or two before the optomechanical instabilities of the reference cavity interrupt the phase relationships. The PDH method has enabled the discovery of gravitational waves, as well as a number of ultrahigh-resolution experiments in laser spectroscopy.[22]

### 2.1.10 Pointing stability

In addition to power and frequency instabilities, lasers and laser systems are susceptible to a third type of non-ideality, namely, beam-pointing instabilities. Figure 2.14, for example, illustrates how a random change in laser pointing results in beam placement on a micro-array plate that is not repeatable to the degree required by the small size of the micro-array elements (wells). Such pointing errors can be due to laser-pointing instabilities or the beam-control subsystem (see Chapter 5); this section addresses the errors unique to the laser.

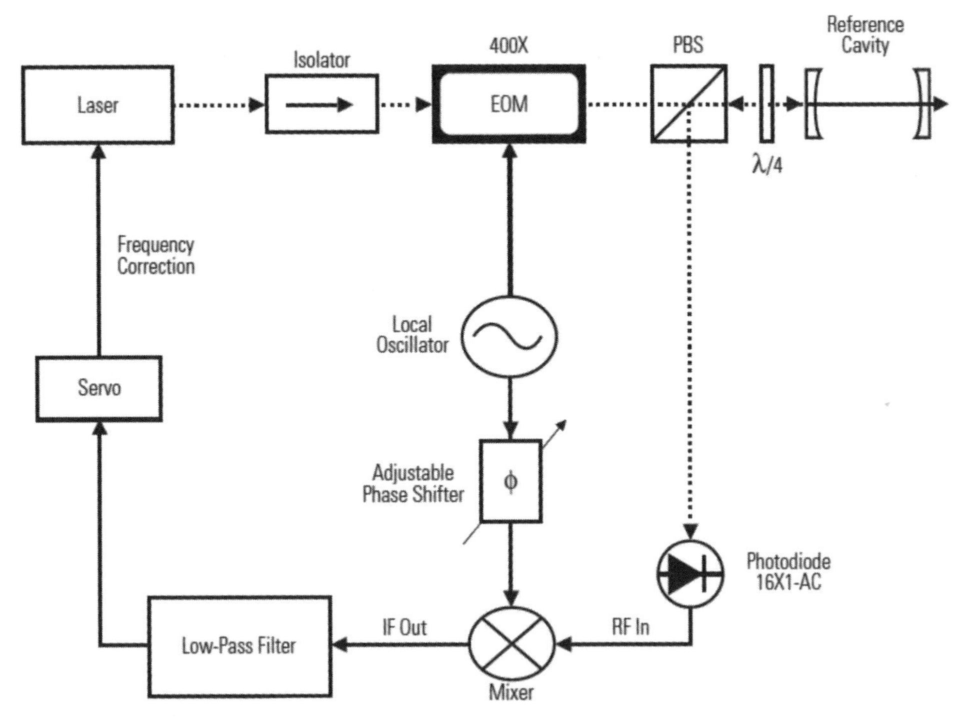


**Figure 2.13** Experimental apparatus using a reference cavity for high-precision laser frequency stabilization. (Reprinted with permission from Newport Corp.; all rights reserved.)

Beam pointing can be classified as one of three types: static (boresight), short-term jitter, and long-term drift. The static boresighting is determined by the initial alignment with respect to a mechanical mounting surface and is not affected by temporal changes in pointing. As we have seen, however, jitter-induced misalignments of the laser-cavity mirrors can result in frequency broadenings, but they can also result in changes in the laser's pointing direction by $\Delta\theta$ with respect to the boresight angle $\theta_b$. Propagating this over the focal length $f$ of a lens gives the change in pointing location $\Delta y = f \times \Delta\theta$. So for a laser with $\Delta\theta \approx 50$ μrad of jitter (full angle) and a lens with $f = 100$ mm, we can expect changes in pointing location on the order of 5 μm, potentially a large number in comparison with the focused spot size or system pointing-stability and beam-position requirements.

Even if the laser is isolated from vibrations, the laser pointing angle will still change based on the internal dynamics of the laser, with changes in the laser's pointing direction by $\Delta\theta \approx 10$–$100$ μrad after a specified warm-up time being common (and shifts in pointing angle being as much as $10\times$ larger during the warm-up period). Such "wiggle noise," if it occurs during the measurement time, increases the effective spot size on a target or at the focal plane of a lens; if it occurs between measurement times—as in obtaining data

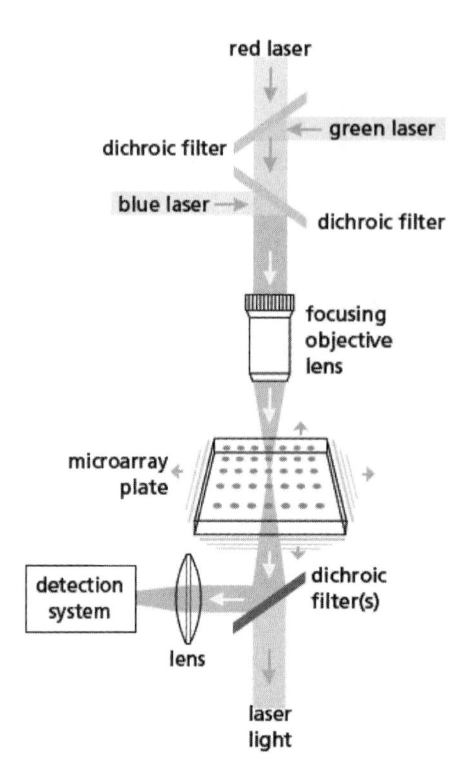


**Figure 2.14** DNA sequencing relies on a high degree of laser-pointing stability to address individual elements (wells) in a micro-array plate. (Credit: CVI Laser, LLC.)

from individual wells in Fig. 2.14—then the location of the beam with respect to the boresight axis has a tolerance or error $\Delta y$.

As with power and frequency stability, short-term jitter and long-term drift thus depend on the measurement time, with drift for most measurements governed by the thermal environment; in such cases, the stability of the thermal environment must be specified. The most likely source of pointing drift will be angular misalignments of the mirrors, a result of temperature gradients across the diameter of the laser causing bending of the laser cavity.[4] Another source for semiconductor, fiber, and solid-state lasers is a change in refractive index of the gain medium due to pump-induced or non-uniform environmental changes in temperature.

In addition to vibration and temperature control, pointing stability can also be controlled via laser selection, with some laser types inherently more stable than others. For example, semiconductor lasers—with their sensitivity to back-reflections—can have large changes in pointing as their refractive index changes with optical feedback. Another example is that of multimode fiber lasers, where the pointing instability must be on the order of 25% of the large multimode beam divergence (see Chapter 3) for it to become significant—a useful criterion for excessive pointing errors of single-mode lasers as well. In highly specialized applications requiring extremely low values of pointing jitter or drift, it may even be necessary to re-design the laser itself, in which case using a flat mirror as the output coupler has the best pointing stability.[23]

Finally, active control of pointing stability might be required if vibration control, temperature control, and laser selection are insufficient. That is, by measuring the pointing angle with a quad-cell detector and providing feedback to fast-steering mirrors, it is possible to compensate for inherent changes in the laser's pointing. This is limited by any additional focusing or beam-expanding optics (Chapter 4), mirror pointing stability (Chapter 5), and quad-cell noise (Chapter 7).

### 2.1.11 Wall-plug efficiency

While considered by some to be a mundane spec, laser wall-plug efficiency—i.e., the ratio of how much (average) optical power $P$ is produced for 1 W of (average) electrical power input, giving $\eta_{WP} = P/P_{elec}$—can be a make-or-break criterion for many laser systems. The obvious examples are high-power industrial, defense, or space-based lasers, where the inefficient conversion of electrical power affects operating costs, the generation of greenhouse gases, and even portability.

Typical laser efficiencies run from <1% for some types of gas lasers to >60% for semiconductor diode lasers, depending on operating conditions. Components for a frequency-doubled solid-state laser are illustrated in Fig. 2.15; the biggest contributors are:

- How far above threshold the laser is operating. As seen in Fig. 2.5, wall-plug efficiency first increases above threshold as the laser creates more photons; it then drops off as the laser generates more heat.
- The operating temperature, where a hotter laser generally has a lower efficiency.[24] As a result, the laser systems engineer must pay close attention to the removal of heat, affecting the wall-plug and overall efficiency of the system (see Section 2.3).

In addition to electrical power consumption, wall-plug efficiency also affects power, frequency, and pointing stability. That is, the heat load $Q = P_{elec} - P$ will be removed from the laser in all cases; what is unknown is

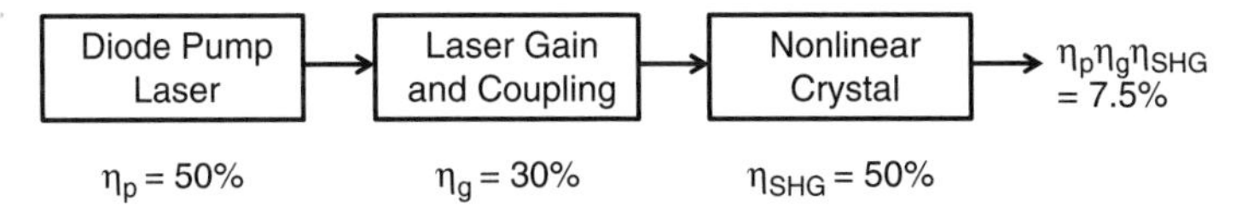


**Figure 2.15** Wall-plug efficiency for a solid-state laser depends on the efficiency of the pump laser, the lasing efficiency of the solid-state crystal, and the losses associated with any wavelength-conversion crystals. See Schepps[25] for more details.

how hot the laser needs to get to do so. A low thermal resistance $R_t$ to the outside world keeps the laser cooler, but the laser systems engineer might also need to utilize thermal management technologies such as fins, fans, water cooling, heat pipes, and so on, to keep the temperature rise $\Delta T = Q \times R_t$ from becoming excessive.[4] As we have seen in Sections 2.1.8 through 2.1.10, the requirements on the temperature rise can be governed by the drift in power stability due to changes in cavity length $L$ and gain-medium refractive index $n$, a frequency shift $\Delta\nu_L/\nu = \alpha_t\Delta T$, or pointing error $\Delta\theta$ due to temperature gradients across the diameter of the laser causing index changes or slight misalignments of the laser mirrors.

### 2.1.12 Polarization

The final laser spec considered in this section is that of beam polarization, i.e., the orientation of the beam's electric field with respect to a reference direction such as horizontal or vertical. Figure 2.16 illustrates the concept for electromagnetic waves whose electric field is oriented vertically. A linearly polarized laser beam is one that has only one orientation; an unpolarized beam is one whose electric-field orientation (and phase) varies randomly along the propagation direction and can thus be measured as a combination of horizontal and vertical polarizations.

There are a number of applications where the polarization of the laser beam is important. Perhaps the most common is the need for a polarized beam for efficient harmonic generation by a nonlinear crystal.[7] Another example is the combination of vertically and horizontally polarized beams to nearly double the power available for applications such as pumping or laser radar. Remote sensing of weather patterns with laser radar might require a laser with only one polarization, however, because ice scatters (depolarizes) a vertical polarization (e.g.) into both vertical and horizontal components—and to a larger degree than water, thus allowing polarization-based measurements that can distinguish between the two.[26]

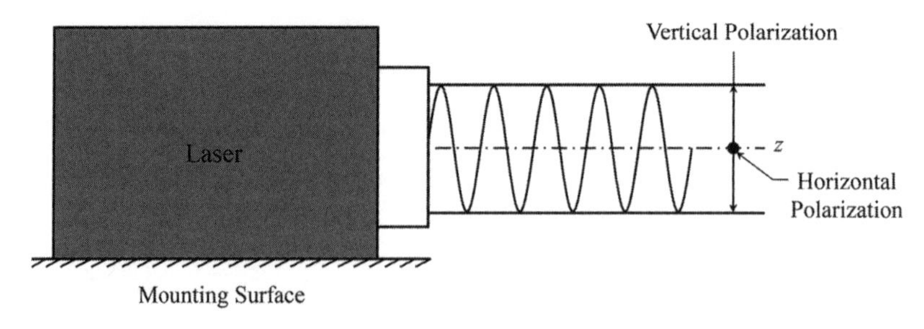


**Figure 2.16** The electric field of a laser's output wavefront can be polarized vertically with respect to the horizontal mounting surface. Horizontal (as illustrated by the solid dot representing an electric-field vector out of the page) or random polarizations are also possible.

As spontaneous emission from a large number of randomly oriented atoms is randomly polarized, the polarization of a laser is determined by asymmetries in the gain (i.e., a polarization-dependent absorption), the gain-medium's refractive indices (i.e., the natural and thermally induced changes in birefringence, giving two refractive indices that depend on the polarization), or polarization-dependent losses in the laser-cavity optics such as a Brewster window (see Section 4.5.5). Depending on how the laser designer "juggles" these parameters, lasers are specified as having either linear or random polarization.

A linear polarization spec requires two pieces of information: the degree of linear polarization, as well as its orientation (including angular tolerance) with respect to the laser's mounting surface. For example, a typical gas laser (Section 2.2.4) may have a polarization extinction ratio $PER \equiv P_v/P_h = 500{:}1$ (for a vertically polarized power $P_v$ and a horizontally polarized power $P_h$), while some types of solid-state lasers (Section 2.2.2)—with polarization-dependent gain and thermally induced changes in birefringence[25] that a gas laser does not have—may have a ratio of only 100:1. In this case, the horizontally polarized power is as much as 1% of the vertically polarized power, possibly placing a lower bound on the precision of any measurements that rely on having a single state of polarization. Independent of the extinction ratio, tolerances on the orientation of a linear plane of polarization can be as large as ±5 deg with respect to the laser's mounting surface.

As we will see in Section 2.2.1, the laser-cavity optics for many semiconductor lasers are the cleaved facets of the laser, and these typically reflect only horizontal polarization with sufficiently low loss to allow lasing. However, polarization-dependent semiconductor gain of either horizontal or vertical orientation can be designed to dominate over the mirror loss (depending on wavelength), with both polarizations available from some vendors.

A fiber laser (Section 2.2.3) is very sensitive to environmental perturbations of the fiber's index, thus requiring a polarization-maintaining (PM) structure in the fiber to guarantee linear polarization. Low-power fiber lasers using such structures are available with a PER = 200:1; random polarizations are also available. High-power fiber lasers are almost always randomly polarized, as the manufacturing applications for which these lasers are commonly used do not require a specific polarization.

Independent of laser type, a randomly polarized laser is one that has a time-varying orientation of its linear polarization. This can have a number of disadvantages in system design. The first is that the output power may be lower than a polarized laser; one vendor, for example, indicates that their linearly polarized laser has an output power of 80 mW, but their randomly polarized version has only 50 mW. The second is that the linear polarization from a randomly polarized beam changes its orientation slowly enough for detectors to measure. As a result, a linear polarizer anywhere in the optical path will produce unwanted changes in power over time, with the power being reduced by 2× as the polarization changes randomly from vertical to horizontal and back again. This interaction of a laser beam—randomly or linearly polarized—with optical components will be explored in more detail in Section 4.5.5.

## 2.2 Laser Types

Given the variety of laser specs of potential importance to the laser systems engineer—wavelength, temporal coherence, spatial coherence, output power, polarization, and so on—we see that laser selection requires the "juggling" of a large number of parameters. The next step down this trail is an understanding of the commonly used types of lasers, and the specifications we can expect to obtain from them.

When people speak of laser "types" they are often referring to the gain medium, four of which are in common usage: semiconductors, solid-state crystals, solid-state fibers, and gases. However, there are other ways of classifying lasers as well, including high power, USP, geometry, and so on. In this chapter, we review the four types based on gain medium, and include subdivisions into power, pulse width, etc. We emphasize commercial lasers that would be used in most applications, and do not review specialized directed-energy weapons such as phase-corrected waveguide lasers, gas lasers such as carbon monoxide (CO), or the lesser-used wavelengths (1153 nm, e.g.) obtained from common lasers such as the helium-neon.

### 2.2.1 Semiconductor lasers

Semiconductor lasers were not sufficiently mature in the mid-1980s to be featured in the "Laser of the Month" columns in *Laser Focus/Electro-Optics* magazine. As a result of numerous improvements over the years, however, they are now the most commonly used, and their many advantages over other types of lasers—size, efficiency, cost, lifetime, etc.—guarantee that they will continue to be so for the foreseeable future. They can be classified into one of four common categories: low-power edge emitters, high-power edge emitters, vertical-cavity surface emitting lasers (VCSELs), and QCLs.

**Low-Power Edge Emitters.** As is almost always the case, the low-power version of a laser is the first to market, and the semiconductor laser was no exception. The geometry of the low-power edge emitter is shown in Fig. 2.17. Light is generated near the semiconductor *p-n* junction (or diode) where a population inversion is created using electrical pumping of electrons into excited states using the top (+) and bottom (–) metal contacts.

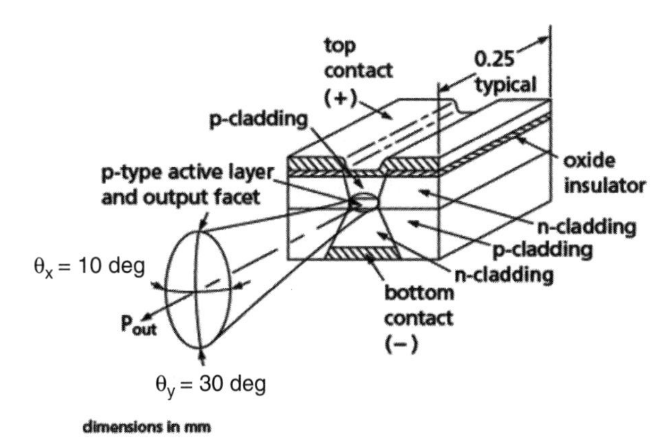


**Figure 2.17** The semiconductor diode laser relies on an electrically pumped *p-n* junction active layer to generate photons and a waveguide to create the laser cavity. (Credit: CVI Laser, LLC.)

Spontaneously emitted photons stimulate more photons as they propagate along the 250-μm length of the laser via total internal reflection (TIR) waveguiding, which defines the laser cavity. The waveguide is on the order of 3 μm wide × 1 μm thick, and light emitted from the smaller dimension diffracts light at a larger angle; light is thus emitted in an elliptical power distribution at the partially reflecting edge (or facet mirror) where some light escapes the cavity.

The wavelengths emitted are controlled by the semiconductor materials used. Referring to Table 2.1, the familiar red wavelengths (620–680 nm) can be created with a combination of aluminum, gallium, indium, and phosphorus (AlGaInP), while aluminum gallium arsenide (AlGaAs) produces the 808-nm wavelength needed to pump certain solid-state lasers (Section 2.2.2). Because of the gain properties of semiconductors, the wavelength depends somewhat on temperature (≈0.3 nm/°C). This can be used to vary (or "tune") the wavelength (Section 2.1.1); alternatively, temperature-controlling thermoelectric coolers (TECs) are sometimes used for wavelength stabilization for applications such as dense wavelength-division multiplexing (DWDM) of closely spaced wavelengths into the same telecommunications fiber.

Depending on wavelength, typical CW output power is on the order of 1–1000 mW with UV wavelengths having lower power and NIR wavelengths (808 and 980 nm) being the "sweet spot" for higher power. Not all wavelengths are available from semiconductor lasers, and this restriction forces consideration of other laser types during the process of laser selection.

A high degree of spatial coherence across the micron-scale dimensions of the waveguide allows diffraction-limited focusing to small spot sizes (see Chapter 4). Figure 2.18 illustrates an example where this spec is

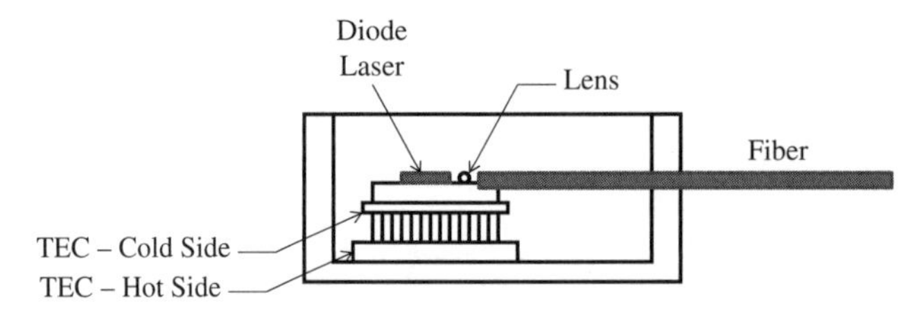


**Figure 2.18** Coupling of a low-power edge emitter into a 10.5-μm diameter fiber for telecommunications applications requires focusing to a small spot.

important, namely, the coupling of the beam into a single-mode fiber (SMF) with a diameter of approximately 10 μm. Such coherence is not necessary for applications such as laser pointers, but is critical for those such as SMF coupling, laser printers, CD and DVD players, etc., which require a small spot.

**High-Power Edge Emitters.** Many applications—pump lasers and manufacturing (direct diode) processes such as welding, for example—do not require a small spot, and high power is an important specification. As shown in Fig. 2.19, output power is increased by using a linear array (or "bar") of lower-power lasers, with as many as 50 diode lasers each emitting $\approx$1 W CW on a 10-mm-wide bar. With poor beam quality of each wide-aperture (100 μm) diode, and the diodes emitting independently of each other, there is little spatial coherence for this type of laser. As a result, bars cannot be focused into a small spot as expected for a coherent beam; instead, the imaging of these sources is more like that of an incoherent "lightbulb."[14]

Even higher power can be obtained by stacking bars on top of each other, with CW output powers of 1–5 kW commercially available. Wall-plug efficiencies for the NIR stacks are greater than 50%—a significant advantage in reducing (but not eliminating) the unavoidable hardware for active water

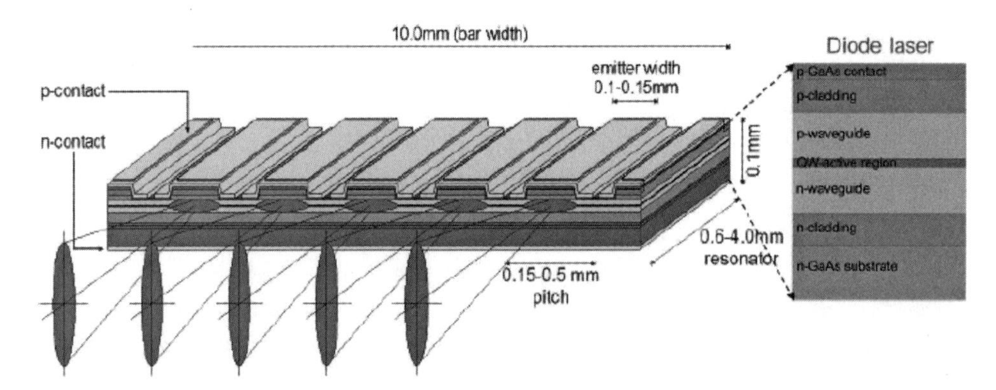


**Figure 2.19** A 1D array (or bar) of low-power edge emitters creates an incoherent source of photons. (Credit: JENOPTIK Diode Lab GmbH.)

cooling. QCW pulsing (Fig. 2.6) is also a common operating mode for their use as pump lasers, in which case passive conductive cooling is usually sufficient. With clever beam-shaping optics, stacks can also be coupled into large-diameter (100–400 μm) multimode fiber (MMF), with NIR wall-plug efficiencies dropping to ≈35% due to the fiber-coupling losses.

In addition to poor spatial coherence, high-power arrays of bars and stacks also have poor temporal coherence. Specifically, the center wavelength of each diode in the array can vary by ±3 nm from the other diodes due to semiconductor manufacturing variations; in addition, each diode will itself have a FWHM linewidth of 3–5 nm. The net result is a large wavelength range and thus a short coherence length—which is not in and of itself a problem for the pumping and manufacturing applications for which these lasers are most-often used.

**Vertical-Cavity Surface-Emitting Lasers (VCSELs).** Going in the other direction, the VCSEL was first developed as a low-power semiconductor laser for optical mice and short-distance laser communications. As shown in Fig. 2.20 (left), it is different from the low-power edge emitter in that light is now emitted perpendicular to the semiconductor wafer on which it is fabricated—an orientation defined as "vertical." Rather than cleaved facets, the cavity mirrors are two stacks of quarter-wave (λ/4)-thick layers known as distributed Bragg reflectors (DBRs); the active region is a *p-n* junction semiconductor emitting red, NIR, and SWIR wavelengths.

The advantage of the vertical, surface-emitting geometry is the low cost due to the removal of expensive fabrication and assembly steps—hence its use in high-volume consumer applications such as optical mice. Specifically, edge-emitting semiconductor lasers must be cleaved from the wafer on which they are fabricated, and the exposed facets must then be coated with high-reflection and antireflection coatings such as aluminum oxy-nitride. In addition, the coupling optics for the elliptical, highly diverging beam of the edge emitter are expensive (see Chapter 4). The VCSEL, on the other hand, does not need

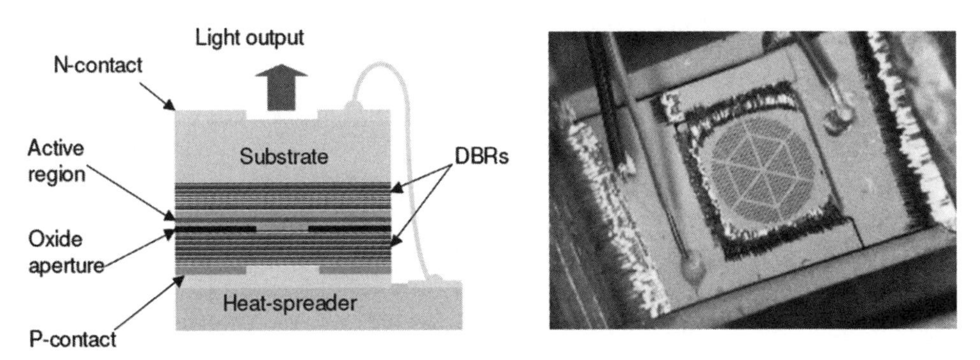


**Figure 2.20** Individual VCSELs (left) and arrays (right). (Reprinted with permission from Princeton Optronics, Inc.)

additional coatings (the DBRs perform the same function), and the coupling optics for the inherently round beam are simpler and less expensive than for the elliptical beam of the edge emitter.

CW output power for low-power VCSELs is ≈1 mW for a single-transverse-mode 4-μm-diameter active region, and up to 3 W for a multi-transverse-mode 350-μm region. Independent of transverse mode, the extremely short cavity length *L*—on the order of one wavelength—ensures single-longitudinal-mode lasing [see Eq. (1.6)] with a DBR-controlled linewidth $\Delta\lambda < 1$ nm. This is the case even under high-speed modulation (10 GHz) for short-distance data communications, a common application of these devices.

As with stacks of high-power edge emitters, incoherent arrays of VCSELs are also available [Fig. 2.20 (right)]. The 5-kW CW power of these arrays is similar to that of edge-emitting stacks; in addition, the wall-plug efficiency is excellent, exceeding 50% for NIR (800–1100 nm) arrays.

Uniformity of the center wavelength of each VCSEL in the array is better than that of an edge-emitting array and may vary by only ±1 nm from the other VCSELs due to DBR manufacturing variations. Important for high-power arrays where a large amount of heat is generated, the wavelength shift with temperature is about 4× lower (≈0.07 nm/°C) than that of an edge emitter. This is determined by the wide longitudinal-mode spacing of the VCSEL, such that the shift of the gain peak to longer wavelengths that dominates edge emitters at higher temperatures is of no consequence for VCSELs; instead, the relatively small changes in both VCSEL thickness and refractive index *n* with temperature ($dn/dT$) control the temperature sensitivity. For the same reason, VCSEL power stability is also very good (<1%).

While initially developed as a low-cost alternative to edge-emitting semiconductor lasers, recent developments in VCSEL design allow high-power SHG as well as moderate-energy USPs. Known as vertical external-cavity surface-emitting lasers (VECSELs), Fig. 2.21 shows that an extended cavity allows a SHG frequency-doubling crystal to be placed between a conventional DBR-based VCSEL and an additional external mirror, creating another cavity in which light can resonate. In this way, the common NIR and SWIR outputs can now be halved to produce a range of visible wavelengths—for example, 532 nm from 1064-nm VCSELs—allowing the use of these lasers for biomedical and display applications. A typical laser-based digital-cinema projector, for example, might use a 6-W red (635 nm), 3-W green (532 nm), and 3-W blue (455 nm) laser for RGB color.

There are two "flavors" of VECSELs: electrically pumped and optically pumped. The electrically pumped VECSELs have up to 6 W of output power with a single-mode beam; the optically pumped devices—also known as optically pumped semiconductor lasers (OPSLs)—have as much as 10 W of

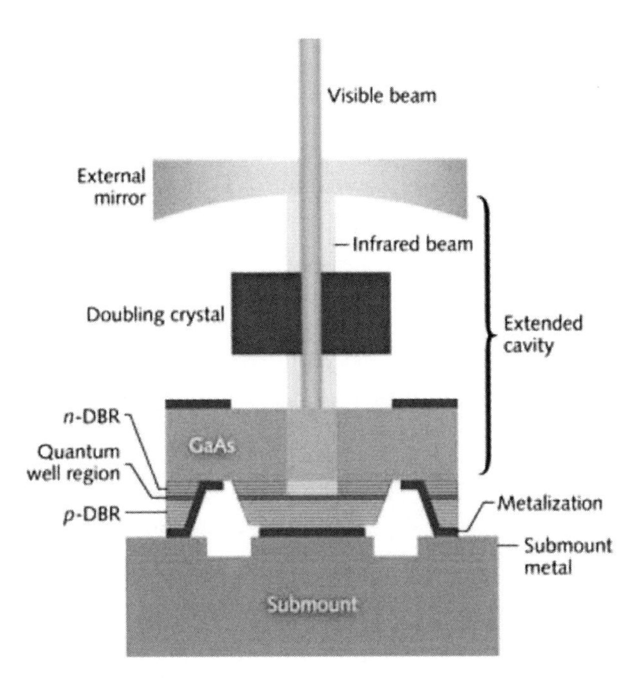


**Figure 2.21** The vertical external-cavity surface-emitting laser (VECSEL) allows for wavelength conversion and USP mode locking. (Reprinted with permission from Necsel IP Inc.)

diffraction-limited output power, a result of being able to uniformly pump a larger area than is possible with electrical ring contacts. The disadvantage of the OPSL is the additional manufacturing cost of a pump laser and its alignment.

Independent of pumping, the range of wavelengths available extends from the UV (355 nm using THG of GaAs-based VECSELs emitting at 1064 nm) to the SWIR (1550 nm using InP-based VECSELs). Not all wavelengths are available in these ranges, as harmonic generation does not allow the efficient generation of orange ($\lambda \approx 590$ nm). In general, wavelength-conversion efficiencies (and therefore output power) depend on wavelength, with 1064-nm lasers having more power than 532-nm SHG devices, which have more power than 355-nm THG VECSELs. Because phase matching is required in wavelength-conversion crystals, wavelength and power stability require temperature stabilization using TECs, thus reducing the overall wall-plug efficiency of the system (see Section 2.3).

In addition to visible wavelengths with high power, VECSELs can also be fabricated with a semiconductor saturable absorber mirror (SESAM) to produce mode-locked pulses as short as 0.1–10 psec[12]—pulse widths not obtainable by directly modulating a VCSEL.[27] While semiconductor-laser pulse energies are inherently low, commercially available products using follow-on power amplifiers at $\lambda = 1064$ nm have an average power of 50 W, a pulse width of 10 psec, a pulse energy of 6.25 μJ, and a peak power of 625 kW at a PRF of 8 MHz.

**Quantum-Cascade Lasers**. The wavelengths available from the semiconductor materials used for both edge emitters and VCSELs is based on the energy bandgap $E_g$ of the materials ($E_g = hc/\lambda$) plus additional wavelength-conversion technologies. In practice, this results in semiconductor lasers emitting at wavelengths from the UV to the SWIR; unfortunately, longer wavelengths such as MWIR and LWIR are not conveniently available from most lasers—a disadvantage for a number of applications such as IR spectroscopy and countermeasures.

What is unique about quantum-cascade lasers is their ability to generate MWIR and LWIR photons. This is illustrated in Fig. 2.22, where the method for creating light is seen to be different from that of *p-n* junction excited states. Specifically, very thin layers of semiconductors known as quantum wells—on the order of nanometers thick—constrain electron energies to certain values (or states) that determine the laser's emission wavelength. When quantum wells are closely stacked next to each other with well energies as shown in Fig. 2.22, an electron that has just given up its energy in the form of a photon can tunnel into the adjacent well where it can again change its energy state. Such a cascade of a single electron can thus emit a number of photons.

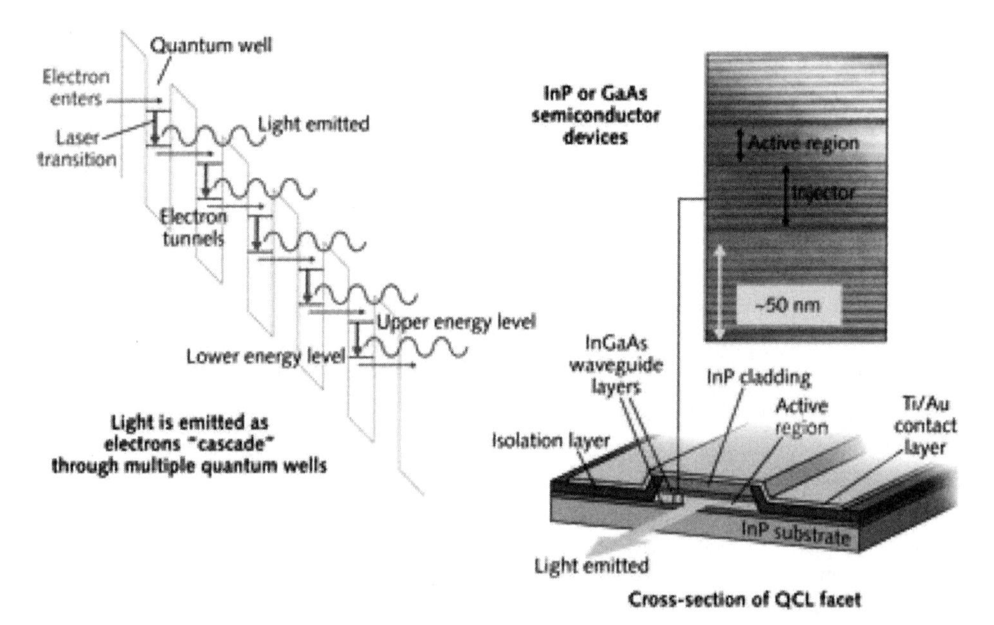


**Figure 2.22** Closely stacked quantum wells allow an electron that has changed its energy state by emitting a photon to cascade through the wells. (Credit: Prof. Jerome Faist, ETH Zurich.) (See color plate.)

The wavelength of a QCL is thus determined not by the bandgap of the semiconductors used but by the energy states of the quantum wells, such that $\lambda = hc/(E_2 - E_1)$ for well energies $E_1$ and $E_2$. Given the state-of-the-art in materials and fabricating quantum wells and tunneling barriers, the "sweet spot" for QCL wavelengths is 4.6 μm. Other MWIR and LWIR wavelengths from 3.5–10.4 μm are also possible, though with a somewhat lower output power and wall-plug efficiency. Room-temperature CW output power for single-mode edge-emitters ranges from 4 W at $\lambda = 4.6$ μm to 2 W at $\lambda = 9.5$ μm; wall-plug efficiency is 5–20% at $\lambda = 4.6$ μm.

QCW-modulated QCLs are also commercially available with higher power using relatively long pulse widths ($\Delta t_p = 10$–500 nsec) at a maximum PRF of 2 MHz. Because MWIR wavelengths are useful for spectroscopic identification of explosives and neurotoxins, external-cavity QCLs are also available with a wide tuning range and a tuning resolution as small as 0.5 nm.

**Summary.** Semiconductor laser options range from low-power, single-transverse-mode devices—edge emitters and VCSELs—that can be focused to a diffraction-limited spot, to high-power arrays that have poor spatial coherence. Wavelength conversion and USPs are also possible with VECSELs, while QCLs emit MWIR and LWIR wavelengths. With the exception of QCLs with a lifetime of approximately 5,000 hours, a general advantage of semiconductor lasers is a lifetime on the order of 10,000 hours and longer—a factor of 10× improvement over conventional sources such as arc lamps. Wall-plug efficiencies are also extremely good, the best of any type of laser. In addition, the cost (unit and operating) can be extremely low; these and other properties of semiconductor lasers are summarized in Table 2.3.

**Table 2.3** Properties of commonly used semiconductor lasers and typical applications.

| Property | Low-Power Edge Emitter | High-Power Edge Emitter | VCSEL | QCL |
|---|---|---|---|---|
| Wavelength | UV → MWIR | 808, 980 nm | VIS → SWIR | SWIR → LWIR |
| Linewidth | $\Delta\nu \approx 1$–100 MHz | $\Delta\lambda \approx 0.5$–5 nm | $\Delta\lambda < 1$ nm | $\Delta\nu \approx 10$ MHz |
| Beam Quality, $M^2$ | $M^2 < 1.2$ | Incoherent arrays | $M^2 < 1.2$; incoherent arrays | $M^2 < 1.3$ |
| Average Power | 1–150 mW | 1 W → 10 kW | 1 mW → 1 kW | 0.1–5 W |
| Wall-Plug Efficiency | >50% | >50% | 10–50% | 5–20% CW |
| Pulse Width, $\Delta t_p$ | 0.1 nsec | 0.1 msec QCW | 0.1–10 psec (VECSEL) | 10–500 nsec |
| Applications | Telecom, DVDs, displays, printing, biomedical | Pump lasers, manufacturing | Datacom, displays, biomedical | Defense, sensing, spectroscopy |

### 2.2.2 Solid-state lasers

In contrast with semiconductor lasers, solid-state lasers use a nonconducting (dielectric) material as the gain-medium host. Commonly used hosts include yttrium aluminum garnet (YAG), sapphire ($Al_2O_3$), and silica ($SiO_2$) glass. These are all selected because they are commonly available materials and can accept the relatively large concentration of dopants necessary for high peak power and pulse energy.

With pulse widths of 5–10 nsec, the peak power of a DPSS laser can be as much as $10^6\times$ larger than the average power. In addition, with long excited-state lifetimes to store energy, pulse energies can be greater than 0.5 J, depending on the number of excited-state atoms (or mode volume). Ultrafast solid-state lasers (10-fsec pulses) are also possible with a large gain bandwidth or low-nonlinearity designs.

Applications for solid-state lasers include biomedical, manufacturing, research, and laser radar for autonomous vehicles or target ranging.[11] Commonly used categories of solid-state lasers include neodymium (Nd)-doped YAG, titanium (Ti)-doped sapphire, erbium (Er)-doped glass, and ytterbium (Yb)-doped YAG disks.

**Nd:YAG Solid-State Lasers**. The most common solid-state laser (Fig. 2.23) uses a YAG crystal doped with ≈1% neodymium (Nd). Many similar solid-state crystals can also be doped with Nd (e.g., $YVO_4$ and YLF) for a limited range of solid-state wavelengths. The nominal wavelength of the Nd:YAG is $\lambda = 1064$ nm, with 2× (532 nm), 3× (355 nm) and 4× (266 nm) wavelengths available via nonlinear harmonic generation.

Solid-state lasers can generally be pulsed to high peak power (via long excited-state energy storage). Pulse widths with Q-switching are on the order of $\Delta t_p = 5$–$50$ nsec, with a pulse energy $Q_p$ up to 100 mJ for commercial Nd: YAG lasers. The advantage of Nd-doping is the high gain and therefore short crystal lengths; with a typical YAG crystal on the order of 10 mm long × 3 mm in diameter, the mode volume is still orders of magnitude larger than that of a semiconductor laser, with correspondingly higher-energy pulses.

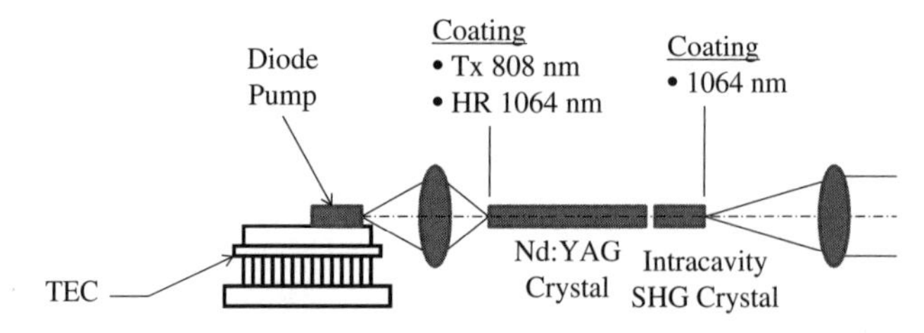


**Figure 2.23** Schematic of a DPSS laser with an intracavity SHG crystal for frequency doubling.

As we have seen in Fig. 2.9, pulse energy and peak power can depend on PRF, and higher pulse rates can have lower-energy pulses with lower peak power. Pulse energy also depends on wavelength; as with VECSELs, visible (532 nm) and UV (266 and 355 nm) wavelengths are generated with nonlinear crystals, a process that is not 100% efficient. Even though the pulse energy is inherently lower based on THG losses, high-energy UV wavelengths produce less thermal damage of work pieces transparent to visible wavelengths—a significant advantage when manufacturing yield is critical to profitability.

The first solid-state lasers were pumped with flashlamps surrounding the crystal; this is an extremely inefficient method—both spatially and spectrally—of creating a population inversion. The use of diode pumping has led to a huge increase in wall-plug efficiency to ≈15% (Fig. 2.15) with near-diffraction-limited beam quality ($M^2$ = 1.2–1.7). Even though the efficiencies are much smaller than those of semiconductor diodes, the much higher pulse energy of the YAG laser is sometimes required.

A relatively recent development in DPSS lasers is the micro-chip laser—the solid-state equivalent of the semiconductor VCSEL. That is, by using a thin layer of Nd:YAG gain material, the benefits of SLM operation can be obtained in a compact package much smaller than a conventional DPSS laser. The disadvantages of these low-gain devices are the low pulse energy (<10 μJ) and peak power (≈10 kW), even though the Q-switch pulse width is <1 nsec.

In addition to pulse energy, PRF, peak power, and beam quality, another unique feature of concern to the laser systems engineer includes the changes in beam quality and focus position with output power (Fig. 2.24). In general, the power of a solid-state laser is limited in the extreme by thermal fracture of the solid-state crystal.[28] Before that point is reached, however, increases in

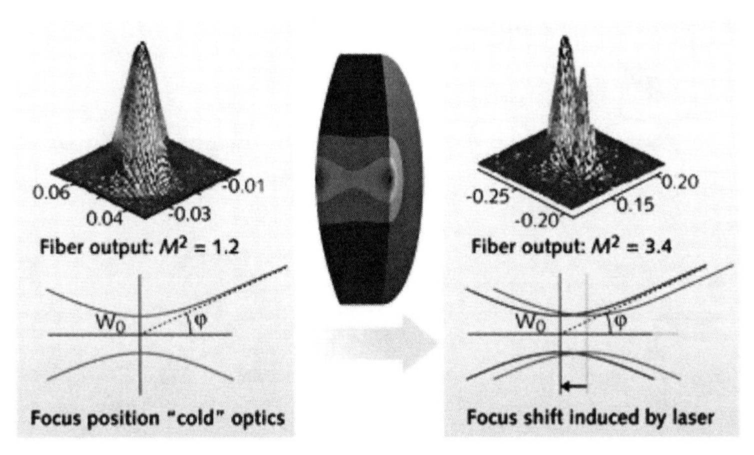


**Figure 2.24** Thermal lensing from a non-uniform temperature distribution changes both the focus position and transmitted beam quality. (Reprinted with permission from the 49th edition of *Laser Focus World*. © 2013 PennWell.) (See color plate.)

pumping to increase the output power also affect the crystal's temperature and thus its refractive index,[4] a condition known as thermal lensing.

As we will see in more detail in Section 4.1, thermal lensing can be mitigated by the laser designer using innovative designs such as pumping wavelengths more closely matched to the output wavelength (for Yb:YAG, e.g., thus reducing thermal dissipation) or a side-pumping geometry to reduce the temperature non-uniformities associated with the pump.[26] In addition, the user of the system can clearly reduce thermal lensing by operating the laser in a restricted power range. Finally, the systems engineer can control thermal lensing through laser selection—Nd:YLF lasers have better beam quality and pointing instabilities in comparison with Nd:YAG[12]—and appropriate cooling and heat sinking. For example, the user's manual for a commercially available Nd:YLF laser[17] states: "The laser will not function properly without adequate cooling. A heat sink needs to be supplied by the user.... The thermal resistance of the heat sink should be under 0.2 °C/W.... A lapped flat heat sink is an ideal mating surface." With appropriate thermal management of the laser temperature, DPSS YAG-based lasers are rugged and reliable—a lifetime of 10,000 hours is common—to the point where they have even been launched into space.[26,29]

**Ti:sapphire Solid-State Lasers**. A qualitatively different solid-state gain medium is titanium-doped sapphire (Ti:sapphire). The advantage of this medium is the extremely large gain bandwidth (670–1100 nm), thus allowing both tunability and mode-locked USPs ranging from 1 psec down to 5 fsec [Eq. (1.14)], or approximately 2 cycles of 800-nm light.

As shown in Fig. 2.25, the disadvantage of all this ultrafast "firepower" is a large and environmentally sensitive laser that cannot be launched into the ceiling of outer space, nor used 24-7 on the floor of the factory. This is due in part to the research community that has typically driven the development of

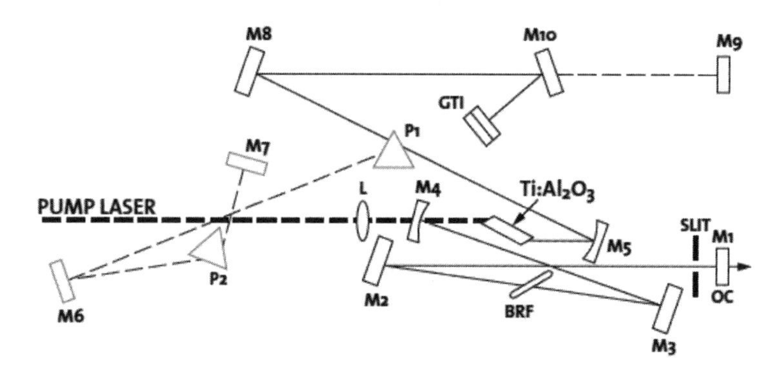


**Figure 2.25** Schematic of an ultrafast Ti:sapphire ($Ti:Al_2O_3$) laser illustrating the number and complexity of the components. (Reprinted with permission from Coherent Inc., Mira Optima 900-D product specs.)

these lasers, and in part by the number and complexity of the components required for generating femtosecond pulses, including low-RIN pump lasers, mode lockers, group-velocity-dispersion (GVD) management, pulse picking, pulse compression, phase stabilization, and chirped-pulse or regenerative amplifiers to increase the pulse energy.

Ti:sapphire lasers are thus extremely powerful research tools for tunable, femtosecond "hero" experiments in the lab—time-resolved research into biological and chemical processes, for example—but are otherwise unacceptable for use in the field or manufacturing plant, a result of their large size, heavy weight, excessive cost, extreme sensitivity to temperature and vibrations, and requirement for frequency-doubled, low-RIN VECSELs or Nd:YLF lasers to pump them. A recent innovation that addresses the environmental sensitivities—which often has graduate students spending many hours of their day realigning mirrors—is the use of soldered optical-component mounts, which reduce the tendency of threaded mounts to drift with temperature and vibration.

So within the context of a nonruggedized laser used in a temperature-controlled lab and mounted on a vibration-isolation table, typical specs for an off-the-shelf Ti:sapphire laser are single-transverse-mode beam quality with a pulse width $\Delta t_p \approx 100$ fsec, pulse energy $Q_p = 40$ nJ, PRF = 75 MHz, and $P_{avg} \approx 4$ W. In general, shorter pulses allow more pulses per second (higher PRFs), and Ti:sapphire lasers follow this trend. For example, Q-switched Nd:YAG lasers may have a useful PRF ≈ 10 kHz (Fig. 2.9), while that for Ti:sapphire lasers may be as large as 80 MHz. The disadvantage is that the higher PRF also means a higher average power for the same pulse energy [Eq. (2.6)], and this additional power can be converted to heat that can damage the sample or work piece if the pulses are not scanned quickly enough (see Chapter 5).

**Er:glass Solid-State Lasers**. Yet another category of solid-state laser is erbium-doped glass (Er:glass, or Er:$SiO_2$). These are primarily motivated by the need for eye-"safer" wavelengths near 1550 nm for laser radar systems such as those used by pilots to determine the range to a distant object. The basic concept is that the time of flight $t_f$ of a pulse moving at the speed of light determines the range $R$, given that $2R = c \times t_f$. In addition, the range resolution $\Delta R = c \times \Delta t_p/2$, illustrating the need for short pulses to identify objects within a plus-or-minus range tolerance.

While low-power semiconductor diode lasers are used to generate an eye-safe (Class 1) wavelength ($\lambda \approx 900$ nm) for range measurement in self-driving cars, the range is limited by the relatively low eye-safe power level. For longer ranges such as those required by pilots, higher pulse energies at $\lambda = 1550$ nm or so may also be Class 1, and a diode-pumped Er:glass laser emitting at $\lambda = 1540$ nm is a common solution for such rangefinders.[30]

Maximum permissible exposure (MPE) for a 10-nsec pulse width at $\lambda = 1540$ nm is on the order of 1 J/cm$^2$. This translates into typical pulse energies of 8–10 mJ for high-end rangefinders, giving these lasers a range $R \approx$ 20 km when combined with appropriate optics (Chapter 4) and detectors (Chapter 7). Fast update rates for range data are not usually required, so the PRF = 1–10 Hz for Q-switched devices. Pulsed laser lifetime is specified in terms of number of pulses (or "shots"), and the mean time-to-failure (MTTF) is $>10^8$ pulses.

Lower-performance Er:glass lasers—in terms of energy, energy stability, and timing jitter—are also used as "flashlights" for scene illumination in active range-gated imaging (see Chapter 7). Whether rangefinder or illuminator, Er:glass lasers are mature products used in difficult tactical environments with a long lifetime over a range of temperature, vibration, and shock specs.

**Yb:YAG Disk Lasers**. A unique geometry similar to the microchip is the disk laser, an increasingly popular addition to the commercially available options for cold-ablation micromachining using USPs.[3] The conventional Nd:YAG laser uses a rod or slab of YAG crystal approximately 10 mm long. The disk laser, on the other hand, uses a thin layer (200 μm) of ytterbium-doped YAG (Yb:YAG) as the gain medium (Fig. 2.26). The benefits are threefold: (1) Yb has much less heat dissipation from nonradiative electron transitions than Nd, making Yb preferred for high-power lasers;[31] (2) the thin layer has a short interaction length for peak-power nonlinearities to accumulate, allowing the generation of USPs with a high peak power useful in manufacturing and micromachining; and (3) the large diameter (and surface area) of the disk in comparison with its thickness allows for low power density (W/m$^2$) and efficient heat transfer, thus minimizing thermal lensing across the disk.

Because of their low nonlinearities, disk lasers are typically used for mode-locked USPs with $\Delta t_p \leq 10$ psec, a peak power $P_{peak} \approx 1$ kW, and near-diffraction-limited beam quality ($M^2 < 1.3$). Given the thin disk (and therefore low gain), the pulse energy is also extremely small, on the order of 10 μJ at

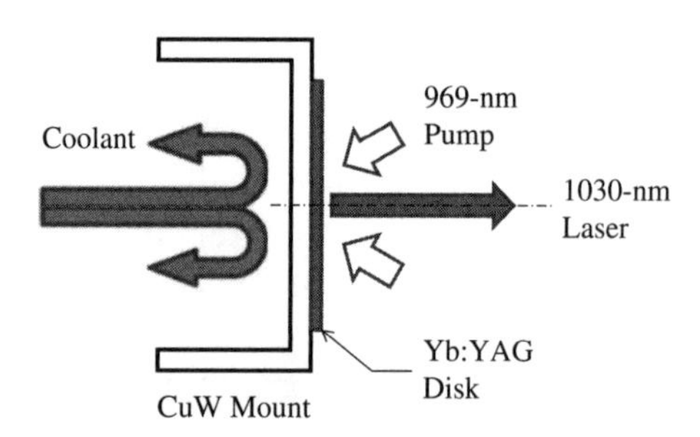


**Figure 2.26** Water-cooled thin-disk lasers and amplifiers allow the generation of picosecond-class pulses with high peak power and essentially zero thermal lensing.

$\lambda = 1030$ nm. Unfortunately, increasing the pulse energy beyond this level initially entailed significant complexity in the form of multipass cells.[32]

As is now a common theme in laser system design, however, low-energy pulses can be amplified in an arrangement known as a master oscillator–power amplifier (MOPA), where the disk geometry is useful for power amplification, independent of the type of master oscillator (i.e., the laser). Using a low-power fiber laser as the oscillator, commercial products using disk power amplifiers offer a $10^6\times$ increase in nanojoule-level fiber-laser pulse energy[33] with output $Q_p \approx 250$ μJ at $\lambda = 1030$ nm and $PRF = 400$ kHz. Not surprisingly, the increase in peak power to 25 MW also allows efficient harmonic generation, with $Q_p \approx 100$ μJ at $\lambda = 515$ nm.

Up to 16 kW of CW power is also available from disk lasers, although with poor beam quality ($M^2 \approx 36$), so appropriate for deep-penetration welding but not focused micromachining (Fig. 2.27). While recent research results show up to 4 kW CW with $M^2 < 1.4$,[33] commercial products have $M^2 \approx 6$ for 1-kW CW and $M^2 \approx 24$ for 2- to 10-kW CW output.[34] Both the pulsed and high-power CW lasers all have open-loop cooling-water requirements; the resulting size of the CW disk systems is on the order of 2 m × 2 m × 1 m.

Beam quality is not a critical laser-system spec for CW disk-laser applications such as welding; however, pointing stability, pulse-to-pulse energy stability, and timing jitter are important for pulsed micromachining applications that require the precise placement—in space and time—of a focused pulse of a known energy density (J/m$^2$) on a work piece. Unfortunately, it is difficult to find these specs quantified in the vendor literature, although with essentially zero thermal lensing across the disk, the

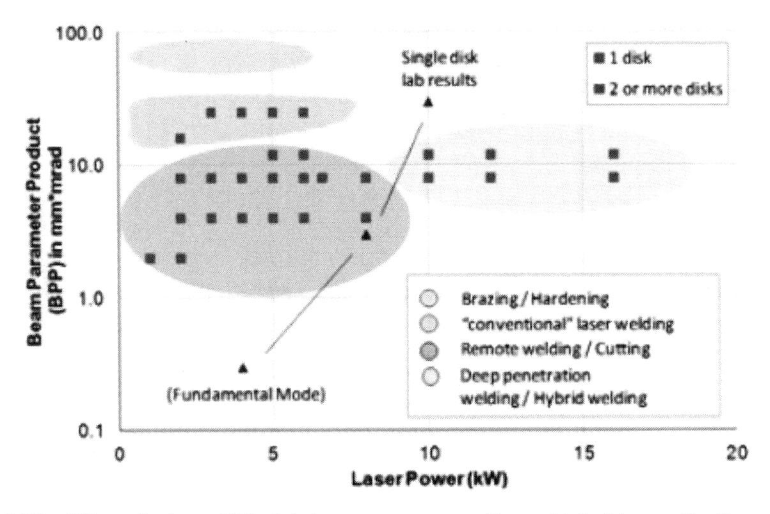


**Figure 2.27** Kilowatt-class CW disk lasers are currently restricted to applications such as welding that do not require good beam quality. (Reprinted from Ref. 33.) (See color plate.)

**Table 2.4** Properties of commonly used solid-state lasers and typical applications. The YAG laser wavelengths are also available with harmonic generation (HG) such as SHG and THG. In general, pulse energy will tend to be smaller at higher PRF.

| Property | Nd:YAG | Ti:Sapphire | Er:Glass | Yb:YAG Disk |
|---|---|---|---|---|
| Wavelength | 1064 nm (+HG) | 700–1000 nm (tunable) | 1540 nm | 1030 nm (+HG) |
| Linewidth | $\Delta\lambda \approx 0.05$ nm | $\Delta\lambda \approx 0.1$–10 nm | $\Delta\lambda \approx 5$ nm | $\Delta\lambda \approx 10$ nm |
| Beam Quality, $M^2$ | $M^2 = 1.2 \rightarrow 5$ | $M^2 < 1.3$ | $M^2 < 1.3$ | $M^2 < 1.3$ (pulsed) $M^2 \approx 10$–35 (CW) |
| Avg. Power | 10 W at 60 kHz | 0.1–1.5 W | 10–100 mW | 1–16 kW CW |
| WP Efficiency | 10–20% | <3% | <1% | 20% |
| Pulse Width, $\Delta t_p$ | 5–20 nsec | <10 fsec | 5–20 nsec | 10 psec |
| Pulse Energy, $Q_p$ | 0.1–100 mJ | 0.1 μJ–40 mJ | 0.1–20 mJ | 0.25 mJ (w/amp) |
| PRF | 10 Hz → 100 kHz | 1 kHz–80 MHz | 1–10 Hz | 0.1–10 MHz |
| Applications | Manufacturing, biomedical, laser radar | Research – Biomedical, chemistry, etc. | Laser radar, range-gated illumination | Manufacturing, defense |

pointing stability and beam-quality variations with output power are expected to be better than those of other solid-state laser types.

**Summary**. Solid-state laser options range from ruggedized high-energy Nd:YAG and eye-safe Er:glass lasers with millijoule-scale pulses and 5- to 10-nsec pulse widths to laboratory research tools such as the Ti:sapphire laser for the ultimate in tunability and for the shortest of USPs. For intermediate-width pulses ($\Delta t_p \approx 0.5$–10 psec) that are cost effective in a manufacturing environment, Yb:YAG disk-based MOPAs are now commonly used for cold-ablation micromachining and have become more "socialized" with higher reliability and operating time. None of the solid-state lasers have the low cost or high wall-plug efficiency associated with semiconductor lasers, but all are useful for meeting a number of laser-system requirements—pulse width, pulse energy, peak power, etc.—which diode lasers cannot meet; these and other properties of solid-state lasers are summarized in Table 2.4.

### 2.2.3 Fiber lasers

Silica ($SiO_2$) fibers were originally developed for low-loss transmission of telecommunications signals and are now the basis of the Internet, which is embedded in everyday life. It was later discovered that these same fibers could be used to make lasers (Fig. 2.28), and the benefits of doing so are twofold:

- A small-diameter fiber has a large surface-to-volume ratio for efficient heat transfer. Neglecting the ends, the surface area available for heat transfer from any cylinder is $A_s = \pi D L_f$ for a diameter $D$ and fiber length $L_f$, while the volume of gain medium in which heat is generated due to nonradiative electron transitions is $V = \pi D^2 L_f/4$. The

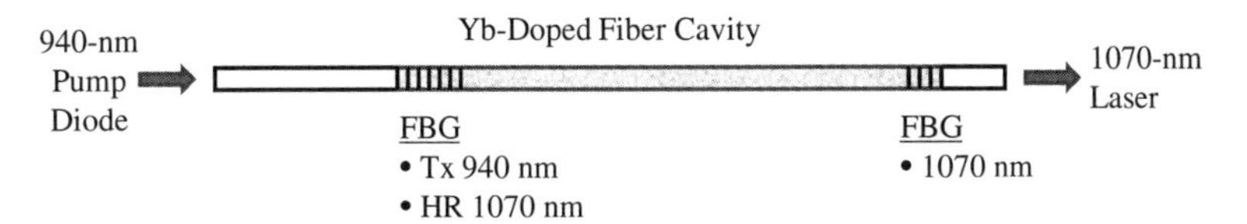


**Figure 2.28** A diode-pumped fiber laser creates the laser cavity using fiber Bragg gratings (FBGs) consisting of small index variations in the UV-photosensitive fiber.

surface-to-volume ratio is thus $A_s/V = 4/D$, illustrating that, by exposing a larger fraction of atoms with gain to the heat sink (air, e.g.), a smaller-diameter fiber is more efficient at transferring heat from its interior.

- The two ends of the fiber—which can be fabricated as fiber Bragg gratings (FBGs) that transmit (Tx) the pump diode but with a high reflectivity (HR) at the laser wavelength to create a laser cavity (Fig. 2.28)—cannot be misaligned with respect to each other, even if the fiber is bent. This is a result of how light propagates in a fiber (i.e., TIR), such that within certain limits on the fiber bending radius, light that is reflected off of the FBG on one end of the fiber will automatically be reflected off of the other. This robustness against FBG "mirror" misalignment makes fiber lasers extremely stable in real-world environments.

While fiber lasers are simple in concept, a number of important details have been developed over the years to increase the range of wavelengths, output power, and pulse energies. With the exception of supercontinuum fibers, peak emission wavelength is in part controlled by the dopant, of which there are three primary options. For $\lambda = 1030$–$1070$ nm—with the exact wavelength determined by the FBGs—Yb is the dopant due to its ability to emit photons with little heat, a huge benefit for high-power fiber lasers. Fiber lasers emitting in the eye-safe band of $\approx$1550 nm, on the other hand, use Er doping, while thulium (Tm)-doped silica lases at $\lambda = 2000$ nm or so. Combinations of these dopants are also used, with Er:Yb co-doping being one option.

Due to its extremely low transmission loss, silica ($SiO_2$)—sometimes also known as glass—is the most common fiber-laser host material, although phosphate fibers are also used due to their ability to retain high levels of doping and thus require shorter lengths of fiber to lase. In addition, fluoride fibers are also used for MWIR wavelengths.

Applications for fiber lasers include super-resolution imaging of biomedical specimens, USP precision micromachining, CW manufacturing (welding, brazing, surface heat treatments, etc.), ultrafast research in biological and physical sciences, and coherent sensing and laser radar that require extremely long coherence lengths. These lasers can be classified into one of four common categories: low power, high power, ultrafast, and supercontinuum.

**Low-Power Fiber Lasers**. This category of fiber lasers relies on the use of single-mode telecommunications fiber and typically has an average power ≤10 W CW. Two variations are common: pulsed (for illumination, e.g.) and high-coherence lasers with less than 10-kHz linewidth for coherent sensing and laser radar.

Pulsed low-power fiber lasers can be used to light up a scene with eye-safe, near-diffraction-limited ($LP_{01}$ fiber mode) pulses at an Er:glass wavelength $\lambda = 1540$ nm with $\Delta t_p \approx 5$–10 nsec and $Q_p \approx 50$–60 μJ at a PRF ≈ 50–500 kHz and an average power ≈4 W. Pulsed illumination for range-gated imaging relies on the peak power; rangefinding or direct-detection laser radar is also a common application with the potential for higher reliability than Er:glass solid-state lasers. Pulsed low-power fiber lasers are available as stand-alone conduction-cooled boxes approximately 50 mm × 150 mm × 150 mm with an operating temperature of –10 °C to +60 °C.

High-coherence low-power fiber lasers use a principle we have already seen a number of times in this book, namely, that a short cavity has a large mode spacing, thus resulting in single-longitudinal-mode emission. The narrow linewidth of this single mode—determined by high-reflectivity, temperature-controlled FBGs [Eq. (1.7)]—then determines the coherence length [Eq. (1.3)], allowing these lasers to be used in sensing applications that require phase stability over a long coherence length, i.e., coherent-detection laser-radar and interferometry measurements.

Available at both 1050-nm and 1550-nm wavelength ranges with a CW output power of ≈100 mW, the SLM linewidth is less than 10 kHz with a frequency stability of 50 MHz over 1 hour with appropriate thermal control of the laser's base temperature. Frequency tuning is also possible with a range of 20 GHz but with well-characterized mode hops. The performance of these lasers can also be susceptible to vibrations, as optical fibers are also extremely sensitive motion sensors, particularly at the level of frequency stability these products are used for.

Low-power fiber lasers—whether pulsed or narrow linewidth—are generally low-maintenance products with turn-key, "plug-and-play" capability. Although not usually ruggedized for field use in terms of thermal, shock, and vibration stability, they have a reliability, size, weight, and power consumption suitable for commercial laboratory instrumentation, with the occasional push into aerospace markets.

**High-Power Fiber Lasers.** At the other extreme are high-power fiber lasers, where recent advances in the product development have been extraordinary. For example, up to 10 kW of CW single-mode power and 100 kW of average multimode power is available from IPG Photonics. Typical applications center on the industrial laser market for materials processing and automobile manufacturing steps such as welding, cutting, drilling, and heat treating that require intense heat. Single-mode lasers can be focused to a small spot for the

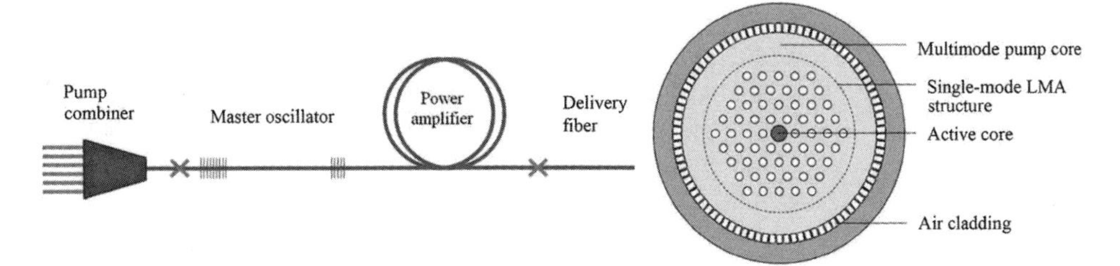


**Figure 2.29** High-power fiber lasers (left) use a large-mode-area double-cladding design (right) to increase pump coupling and decrease fiber nonlinearities. [Reprinted from K. P. Hansen et al., "Airclad fiber laser technology," *Optical Engineering* **50**(11), 111609 (2011).]

high power density required for cutting or drilling, while multimode lasers are best for heating a larger area during welding or heat treating.

The peak power for fiber lasers based on single-mode telecommunications fiber with a 10.5-μm active-core diameter—with 10 kW being the highest-possible power—is limited by fiber nonlinearities [stimulated Raman scattering (SRS), which depends on both the peak power density ($W/m^2$) and the fiber length]. For high-power fiber designs, nonlinearities can be minimized by the use of a double-clad fiber (Fig. 2.29). In addition, a fiber laser must not only create light efficiently, but it must also be pumped with low loss. For single-mode telecommunications fibers, this requires a single-mode pump diode, a huge design limitation in obtaining higher power levels. As a result, double-clad fibers are used for high-power lasers, where a large mode area (LMA) reduces power-density-limiting nonlinearities and a second outer cladding allows pumping with a multimode diode laser.

The architecture shown in Fig. 2.29 is that of a MOPA using a fiber laser as the master oscillator and a fiber amplifier to increase the power. Unfortunately, LMA fibers for the power amplifier tend to go multimode with very little perturbation (e.g., bending losses and refractive index non-uniformities due to temperature gradients); special techniques are thus used to keep high-power single-mode fiber from becoming multimode, or multimode fiber from becoming excessively multimode. Alternatively, rod amplifiers approximately 1–2 mm in diameter with a 100-μm active core are also common, avoiding the macro- and microbending instabilities of fiber.

Single-mode CW power up to 1 kW with ±0.5% power stability is available for water-cooled, Yb-doped silica fiber lasers emitting at $\lambda \approx$ 1070 nm, although up to 10 kW is available using a MOPA design. Multimode ($M^2 > 30$) CW power up to 100 kW is also available by incoherently combining lower-power lasers. The wall-plug efficiency—which cannot be as high as the pump diodes themselves—is still extremely good, with values exceeding 45% due to the high efficiency of the diode pump as well as the almost complete conversion of absorbed 940-nm pump photons into 1070-nm Yb-output photons, and very little nonradiative energy (heat).

The commonly used 1070-nm wavelength is not optimal for many of the manufacturing and materials processing tasks for which high-power fiber lasers are used. As a result, Er-doped ($\lambda \approx 1550$ nm) and Tm-doped ($\lambda \approx$ 2000 nm) silica fiber lasers are also available with single-mode CW power up to $\approx$100 W. In addition, SHG conversion to $\lambda = 535$ nm (green) is also available with up to 500 W of CW and QCW power.[35]

High-power fiber lasers are also available with QCW and nanosecond pulse widths. By modulating the pump diodes at a 10-Hz rate, QCW switching with 10-msec pulses and a 10% duty cycle increases the peak power by a factor of 10 over the average power; average power ranges from 150–900 W. Nanosecond pulsing uses Q-switching to obtain a pulse width $\Delta t_p = 100$–500 nsec and a pulse energy $Q_p = 1$ mJ at a PRF = 20–50 kHz. Beam quality varies from $M^2 = 1.6$ for 1-mJ pulse energy ($P_{avg} = 20$ W) to $M^2 = 5$ for 2-mJ pulse energy ($P_{avg} = 100$ W). Picosecond-pulsed fiber lasers are also available, as discussed in the next section.

**Ultrafast Fiber Lasers.** Of the recent developments in laser and laser systems design, ultrafast fiber lasers are also among the most important. Given the high peak power associated with moderate-energy USPs, these lasers are being used in a number of new applications such as cold-ablation micromachining and multiphoton biomedical imaging.[36] Ultrafast fiber lasers are even a key component in sub-diffraction-limited stimulated emission depletion (STED) microscopy, for which the 2014 Nobel Prize in Chemistry was awarded.[37]

With the addition of a passive mode locker such as a SESAM, the same double-clad fiber design that allows high CW power is also used in ultrafast fiber lasers. A typical MOPA architecture is shown in Fig. 2.30, where the laser oscillator consists of Er-doped silica fiber for emission at $\lambda \approx 1560$ nm. The figure shows that the oscillator is mode locked using a saturable-absorber mirror (SAM), a separately pumped power amplifier with an optical isolator

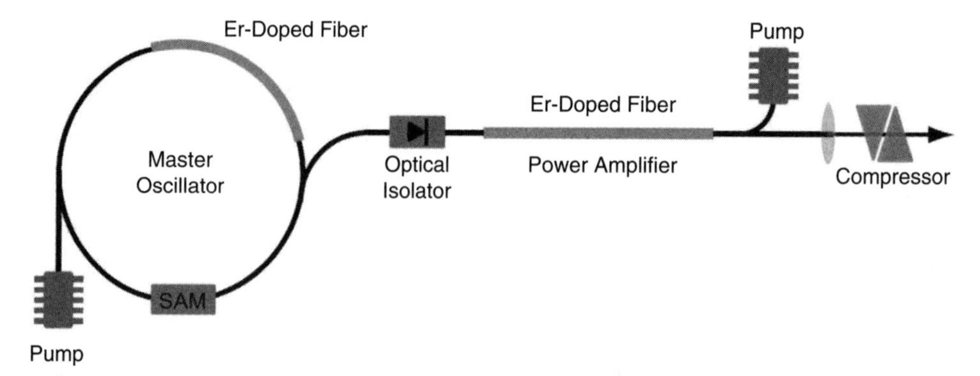


**Figure 2.30** Schematic of an ultrafast fiber laser for generating and amplifying USPs. [Adapted from M. Lang et al., "Technology and applications of ultrafast fiber lasers," *Proc. SPIE* **8330**, 833007 (2012).]

**Table 2.5** Comparison of nanosecond, picosecond, and femtosecond pulse-width lasers emitting at $\lambda \approx 1050$ nm. The nanosecond data are for Nd:YAG solid-state lasers, while the picosecond and femtosecond data are for Yb:silica ultrafast fiber lasers.[38]

| Laser Class | Avg. Power | Pulse Width | Pulse Energy | Peak Power | PRF |
|---|---|---|---|---|---|
| Nanosecond | 10 W | 5 nsec | 10 mJ | 2 MW | 1 kHz |
| Picosecond | 20 W | 10 psec | 100 μJ | 10 MW | 0.2 MHz |
| Femtosecond | 1 W | 450 fsec | 10 μJ | 22 MW | 0.1 MHz |
| Femtosecond | 20 W | 350 fsec | 100 μJ | 280 MW | 2 MHz |
| Femtosecond | 40 W | 500 fsec | 400 μJ | 800 MW | 0.1 MHz |

to prevent amplified spontaneous emission (ASE) from back-propagating into the oscillator, and a prism-pair compressor for pulse-width reduction via dispersion compensation.[12]

Pulse widths for most applications of ultrafast fiber lasers range from $\Delta t_p = 0.1$–$10$ psec; pulses as small as 20 fsec and as large as 100 psec are also available. Table 2.5 shows that the transition from picosecond to femtosecond pulse widths with the same average power generally results in higher peak power; within the femtosecond class, the peak power increases as pulse energy increases, since the pulse widths are more or less the same. Er-doped (1560 nm), Tm-doped (2000 nm), and frequency-doubled (515 and 780 nm) wavelengths are also available with specs that differ from those listed in the table.

Designing these (and other) pulsed lasers into a laser system is more difficult than implied by Table 2.5. The problem is that a PRF that differs from what is listed in the vendor's spec sheet will have a different pulse energy, typically dropping at a higher PRF as there is less time for energy to accumulate before being released (Fig. 2.31). As a result, ultrafast-scale pulse width does not guarantee high peak power for nanosecond or picosecond pulses, as the peak powers given in Table 2.5 will be lower as the PRF

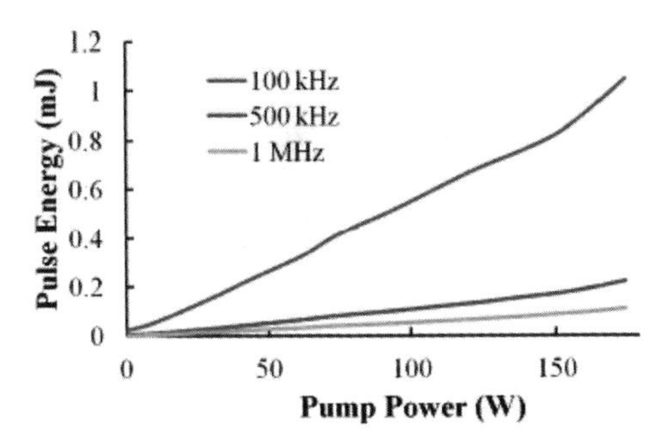


**Figure 2.31** With the same average pump power, pulse energy decreases as PRF increases per Eq. (2.6). [Reprinted with permission from P. Wang et al., "All fiber-based Yb-doped high energy, high power femtosecond fiber lasers," *Optics Express* **21**(24), 29854–29859 (2013).] (See color plate.)

increases—oftentimes out of proportion to the increase in PRF, as the available pulse energy changes nonlinearly at sufficiently high PRF (see Fig. 2.9). The average power can also reach a maximum at a higher PRF, as the drop in pulse energy is not compensated by the increase in PRF required by Eq. (2.6) to keep the average power constant, so what is required to use pulsed lasers in a system are design curves showing these trends, not data points from a spec sheet.

Power and pointing stabilities are also critical for micromachining and biomedical imaging, which rely on multiphoton absorption. These are shown in Figs. 2.32 and 2.33, illustrating the utility of this type of laser for these applications.

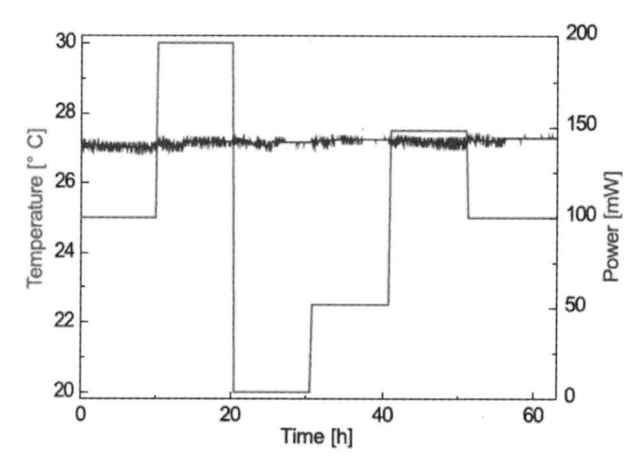


**Figure 2.32** Power stability of an ultrafast fiber laser for temperature changes of ±5 °C. (Reprinted with permission from TOPTICA Photonics AG.)

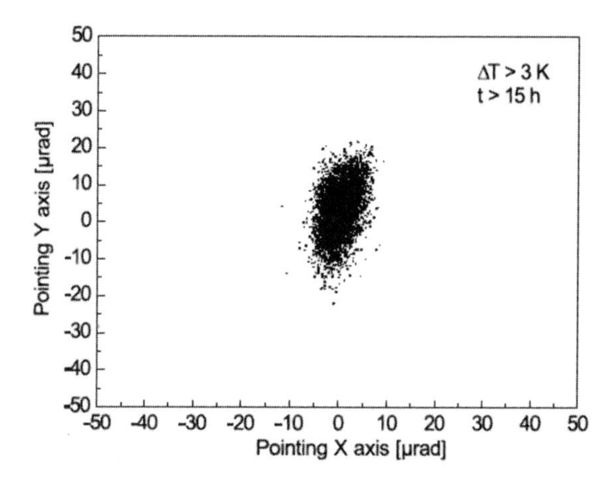


**Figure 2.33** Pointing stability of an ultrafast fiber laser over a 15-hour period with an environmental temperature change $\Delta T > 3$ °C. (Reprinted with permission from TOPTICA Photonics AG.)

**Supercontinuum Fiber Lasers.** While laser linewidth can vary from kilohertz for high-coherence fiber lasers to nanometers for high-power semiconductor lasers, applications such as spectral-domain optical coherence tomography (OCT) require a much wider bandwidth—on the order of hundreds of nanometers. In the past, a wide spectral emission had been considered to be "out of scope" for lasers, and LEDs were used for OCT and other applications. More recently, it was understood that a broadband ("white light") laser has many benefits—spatial coherence and diffraction-limited brightness, e.g.—even if a long coherence length is not one of them.

A typical spectrum for a broadband, supercontinuum fiber laser extends from 400 nm to 2400 nm (Fig. 2.34). This spectrum is obtained not by the bandwidth of the gain medium, but by a combination of chromatic dispersion and a nonlinear process known as Raman self-scattering, which generates wavelengths other than what is initially propagating down a fiber.[39] Nonlinearities depend on the power density, i.e., a high peak power (and thus a short pulse width) and a small mode area. A supercontinuum is thus generated using USPs ($\approx$5 psec) propagating in a low-loss, highly nonlinear photonic crystal fiber (PCF) with a core size even smaller than that of SMF.

Total output power over the entire spectrum is somewhat less than that of the ultrafast laser that feeds into the nonlinear fiber, and ranges from 0.2 W to 20 W but with significantly smaller values over a specific spectral band (VIS, e.g.). The in-band power can be estimated by integrating the power spectral density (mW/nm) curve in Fig. 2.34 over the bandwidth $\Delta\lambda$; alternatively, some vendors have measured these numbers, and their data sheets list the total power in a given band.

Beam quality is essentially diffraction limited with $M^2 < 1.1$. Unless pulse pickers are used to reduce the PRF, the pulse rate matches that of the mode-locked "seed" laser—also usually a fiber laser—at $PRF = 20$–$80$ MHz. As expected for a stable fiber cavity, power stability ($\pm$0.5%) and beam-pointing stability (<50 $\mu$rad) are good—and thus useful for OCT imaging.

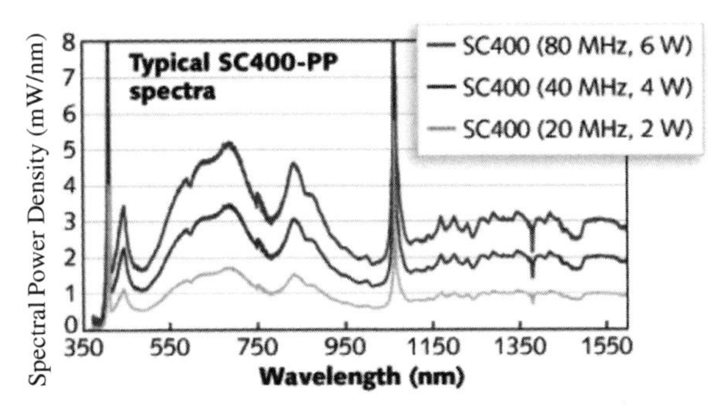


**Figure 2.34** Output spectrum of a supercontinuum fiber laser. (Reprinted with permission from Fianium Corp.)

**Table 2.6** Properties of commonly used fiber lasers, and typical applications. Some wavelengths are also available with harmonic generation (HG) such as SHG and THG. In general, pulse energy will tend to be smaller at higher PRF.

| Property | Low-Power | High-Power | Ultrafast | Supercontinuum |
|---|---|---|---|---|
| Wavelength | 1070 nm (+HG)<br>1550 nm (+HG)<br>2000 nm | 1070 nm (+HG)<br>1550 nm (+HG)<br>2000 nm | 1070 nm (+HG)<br>1550 nm (+HG)<br>2000 nm | VIS → SWIR;<br>MWIR |
| Linewidth | $\Delta\nu < 10$ kHz → 100 MHz | $\Delta\lambda \approx 1$–10 nm | $\Delta\lambda \approx 10$–100 nm | $\Delta\lambda \approx 2000$ nm |
| Beam Quality, $M^2$ | $M^2 < 1.2$ | $M^2 = 1.2 \rightarrow 30$ | $M^2 < 1.3$ | $M^2 < 1.2$ |
| Avg. Power | 1 mW–100 W | 100 W–100 kW | 0.2–40 W | 0.2–20 W |
| WP Efficiency | 0.5–1.5% | >45% | 1–2% | 5–10% |
| Pulse Width, $\Delta t_p$ | 5–10 nsec | 0.1–0.5 μs QCW | 0.1–10 psec | 0.1–10 psec |
| Pulse Energy, $Q_p$ | 100 μJ | 1–2 mJ | 10–400 μJ | N/A |
| PRF | 10–750 kHz | 20–50 kHz | 0.1–20 MHz | 0.1–80 MHz |
| Applications | Coherent sensing, laser radar | Manufacturing, defense | Biomedical, manufacturing | Sensing, defense |

MWIR supercontinuum lasers using fluoride-based fibers such as ZBLAN are also available. These can be useful for IR countermeasures to protect commercial and military flights against missile threats, in competition with semiconductor QCLs.

**Summary**. Fiber laser options range from low-power lasers with an extremely narrow bandwidth to high-power lasers with the highest average power. Pulsed peak power can also exceed 1 GW, which can be used to generate supercontinuum, white-light lasers with a 2000-nm spectral bandwidth.

Fiber lasers are generally alignment free and allow high-power fiber delivery, with low-maintenance, low-infrastructure—i.e., no water cooling due to excellent heat transfer from small-diameter fibers—high-reliability lasers having "plug-and-play" capability useful for many products, though not typically ruggedized to the degree that Er:glass rangefinders are. Their many applications include high peak power for cold micromachining and high average power for industrial-scale throughput, as the higher power can be distributed over a larger area and maintain the same power (or energy) density ($W/m^2$ or $J/m^2$) on which so many processes depend. These and other properties of fiber lasers are summarized in Table 2.6.

### 2.2.4 Gas lasers

While ruby solid-state lasers were the first to be built, HeNe gas lasers were not far behind and quickly surpassed ruby as the "go to" laser type. The reason is that the helium-neon gas mixture is electrically pumped, so a large and expensive flashlamp to optically pump a population inversion is not needed as it is for ruby lasers. The resulting products were also less prone to thermal lensing and had the best beam quality of any other commercially available laser at the time.

One of the biggest disadvantages of most gas lasers is the huge amount of current it takes to electrically pump a low-density gas medium; the resulting wall-plug efficiencies are extremely low, on the order of 0.1% or lower. Because of their low efficiency, large size, and potentially costly maintenance requirements, many gas lasers are being replaced by semiconductor, solid-state, and fiber lasers; nonetheless, there are some applications that rely on the unique benefits of gas lasers, which can be classified into one of four commonly used categories: helium, excimer, carbon dioxide ($CO_2$), and ion. Typical applications are HeNe lasers for interferometry, excimer lasers for semiconductor photolithography and eye surgery, and carbon dioxide lasers for manufacturing.

**Helium Lasers.** The construction of a HeNe laser is shown in Fig. 2.35. Typical of the gas lasers is a glass tube to contain the gas medium and support the two mirrors that define the laser cavity, a bore to contain the electrical discharge between anode and cathode that pumps the neon into a population inversion, and a high-voltage (or high-current) power supply.

The most common output wavelength is 633 nm (red), but 3.39 μm is also used for interferometric measurement of optical components that transmit at this MWIR wavelength. Other wavelengths are also available, including 543 nm (green), 594 nm (yellow), and 612 nm (orange). Semiconductor lasers of smaller size and cost may be available as a replacement for some of these wavelengths (see Table 2.1).

CW output power is on the order of 1–50 mW with extremely good beam quality ($M^2 < 1.1$). The output spectrum is typically multi-longitudinal mode, with an axial mode spacing $\Delta\nu_a = c/2nL = 3 \times 10^8$ m/sec/(2 × 1 ×

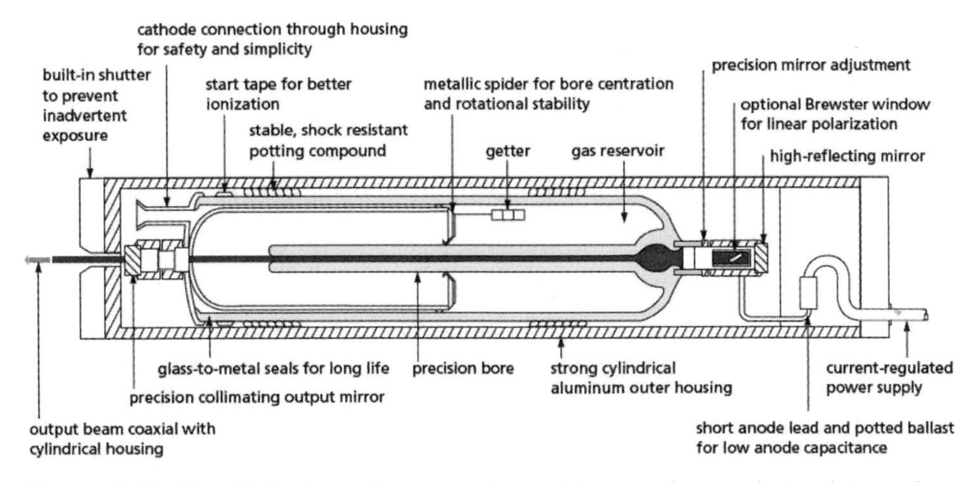


**Figure 2.35** The HeNe laser is a complex yet inexpensive product using a glass containment tube and a high voltage to create a population inversion. (Credit: CVI Laser, LLC.)

0.25 m) = 600 MHz for a HeNe laser with $L = 250$ mm; there are thus 2 to 3 modes that fit within the gain bandwidth $\Delta\nu_g \approx 1.4$ GHz for the inhomogeneous helium-neon medium, giving a total linewidth $\Delta\nu \approx 1.2$ GHz and a minimum coherence length $d_c = c\tau_c = c/2\Delta\nu = 125$ mm—more than sufficient for using these lasers in an interferometer for measuring many optical components (see Fig. 1.5).

The required infrastructure for using a HeNe laser is straightforward: 115 or 230 VAC, with no cooling requirements other than an operating temperature range of –20 °C to +40 °C. Disadvantages of the HeNe are the low wall-plug efficiency (~0.1%) and the possibility of breaking the glass tube if shock loading exceeds 25 g for ≥10 msec.

In addition to the HeNe, the helium-cadmium (HeCd) laser has been developed for applications that require its 325-nm (UV) and 442-nm (blue) wavelengths. These applications typically involve exposure to photosensitive materials and include, e.g., optical fibers for creating the FBGs used in fiber lasers, holographic films, and stereolithography of polymers to create 3D structures. Pointing stability of the HeCd laser is better than 20 μrad with a temperature control of ±2 °C—useful for creating the high-precision features that rely on the short wavelengths of the HeCd.

**Excimer Lasers.** It is not well known that the excimer laser is an essential technology for most of the conveniences (and inconveniences) of modern-day life, given that it is a key component in the semiconductor photolithography process used to manufacture the computer and memory chips that go into the entire array of consumer electronics products. The reason is simply that the excimer laser's UV wavelength is currently the shortest of any commercially available source, allowing the smallest-possible feature size in the silicon transistors that Dr. Moore predicted would continue to increase in density at an exponential rate.[40]

In addition to the uniform exposure of small areas of a silicon wafer, excimer lasers are also used to obtain focused spots for refractive eye surgery processes such as LASIK, i.e., removing material from the cornea to re-shape the surface. In this case, the short wavelength allows high-precision "sculpting," while the large photon energy ($E_p = hc/\lambda$) allows cold ablation with little thermal damage even for long (nanosecond-duration) pulses.

The 193-nm wavelength commonly used for both photolithography and LASIK is obtained with an argon-fluoride (ArF) excimer laser. Other wavelengths are also available, including 157 nm ($F_2$), 248 nm [krypton-fluoride (KrF)], and 308 nm [xenon-chloride (XeCl)]. These are hazardous, corrosive gas mixtures and require care with meeting regulatory safety requirements on the use of excimer lasers.

Other critical specifications depend on the application, roughly divided into photolithography and micromachining (including cornea ablation).

Photolithography specs are the most demanding and include pulse-to-pulse energy stability to ensure low variations in total dose to which a photoresist is exposed, a subpicometer linewidth to reduce the chromatic dispersion of the optical subsystem, and power distribution across the beam that allows a high degree of spatial uniformity across the wafer area being exposed. Vendors such as Cymer and Lambda Physik[15] supply these large and expensive boxes to their limited customer base.

More common are the excimer lasers used for refractive eye surgery and manufacturing operations such as micromachining of flat-panel displays and high-brightness LEDs. These are inherently pulsed lasers, with a pulse width $\Delta t_p = 5$–$25$ nsec, pulse energy $Q_p = 1$–$100$ mJ, PRF = 200–1000 Hz, and average power of 1–10 W.

Pulse-to-pulse energy stability of less than 1–3% RMS is also a critical spec for these lasers, as energy variations affect the micromachining depth and therefore the number of pulses required to complete a manufacturing step. Energy stability is particularly important for small-depth-of-cut applications such as eye surgery, where errors made with too powerful a pulse cannot be reversed and a large number of low-energy pulses at a high PRF are preferred over a small number of higher-energy (and higher energy-variation) pulses.

Unusual features of using excimer lasers in a laser system—whether photolithography or micromachining—include large, rectangular beam dimensions (3 mm $\times$ 6 mm, e.g.), nitrogen purging of the beam path to remove UV-absorbing air, the lifetime of the optical components whose transmission can quickly drop due to UV photodarkening, and the potential for "sunburn" of the skin and cornea of the operators. In addition, required infrastructure can include water cooling for high-PRF systems with $\geq$10 W of average power; dynamic gas replenishment will also be required at a surprisingly fast rate, as the number of shots is $\approx 50 \times 10^6$ (wavelength dependent) and is quickly exceeded when operating at a 1-kHz PRF. Overall lifetime of an excimer laser exceeds $10^9$ shots, with a reliability useful for 24-7 manufacturing environments.

**Carbon Dioxide Lasers**. We have seen a number of types of lasers—high-power semiconductor, Yb:YAG disk, high-power fiber, ultrafast fiber, and excimer—that are useful for manufacturing, but there is yet another type that has a unique niche, namely, the carbon dioxide ($CO_2$) laser with its LWIR (10.6 μm) wavelength. This wavelength is useful for specific manufacturing applications such as ink-free marking of plastics with product expiration dates, as well as engraving, welding, and cutting of metals (steel, e.g.) that absorb 10.6-μm photons. One disadvantage of this long wavelength is that the resolution of the mark or cut is larger by a factor of $10.6/0.193 \approx 55$ in comparison with an ArF excimer laser.

Nonetheless, the lack of precision does not exclude its use, and both pulsed and CW versions are available. Short-pulse $CO_2$ lasers are based on a transversely excited atmospheric (TEA) architecture, where the electrical pumping of the $CO_2$ across the small transverse dimension allows a pulse energy of 150 mJ to accumulate in 50 nsec for a multimode beam, with pulse energies as high as 5 J available in a 100-nsec pulse width at a 12 Hz PRF. These are not clean pulses—microsecond "tails" are common—but they are nonetheless useful for low-precision manufacturing. Long-pulse $CO_2$ lasers are also available, using QCW gain switching with $\approx$20% duty cycle and 0.1- to 1-msec pulse widths for a peak power $\approx 5\times$ the average power.

Despite their relatively high wall-plug efficiency—10 to 20% is common—$CO_2$ lasers can use flowing-gas convection cooling to augment heat transfer for high-pulse-energy and high-CW-power products, with subsequent water cooling to remove heat from the hot gas. Gas cooling can be transverse flow (which may or may not be used in conjunction with transverse excitation), slow axial flow, or fast axial flow. Fast axial flow is used for the heavy-duty industrial "beasts" preferred by auto manufacturers, with CW output power up to 20 kW. Independent of flow geometry, contaminant-free gas must be supplied on each heating cycle, and gas replenishment at a rate of tens of liters per hour can be a major factor in total operating costs.

Diffusion-cooled slab lasers are another product option, and these are capable of handling up to 2 kW of laser output power, with negligible requirements on replacing cooling gases (1–2 years for a 10-liter bottle, e.g.). A similar design for average powers up to 500 W is the sealed $CO_2$ laser, where laser gases do not need to be supplied (even though cooling water may be required). Such turn-key lasers are available with 10–500 W of average power, beam quality $M^2 < 1.2$ up to 400 W, power stability of ±5% after warm-up, and a lifetime exceeding 10,000 hours before gas replacement. Even at the lower powers, however, fibers that transmit at 10.6 μm are not yet available, so it is common to see sealed $CO_2$ lasers in manufacturing plants being moved on robotic arms in a dazzling display of dexterity.

**Ion Lasers.** Ion lasers are largely being replaced by other types of lasers, and we briefly review in this section the reasons for this and the remaining applications.

Also known as noble-gas lasers, ion lasers use argon (Ar), krypton (Kr), or Ar-Kr mixed-gas fills of a glass plasma-containment tube similar to that of a HeNe laser. Shown in Fig. 2.36 for a high-power (1–20 W) ion laser are external mirrors that define the cavity length, Brewster's-angle windows for polarization control, a water-cooled ceramic-bore structure to ensure a high current density for the gas discharge path, and an electromagnet to increase the ion population inversion.

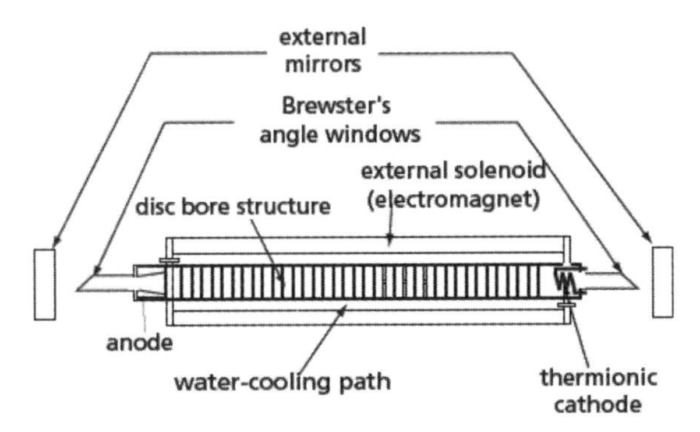


**Figure 2.36** Illustration of a high-power water-cooled ion laser. The cavity length *L* is on the order of 1 m, allowing multifrequency lasing. (Credit: CVI Laser, LLC.)

Ion lasers are available in both multiline (multiple longitudinal mode) and single-line options. With an inhomogeneous gain bandwidth that is around 5× that of the HeNe ($\Delta\nu_g \approx$ 6–8 GHz) and a mode spacing that is smaller than the HeNe due to the longer cavity length, there may be as many as 30 modes with enough gain to lase. The normal range of wavelengths for the Ar-ion laser is UV (335–365 nm) and blue-green (450–520 nm), with 488 nm and 514.5 nm emitting the most power. The 514.5-nm wavelength is a good match for pumping Ti:sapphire lasers, but the ion lasers are rarely used anymore as they have been replaced by lower-noise, frequency-doubled VECSELs and Nd:YLF lasers. Single-wavelength selection requires the use of an intracavity etalon and tuning prism, which the vendors offer as options.

Krypton-ion lasers have lower power than Ar-ion but emit photons over a wider spectrum; the 647.1-nm wavelength carries the highest output power.

While the beam quality, SLM linewidth (≈100 MHz), power stability, and noise of ion lasers are generally excellent, their disadvantages include their large size, low wall-plug efficiency and therefore high power consumption and continuous water cooling at high flow rates (≥10 liters/min), and limited lifetimes.

Despite these disadvantages, the applications that still rely on ion lasers include the ever-popular laser light show, where mixed-gas ion lasers output multiwavelength RGB to produce a variety of hues and colors. In addition, SHG of Ar-ion output is available with up to 1 W of power at $\lambda =$ to 257.2 nm, used for the fabrication of fiber lasers requiring $\lambda/4$ FBG feature sizes, and the average power levels from FHG of Nd:YAG to $\lambda = 266$ nm are not competitive for volume manufacturing. This high CW power at UV wavelengths is also useful for DVD mastering requiring spot sizes <400 nm, where the pulses required for THG of Nd:YAG and VECSEL lasers are not compatible with the modulation required for digital data; the narrow linewidth and high power of a single-line ion laser is also useful for holographic instrumentation requiring long coherence lengths.

**Table 2.7** Properties of commonly used gas lasers, and typical applications.

| Property | Helium | Excimer | $CO_2$ | Ion |
|---|---|---|---|---|
| Wavelength | 325, 442 nm (HeCd); 633 nm, 3.39 μm (HeNe) | 157, 193, 248 nm | 9.3, 10.6 μm | 488, 514.5 nm (Ar); 647.1 nm (Kr) |
| Linewidth | $\Delta\nu \approx 1$ GHz | $\Delta\lambda \approx 1$–10 pm | $\Delta\lambda \approx 1$ nm | $\Delta\nu \approx 100$ MHz |
| Beam Quality, $M^2$ | $M^2 < 1.1$ | $M^2 = 1.2 \rightarrow 30$ | $M^2 = 1.2 \rightarrow 5$ | $M^2 = 1.2$–$1.7$ |
| Average Power | 1–100 mW | 1 W → 1 kW | 10 W → 20 kW | 0.01–25 W |
| WP Efficiency | 0.1% | 0.2–2% | 5–20% | 0.1% |
| Pulse Width, $\Delta t_p$ | N/A | 5–25 nsec | 50–100 nsec | N/A |
| Pulse Energy, $Q_p$ | N/A | 1 mJ → 1 J | 1 mJ → 5 J | N/A |
| PRF | N/A | 0.2–2 kHz | 10–400 Hz | N/A |
| Applications | Optical testing, holography, stereolithography | Photolithography, eye surgery, manufacturing | Manufacturing, optical testing | Manufacturing, holography, displays |

**Summary.** By allowing for direct electrical pumping, gas lasers had an advantage over lamp-pumped solid-state lasers in the early years of laser development. While at one time accounting for half of the dollars spent on lasers, gas lasers are being replaced by semiconductor, solid-state, and fiber lasers, except for the wavelengths (UV and LWIR) with which these lasers cannot compete with sufficient power for industrial processes such as photolithography and micromachining. The factors driving laser systems away from many gas lasers include their large size, poor wall-plug efficiency, and operating infrastructure such as water cooling and gas replenishment. These and other properties of gas lasers are summarized in Table 2.7.

## 2.3 Laser Selection

While there has been some discussion of the operating principles of various types in lasers in the previous section—see Hecht for more details on many of these types[41]—the key goal of this chapter is the selection of a laser to meet customer system requirements.

As a first step in this direction, it is often the case that laser wavelength will be the primary driver of laser selection (Table 2.8). A fluorescence microscope, for example, will need to lase at fluorophore excitation wavelengths, while a manufacturing system may have to trade off the costs and benefits of $CO_2$ lasers at $\lambda = 10.6$ μm versus fiber lasers at $\lambda = 1070$ nm. These trades will involve a number of technical components besides wavelength—spatial coherence, power stability, beam quality, wall-plug efficiency, and so on—and will also entail programmatic metrics such as schedule, risk, and cost trades.

**Table 2.8** Laser types categorized by wavelength band.

| Wavelength (μm) | Band | Laser Types |
|---|---|---|
| 0.1–0.4 | UV | Diode, excimer, ion, HeCd, Nd:YAG (3×), Nd:YAG (4×) |
| 0.4–0.7 | VIS | Diode, fiber (2×), HeNe, ion, Nd:YAG (2×), VCSEL |
| 0.7–1 | NIR | Diode, fiber (2×), Ti:sapphire, VCSEL |
| 1–3 | SWIR | Diode, disk, Er:glass, fiber, Nd:YAG, VCSEL |
| 3–5 | MWIR | HeNe, QCL |
| 8–12 | LWIR | $CO_2$, QCL |

Before getting to the programmatic trades, it is important to first take a look at the "big picture" on technical metrics. That is, while a laser may have individual technical specs such as wall-plug efficiency, what is important is the *system* wall-plug efficiency, not just that of the laser by itself. For example, we saw in Fig. 2.18 that a diode laser may require a TEC to stabilize its temperature and thus reduce its wavelength drift. TECs, however, are extremely *in*efficient at generating cooling capacity and will therefore reduce the wall-plug efficiency of a system that uses this type of laser, even though the diode is itself extremely efficient.

For example, the specs for a COTS diode list an electrical power consumption for the laser of 2.5 W; in addition, the specs for the TEC are 0.8 A at 0.9 V, or an additional power consumption of 0.72 W. Whatever the wall-plug efficiency of the diode is, the efficiency of the diode-plus-TEC system is thus smaller by a factor of $(2.5 + 0.72)/2.5 = 1.3$. More generally, for a given laser efficiency $\eta_{WP}$, the heat load that the TEC must remove is $Q = P_{elec} - P = (1 - \eta_{WP})P_{elec}$, and the electrical power consumption of the TEC is $P_{TEC} = Q/\eta_{TEC}$. The electrical conversion efficiency of the system is therefore $\eta_{sys} = P/(P_{elec} + P_{TEC})$; for a 50%-efficient diode laser with $P = 1$ W and cooled with a 5%-efficient TEC, this works out to a system efficiency $\eta_{sys} = 4.5\%$, or more than a factor of 10× reduction from that of the laser by itself.

Other laser types—disk or $CO_2$ lasers, for example—will have other types of auxiliary heat-transfer equipment such as cooling water, whose electrical power consumption depends on the water pumps, and the system efficiency will change in the same manner. In addition to cooling hardware, there may also be power supplies, control circuits, and so on, whose net effect is to reduce the efficiency of generating photons from electrical power.

In addition to power consumption, system size (volume) and weight—not just that of the laser—are often important technical requirements. Additional examples of laser versus system specs include:

- As we will see in Chapter 4, the beam divergence of the system can be increased to well beyond the laser's beam-quality spec, depending on the optical subsystem.
- As we will see in Chapter 5, the pointing instability can be made significantly worse, depending on the beam-scanning subsystem.

- As we will see in Chapter 7, efficient photon detection can be traded against the efficiency with which photons need to be created by the laser.

And then there are the programmatic metrics for laser system performance. These include:

- Lifecycle costs (cost of ownership) – Included are nonrecurring engineering (NRE), unit cost, operating costs, and maintenance costs such as component replacement and/or replenishment.
- Cost per watt – As an input-output metric for comparing systems, the unit cost ($ or otherwise) per watt of the laser is sometimes used. This is an incomplete metric for a number of reasons, including the fact that it is the total watts of the system that are important, not just that of the laser. In addition, this metric often ignores operating and maintenance costs, and what is ultimately important for commercial applications is total cost of ownership (CoO) per unit increase in revenue.
- Operating infrastructure – This includes auxiliary equipment such as gas supplies, de-ionized cooling water and filters for a closed-loop chiller, massive power supplies, and so on, affecting ease of use. This can also include personnel: do you need to hire a Ph.D. to run the laser—as was often the case in the early days when the Immutable Laws of Lasers were formulated—or is a laser-capable technician sufficient?
- Reliability – A laser that cannot run on a 24-7 schedule in an industrial environment is not reliable; one that works forever on the intermittent schedule of graduate-student research is. Reliability is measured by "downtime," so even daily "tweaking" of a Ti:sapphire or ion laser can be considered a loss in reliability (and therefore productivity). In the industrial environment, even though downtime might not have large explicit costs, it can lead to a huge loss of revenue as repairs are made.
- Throughput – A related metric is the productivity of the laser when it is operating reliably. This is not always straightforward, as there will be both costs and benefits associated with its use. For example, a part manufactured with a picosecond laser will have fewer postprocessing steps (polishing or de-burring, e.g.) due to the small HAZ, but will also be more expensive and machine at a slower rate than a nanosecond laser.
- Maintenance – Even if the laser is reliable, how frequent and how long are the maintenance cycles? Is the Maytag repairman a good model for the maintenance of the laser, or is the vendor's maintenance technician instead living at your facility?
- Lifetime – Even if the laser is reliable and low maintenance, how long will it last? This depends on how "lifetime" is defined—perhaps power degradation, and if so, to what degree? Or perhaps the number of shots from a pulsed laser? And how does the definition affect the maintenance cycle for replacing gases, for example?

A common systems-engineering tool for summarizing both technical and programmatic metrics is the trade table. Examples are shown for micromachining applications in Table 2.9 for picosecond lasers and Table 2.10 for femtosecond lasers, where technical specs such as pulse width, pulse energy,

**Table 2.9** Trade table for comparing picosecond laser specs for micromachining applications. [Reprinted with permission from R. Schaeffer, PhotoMachining Inc. and *Industrial Laser Solutions* (2014). Copyright © PennWell Corp. 2014.]

| COMPANY | PULSE WIDTH (PS) | E/PULSE (MJ) | REP RATE (MHZ) | OUTPUT POWER (W) | L (NM) | HARMONICS (2, 3, OR 4) | TECHNOLOGY BASE | STRENGTHS | FUTURE PLANS |
|---|---|---|---|---|---|---|---|---|---|
| ADVANCED OPTOWAVE | 0.8–10 | Up to 100 | 0–2 | Up to 10 50W/Q1 | 1064–1030 | 2, 3, 4 | Hybrid fiber, free space | Compact, cost-effective, turnkey | Optimal solutions for customers |
| AMPHOS | 0.5–10 | Up to 1000 | 0.1–40 | 100, 200, 400, 1000 | 1030 | 2 | Yb:Innoslab | High power, flexibility in pulse parameters | More compact, higher power, lower cost |
| ATTODYNE | < 10 | Up to 200 | 0–1 | < 10 | 1064 | 2, 3 | Hybrid fiber, free-space multipass MOPA | Compact, Affordable, Turnkey | Higher Power (50W), Smaller footprint, lower cost |
| EDGEWAVE | 0.7–11 | Up to 2000 | 0.05–20 | Up to 400 | 1064 1030 | 2, 3 | Nd Yb | High power, small size, scalable, affordable | Scaling of pulse energy beyond 1mJ, increasing pulse control |
| EKSPLA | < 11 | 300 | 0–1 | Up to 60 | 1064 | 2, 3 | Fiber oscillator, DPSS amplifier | Small, low cost | Future expansion into fiber femtosecond |
| EOLITE (ESI) | 50 | 50 | 0.1–3 | 60 | 1030 | 2, 3 | Rod-fiber | Compact | High average power, energy |
| LUMERA (COHERENT) | 10 | 250 | 0–2 | Up to 100 | 1064 | 2, 3 | Vanadate | Expertise in UV and picosecond lasers | Scaled to 150W |
| PHOTONICS INDUSTRIES | < 15 | 5 mJ | 0–2 | 50 | 1064 | 2, 3, 4 | DPSS | Small, robust | Higher power, lower cost |
| POWERLASE (EO TECHNICS) | < 10 | 200 | 0.1–1 | 200 | 1064 | No | Hybrid fiber, free space | 2mJ in a burst | 2 and 3 harmonics, 1mJ per pulse |
| ROFIN STARPICO | 12–15 | 100 | 0–20 | 15 | 1064 | 2 | Hybrid-fiber oscillator, bulk amplifier | Provides complete turnkey solutions, not just lasers | Higher power, lower cost, higher energies |
| SPECTRA-PHYSICS | < 1–13 | >50 | 0–1 | > 10 | 1040 | 2 | Yb DPSS | Highly dependable, high reliability, responsive global support, stable partner, customer focus | Products 'disruptive' in capability, performance, and cost |
| TALISKER (COHERENT) | 12 | 200 | 0–1 | 25 | 1064 | 2, 3 | Fiber oscillator, DPSS regenerative amplifier | Quality, performance, reliability, UV lifetime, worldwide service | "To address the needs of customers." |
| TIME-BANDWIDTH (JDSU) | 10 | 250 700 (Burst) | 0–8.2 | 50 | 1064 | 2, 3 | MOPA SESAM® | 15+ years' experience, world-class technology | Higher power, higher repetition rate, faster scanning |
| TRUMPF | 0.8–20 | Up to 500 | 0–1 | Up to 150 | 1064 | 2, 3 | Fiber disk, hybrid | Many technologies, huge expert team, worldwide support | "We do what customers require." |

PRF, etc., are given; also listed are some programmatic metrics under the columns Strengths and Future Plans. The specs listed in Tables 2.9 and 2.10 will, of course, improve over time; the concept illustrated by the trade tables is

**Table 2.10** Trade table for comparing femtosecond laser specs for micromachining applications. [Reprinted with permission from R. Schaeffer, PhotoMachining Inc. and *Industrial Laser Solutions* (2014). Copyright © PennWell Corp. 2014.]

| COMPANY | PULSE WIDTH (FS) | E/PULSE (MJ) | REP RATE (MHZ) | OUTPUT POWER (W) | L (NM) | HARMONICS (2, 3, 4, OR 5) | TECHNOLOGY BASE | STRENGTHS | FUTURE PLANS |
|---|---|---|---|---|---|---|---|---|---|
| AMPHOS | < 1ps | > 300 > 3000 | 0.1–40 | 100, 200, 400, 1000 | 1030 | 2 | Yb:YAG Innoslab | High power, flexibility in pulse parameters | More compact, higher power, lower cost |
| AMPLITUDE | 300 up to 10ps | 100 to 2 mJ | Up to 40 | > 30 | 1030 | 2, 3, 4 | Yb:YAG | Focus on USP only, fiber and solid-state | Higher power |
| CLARK-MXR | 10 up to 8ps | Up to 2.5mJ Up to 10mJ | 1–6KHz, < 25MHz | 2.5 20 | 775 1035 | Custom | Ti:SA fiber | 26 years' experience in USP | Confidential |
| EDGEWAVE | 700 | 100 | 0.1–20 | 200 | 1030 | 2 | Nd:YAG Innoslab | High average power, compact size, cost-effective | Power scaling to 1kW, energy scaling |
| IMRA | 350–2 ps | Up to 50 | 0.1–5 | Up to 20 | 1041–1045 | 2, 3 | Fiber | Solid engineering, field-proven experience in fiber femtosecond products | Best fiber-based USP laser products, full solutions for industrial laser processing |
| JENOPTIK | 350–800 | Up to 50 | 0–0.5 | Up to 10 | 1025 | 2 | DPSS disk | Industrial femtosecond since 2006, worldwide service and application support | Grow USP portfolio |
| KMLABS | < 200 | Up to 10mJ | Up to 1 | Up to 10 | 1030–1070 | 2, 3 | Ti:SA Yb:YAG | Understand short pulses, clean pulses, high performance | Higher power, lower cost |
| LIGHT CONVERSION | < 200 up to 10ps | 200–2000 | Up to 1 | Up to 15 | 1028 | 2, 3, 4, 5 | DPSS oscillator, diode-pumped regenerative amplifer | Robust | Higher-power, smaller-footprint harmonics |
| RAYDIANCE | 400–800 | Up to 100 | Up to 1 | 20 | 1553 | No | Monolithic fiber | Robust, industrial, complete manufacturing solutions | Higher power, lower cost, 1030nm wavelength, harmonics |
| ROFIN STARFEMTO FX | 300 up to 10ps | 200 | Up to 1 | 10 | 1552 | 2, 3 | Complete bulk-based system | Provides complete turnkey solutions, not just lasers | Higher power, lower cost, higher energies |
| SPECTRA-PHYSICS | 30 (Ti:SA) 200–400 (Yb) | nJ – 12mJ | 1KHz–8MHz | Various up to 50 | 680–1300 | 2, 3, 4 | DPSS, Ti:sapphire, fiber, etc. | Innovation, dependability | Products "disruptive" in performance—power, pulse width, wavelengths |
| TRUMPF | 800 | Up to 200 | 0–0.8 | Up to 80 | 1030 | - | Fiber disk, hybrid | Many technologies, huge expert team, worldwide support | "We do what customers require." |

thus that of a common systems-engineering tool, not an up-to-date listing of the current product specs from different vendors.

In interpreting tables such as these—as well as spec sheets from vendors—it is critical to keep in mind that "...not all specifications may be obtained simultaneously."[42] For example, when a range of pulse energies and PRFs is listed, we have already seen that the higher PRF may have a lower pulse energy, so it should not to be expected that the high energy will be obtained with the high PRF. Similarly, the importance of operating conditions has been pointed out by another laser vendor:[43] "...specifications may include the laser's output power, beam pointing and spatial beam profile under different operational conditions such as different pulse repetition rates or different trigger patterns. Measuring these second order characteristics is complex and requires great care. The performance requirements depend critically on the specific application and how the laser is used." A biomedical laboratory microscope, for example, is just as much of a laser system as a fielded "box" for 24-7 manufacturing, but the difference in operational conditions can dramatically affect the process of laser selection.

Also influencing laser selection are the other hardware components, i.e., the optical, beam scanning, and detector subsystems. Before proceeding to these topics, we first take a deeper look at beam propagation and quality in Chapter 3.

## 2.4 Problems

**2.1** Does the laser wavelength increase or decrease as the cavity length is changed (either thermally or with a piezoelectric stretcher)? By how much?

**2.2** What is the slope efficiency of a current-driven laser whose output power is given by Eq. (2.2)?

**2.3** In Fig. 2.7, what is the peak power in comparison with the average power if the rectangular pulse width $\Delta t_p$ equals the pulse period $T_p$? What is the duty cycle in this case?

**2.4** Using the data from Fig. 2.9, plot the average power versus PRF. Is there an operating point at which the average power is a maximum?

**2.5** A thulium-doped fiber laser emitting at a wavelength $\lambda = 2$ μm has a peak power of 200 MW, a pulse energy of 12 μJ, and an average power of 24 W. What is the photon energy $E_p$, the number of photons in a pulse, the PRF, and the rectangular pulse width $\Delta t_p$?

**2.6** An eye-safe erbium-doped fiber laser used for laser radar has a peak power of 4 kW, a 50-kHz repetition rate, and a 10-nsec pulse duration. What is the average power? If the electrical power required to run the laser is 1 W, what is the wall-plug efficiency? Is this reasonable?

**2.7** How does the laser frequency $\nu$ change when the laser's refractive index changes? How does it change when both the length and refractive index change?

**2.8** Show that a cavity length change $\Delta L = \lambda/2n$ shifts the laser frequency by one mode spacing, or $\Delta \nu_L = c/2nL$.

**2.9** A Yb:YAG disk laser has a gain bandwidth $\Delta\lambda_g = 9$ nm at $\lambda = 1030$ nm. Does this allow the generation of ultrashort pulses? If so, how short?

**2.10** For a given pump power in Fig. 2.31, does the average power of the laser follow the trend given by Eq. (2.6)?

**2.11** Which can create a higher peak power: a pulsed disk laser or an ultrafast fiber laser?

**2.12** A laser systems engineer is selecting a HeNe laser for use in an interferometer and needs a laser with a longer coherence length. Is it better to select the HeNe with the longer or shorter cavity length $L$?

**2.13** An excimer laser has an output beam that is 6 mm × 3 mm in size; the beam divergence is 1 mrad × 2 mrad. Is the spatial coherence across this beam diffraction limited?

**2.14** Show that for a 50%-efficient diode laser with $P = 1$ W and cooled with a 5%-efficient TEC, the diode-plus-TEC system efficiency $\eta_{sys} = 4.5\%$.

**2.15** What are the trades in selecting an excimer laser emitting at $\lambda = 248$ nm versus an Ar-ion laser emitting at $\lambda =$ to 257.2 nm? What about the comparison of the Ar-ion with the FHG of a fiber laser?

## Notes and References

1. T. Eddershaw, "High power systems shown at Laser Munich," *Laser Systems Europe* **28**, p. 8, Autumn (2015).

2. See, e.g., H. Helvajian, A. Pique, M. Wegener, and B. Gu, Editors, *Laser 3D Manufacturing II, Proc. SPIE* **9353** (2015) [doi: 10.1117/12.2193206].

3. J. König and T. Bauer, "Fundamentals and industrial applications of ultrashort pulsed lasers at Bosch," *Proc. SPIE* **7925**, 792510 (2011) [doi: 10.1117/12.878593].

4. K. J. Kasunic, *Optomechanical Systems Engineering*, John Wiley & Sons, Hoboken, New Jersey (2015).

5. H. J. Onisto, R. L. Cavasso-Filho, A. Scalabrin, D. Pereira, and F. C. Cruz, "Frequency doubled and stabilized all-solid-state Ti:sapphire lasers," *Optical Engineering* **41**(5), 1122–1127 (2002) [doi: 10.1117/1.1466850].

6. The wavelength λ is shorter because the speed of light in the high-index material is slower by a factor of *n*, and the oscillation frequency ν is the same. Quantitatively, both the numerator and denominator in Eq. (1.1) must be smaller by the same factor to maintain the same frequency. In addition, the index will be dispersive; i.e., it will vary somewhat with wavelength.
7. R. Paschotta, *Field Guide to Lasers*, SPIE Press, Bellingham, Washington (2008) [doi: 10.1117/3.767474].
8. B. Saleh and M. Teich, *Fundamentals of Photonics*, Second Edition, John Wiley & Sons (2007).
9. Because the pulse energy usually starts from zero, this equation is often written as $P_{\text{peak}} = Q_p/\Delta t_p$ for rectangular pulses.
10. S. Cundiff, "Autocorrelation," Univ. of Colorado Physics 7660 Course Notes, http://jila.colorado.edu/cundiff/courses/phys7660.
11. E. Garmire, "Nonlinear optics in daily life," *Optics Express* **21**(25), 30532–30544 (2013).
12. R. Paschotta, *Field Guide to Laser Pulse Generation*, SPIE Press, Bellingham, Washington (2008) [doi: 10.1117/3.800629].
13. P. Janssens and K. Malfait, "Future prospects of high-end laser projectors," *Proc. SPIE* **7232**, 72320Y (2009) [doi: 10.1117/12.808106].
14. K. J. Kasunic, *Optical Systems Engineering*, McGraw-Hill, New York (2011).
15. D. Basting, K. Pippert, and U. Stamm, "History and future prospects of excimer laser technology," *RIKEN Review*, No. 43, pp. 14–22 (2002).
16. Daylight Solutions, "Aries High-Power Lasers," data sheet, www.daylightsolutions.com.
17. JDSU, "Continuous Wave (CW) Single-Frequency IR Laser – NPRO 125/125 Series," data sheet, www.jdsu.com.
18. G. P. Agrawal, *Fiber-Optic Communication Systems*, Second Edition, John Wiley & Sons, Hoboken, New Jersey (1997).
19. P. C. D. Hobbs, *Building Electro-Optical Systems*, Second Edition, John Wiley & Sons, Hoboken, New Jersey (2009).
20. The ring geometry removes the possibility of spatial hole burning, as a traveling wave propagates around the cavity and does not allow a resonant standing wave to develop.
21. Thorlabs, "HRS015 Stabilized Red HeNe Laser User Guide," www.thorlabs.com. This laser also has a CW power stability of ±0.1% over a

1 minute period or ±0.3% over 8 hours if the environmental temperature is controlled per the manufacturer's specs.

22. E. D. Black, "An introduction to Pound–Drever–Hall laser frequency stabilization," *American Journal of Physics* **69**(1), 79–87 (2001).
23. A. E. Siegman, *Lasers*, University Science Books, Sausalito, California, pp. 767–769 (1986).
24. An exception is that wavelength-conversion crystals are often temperature tuned, requiring a slight heating of the crystal in an oven. For more details, see Ref. 31.
25. R. Scheps, *Introduction to Laser Diode-Pumped Solid State Lasers*, SPIE Press, Bellingham, Washington (2002).
26. C. Weimer, R. Schwiesow, and M. LaPole, "CALIPSO: lidar and wide-field camera performance," *Proc. SPIE* **5542**, 74–85 (2004) [doi: 10.1117/12.561613].
27. P. Vasil'ev, *Ultrafast Diode Lasers: Fundamentals and Applications*, Artech House, Norwood, Massachusetts (1995).
28. T. Y. Fan, "Heat generation in Nd:YAG and Yb:YAG," *IEEE Journal of Quantum Electronics* **29**(6), 1457–1459 (1993).
29. N. W. Sawruk, P. M. Burns, R. E. Edwards, T. Wysocki, A. Van Tuijl, V. Litvinovitch, E. Sullivan, and F. E. Hovis, "ICESat-2 laser technology readiness level evolution," *Proc. SPIE* **9342**, 93420L (2015) [doi: 10.1117/12.2080531].
30. N. Zafrani, Z. Sacks, S. Greenstein, I. Peer, E. Tal, E. Luria, G. Ravnitzki, D. David, A. Zajdman, and N. Izhaky, "Forty years of lasers at ELOP—Elbit Systems," *Optical Engineering* **49**(9), 091004 (2010) [doi: 10.1117/1.3486204].
31. W. Koechner, *Solid-State Laser Engineering*, Sixth Edition, Springer-Verlag, Berlin (2008).
32. D. H. Sutter, J. Kleinbauer, D. Bauer, M. Wolf, C. Tan, R. Gebs, A. Budnicki, P. Wagenblast, and S. Weiler, "Ultrafast disk lasers and amplifiers," *Proc. SPIE* **8235**, 82350X (2012) [doi: 10.1117/12.906905].
33. V. Kuhn, T. Gottwald, C. Stolzenburg, S.-S. Schad, A. Killi, and T. Ryba, "Latest advances in high brightness disk lasers," *Proc. SPIE* **9342**, 93420Y (2015) [doi: 10.1117/12.2079876].
34. TRUMPF Laser GmbH, "TruDisk" data sheet, www.trumpf-laser.com. The conversion of beam quality in units of $M^2$ to units of mm-mrad is reviewed in Chapter 3.

35. V. Gapontsev, A. Avdokhin, P. Kadwani, I. Samartsev, N. Platonov, and R. Yagodkin, "SM green fiber laser operating in CW and QCW regimes and producing over 550 W of average output power," *Proc. SPIE* **8964**, 896407 (2014) [doi: 10.1117/12.2058733].

36. I. Pastirk, A. Sell, R. Herda, A. Brodschelm, and A. Zach, "Ultrafast fiber lasers: practical applications," *Proc. SPIE* **9467**, 946728 (2015) [doi: 10.1117/12.2176347].

37. S. W. Hell, "Nanoscopy with focused light," *Proc. SPIE* **8882**, 888203 (2013) [doi: 10.1117/12.2032261].

38. Data for the first femtosecond entry in this table are for the IMRA America "DE0210" laser; for the second femtosecond entry the Amplitude Systèmes "Tangerine" laser; and for the third femtosecond entry the PolarOnyx "Uranus mJ" laser.

39. G. P. Agrawal, *Nonlinear Fiber Optics*, Fifth Edition, Academic Press, San Diego (2013).

40. In an unusual twist of technology development, the next generation of lithography sources will not themselves be lasers, but will instead rely on pulsed $CO_2$ lasers to create photons with a wavelength of only 13.5 nm from $CO_2$-evaporated tin.

41. J. Hecht, *The Laser Guidebook*, Second Edition, McGraw-Hill, New York (1992).

42. LightMachinery Inc., "Impact-4000," spec sheet, www.lightmachinery.com.

43. W. Wiechmann, "Diode-pumped Q-switched 355-nm lasers," *Laser Technik Journal* **2**(3), 35–37 (2005).

# Chapter 3
# Beam Propagation

While lasers have a number of "wow!" factors that make them popular in the press, perhaps the most unusual—and least understood—property is that of Gaussian beam propagation. While the mathematics is straightforward, it is difficult to physically explain why, for example, a beam waist placed at the front focal length of a lens images to...the back focal length of the lens!

This counter-intuitive result is not obvious only because our intuition is usually developed using conventional objects, where an incoherent source placed at the front focal length of a lens images to infinity, producing collimated beams. In this chapter, we will take a look at the unique properties of Gaussian beams—some of which can be traced back to the wavefront curvature incident on the lens—but we first need to understand the general concepts of Gaussian beam propagation (Section 3.1) and their real-world imperfections (Section 3.2).

## 3.1 Gaussian Beams

There are many different types of laser beams: Gaussian, Hermite–Gaussian, Laguerre–Gaussian, super-Gaussian, Bessel, Airy, vortex, etc. The most fundamental is the Gaussian, which is an ideal paraxial beam with a Gaussian irradiance distribution $E(r,z)$ whose size $w(z)$ in Fig. 3.1 depends on the propagation distance $z$ from the laser waist at $z = 0$:[1]

$$E(r,z) = E_o(z)e^{-2r^2/w^2(z)} \qquad [\mathrm{W/m^2}] \tag{3.1}$$

where $r$ is the radial coordinate, and $E_o(z)$ is the peak (on-axis) irradiance in units of $\mathrm{W/m^2}$.

Figure 3.1 shows that as the beam propagates away from the waist, the distribution gets wider, and thus the peak irradiance gets smaller. The curvature $C(z)$ of the wavefronts also changes in a non-obvious way, from zero curvature (planar wavefronts) at the waist, to zero curvature at infinity, and a maximum curvature in between at a distance known as the Rayleigh range $z_R = \pi w_o^2/\lambda$ [where the radius of curvature $R(z) = 2z_R$]. For distances

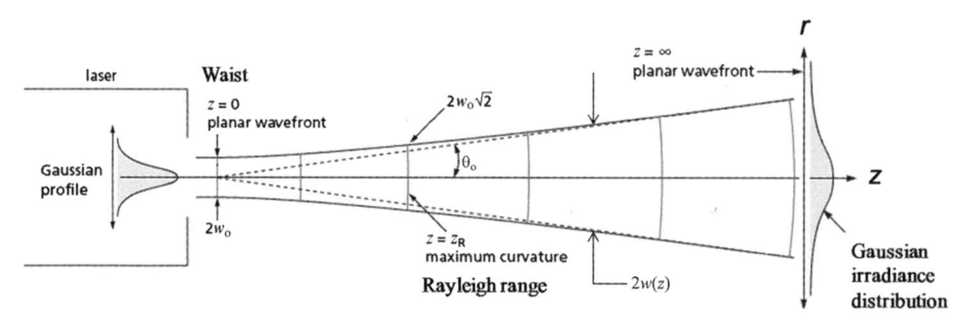


**Figure 3.1** Propagation of a Gaussian beam includes a beam waist of diameter $2w_o$ at $z = 0$, a Rayleigh range $z_R$, and a far-field distance $z \geq 5z_R$. (Credit: Adapted from CVI Laser, LLC.)

$z \geq 5z_R$, the far-field half-divergence angle $\theta_o = \lambda/\pi w_o$, at which point the beam size $w(z) \approx \theta_o z$ (Fig. 3.2); physically, the ratio $\lambda/w_o$ indicates that the beam divergence is governed by wavefront diffraction, and not geometrical optics.

The equations describing the beam size $w(z)$ and the wavefront radius of curvature $R(z) = 1/C(z)$ are given by Eq. (3.2) and Eq. (3.3), respectively:[1]

$$w(z) = w_o\left[1 + \left(\frac{\lambda z}{\pi w_o^2}\right)^2\right]^{1/2} \qquad [\text{mm}] \tag{3.2}$$

$$R(z) = z\left[1 + \left(\frac{\pi w_o^2}{\lambda z}\right)^2\right] \qquad [\text{mm}] \tag{3.3}$$

where $R(z)$ shows two competing dependencies on the propagation distance $z$—that proportional to $z$, and that inversely proportional. The sum of these

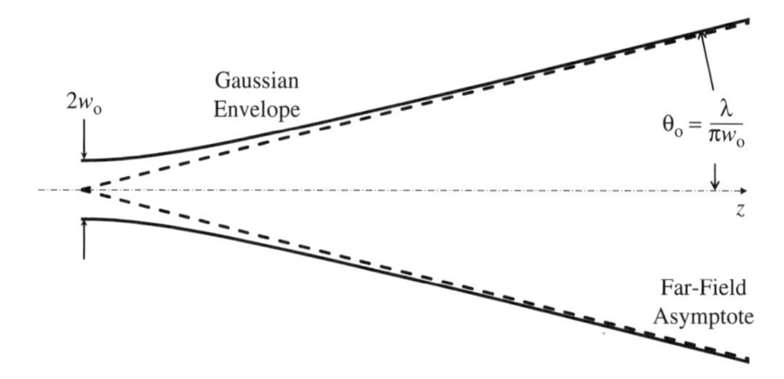


**Figure 3.2** The far-field half-divergence angle $\theta_o$ of a Gaussian beam depends on the wavelength $\lambda$ and the waist size $w_o$, such that a smaller waist diverges at a larger angle.

two terms illustrates mathematically why a Gaussian beam has planar wavefronts at both the waist and in the far field [that is, $R(z) = \infty$ at $z = 0$ and at $z = \infty$], and a minimum radius of curvature in between.

The waist—defined as the smallest beam radius created by the laser with a planar wavefront—has a size $w_o$ and location determined by the laser cavity design (Fig. 3.3). While we do not go into the specifics of laser design in this book—many other references are available for these details[1]—the location of the waist is often (though not always) specified near the output mirror. In addition, the beam diameter specified by laser manufacturers is often (though not always) given at the waist. In general, the beam diameter $D_b(z) = 2w(z)$, and the waist diameter $D_o = 2w_o$; given that a Gaussian profile extends out to infinity in the radial direction, however, how do we define the waist size $w_o$ or beam diameter $D_b(z)$?

As illustrated in Fig. 3.4, there are a number of options for defining the diameter $D_b(z)$ of a Gaussian beam:

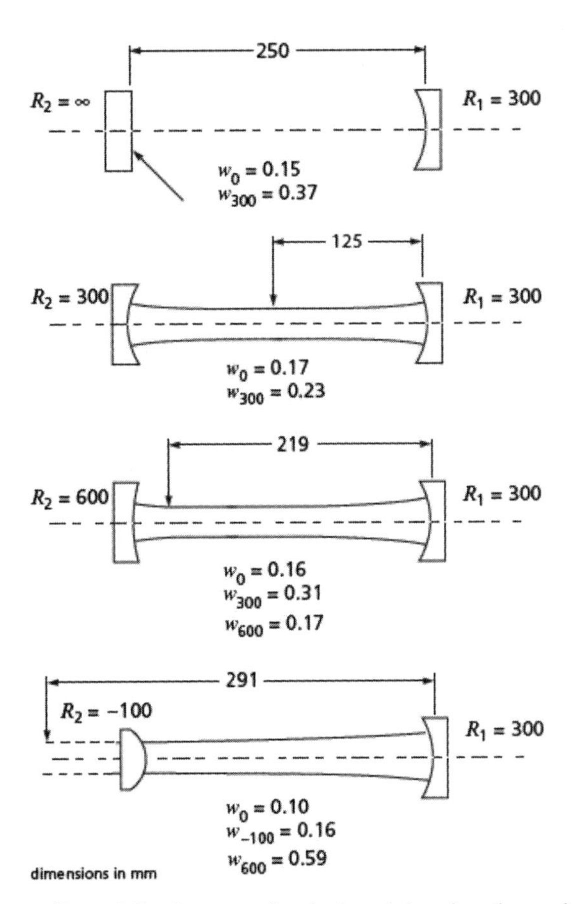


**Figure 3.3** The specifics of the laser cavity design determine the waist size $w_o$ and its location with respect to the laser output mirror. (Credit: CVI Laser, LLC.)

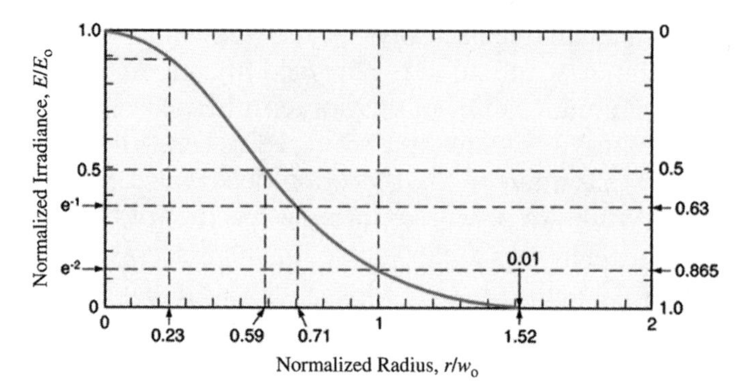


**Figure 3.4** The Gaussian beam waist $w_o$ can be defined based on the 50% point, the 1/e point, the 1/e$^2$ point, etc., of the peak irradiance. (Reprinted with permission from Newport Corp., all rights reserved.)

- The 50% point from the maximum irradiance for a Gaussian (FWHM),
- The 1/e$^2$ point (13.5%) from the maximum irradiance for a Gaussian, or
- The "D86" diameter, encircling 86% of the beam energy.

The 1/e$^2$ radius is commonly used for the waist size $w_o$ and beam diameter of a Gaussian or near-Gaussian profile, and is often used for first-order propagation and focusing as well.[2]

For non-Gaussian beams with arbitrary profiles such as a hyper-Gaussian (see Section 4.4), a more general beam-width definition is based on the variance $\sigma_o^2$ (or second-moment) method, which weights the irradiance profile quadratically with radius (per ISO Standard 11146), and can be converted to a waist size. It can be shown, for example, that the 1/e$^2$ waist size $w_o = 2\sigma_o$ for an ideal $TEM_{00}$ Gaussian beam, while a non-diffraction-limited beam that diffracts energy into a surrounding "pedestal" will have a waist $W_o \equiv 2\sigma_o > w_o$—see Ref. 1 and Sections 3.2 and 4.2.4.

In addition to waist size and wavefront curvature, Gaussian beams also have a property known as the Rayleigh range $z_R$, which depends on the beam area in comparison with the wavelength:[1]

$$z_R = \frac{\pi w_o^2}{\lambda} \quad \text{[mm]} \tag{3.4}$$

Not surprisingly, the Rayleigh range has some unique features that make it an interesting place:

- As shown in Fig. 3.1, the 1/e$^2$ beam diameter is 1.4× larger than the waist diameter (i.e., $D_{1/e^2} \equiv 2w = 2^{1/2} \times 2w_0$) at the Rayleigh range.
- The Rayleigh range is where the wavefront has the most curvature. The wavefront is planar (has zero curvature) at the waist where the

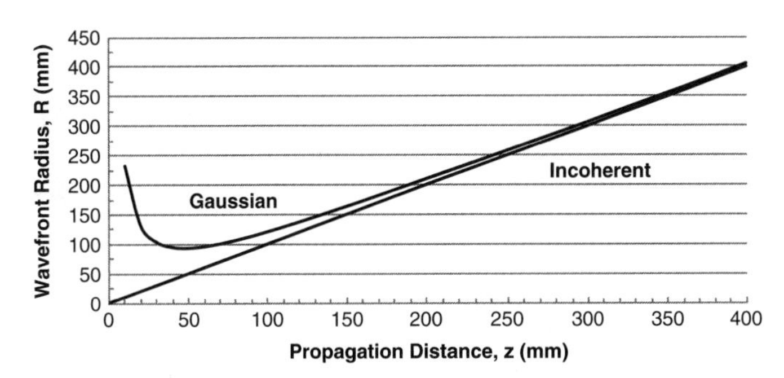


**Figure 3.5** Comparison of the wavefront radius of curvature $R(z)$ emitted by each point of an incoherent source [for which $R(z) = z$] and Gaussian beams [with $R(z)$ given by Eq. (3.3)].

wavefront started from, and it becomes zero again as the wavefront propagates out to infinity.

- Between the waist and the Rayleigh range, the curvature gets bigger until the wavefront reaches the Rayleigh range, where the curvature $C(z)$ reaches its largest value and $R(z) = 2z_R = 1/C(z)$ is smallest at $z_R$ (Fig. 3.5). Past the Rayleigh range, the curvature decreases as it approaches zero (planar) as $z \to \infty$.

As we will see in Sections 3.3 and 4.2.1, this interesting property of coherent wavefronts—unique to Gaussian beams—is the reason for the unusual imaging and focusing properties of these beams.

## 3.2 Beam Quality

Real-world imperfections—unavoidable consequences of entropy and engineering tolerances—result in beams propagating differently from the ideal Gaussian beam propagation described in Section 3.1. A "Gaussian" irradiance distribution, for example, may actually be an incoherent superposition of non-Gaussian beams with the correct weighting to give a near-Gaussian irradiance profile, and phase differences between the incoherent beams guarantee that the beams propagate differently from a pure Gaussian with the same irradiance profile. The purpose of this section is to introduce the concept of beam quality as a way of quantifying the propagation of these non-ideal beams.

Examples of non-ideal beams are illustrated in Fig. 3.6, where phase errors across a wavefront of sufficient magnitude result in what are known as Hermite–Gaussian transverse electromagnetic ($TEM_{pq}$) modes (or spatial profiles) for rectangular geometries. A diffraction-limited $TEM_{00}$ beam—i.e., one with no phase variations across the wavefront—is the "gold standard" of beam quality and is described by the irradiance distribution given by Eq. (3.1) and a beam quality (or beam propagation factor) $M^2 = 1$.

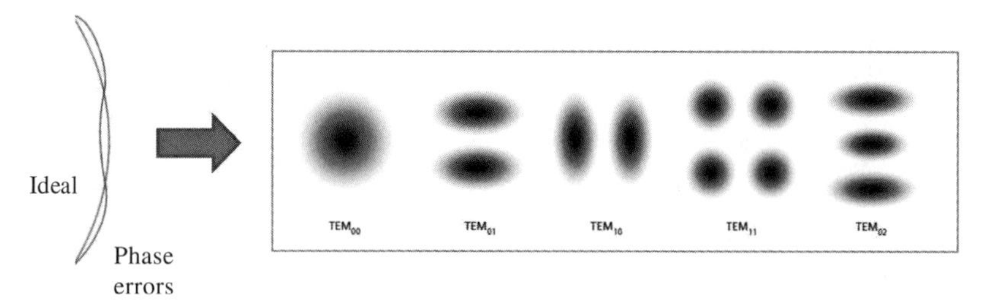


**Figure 3.6** A non-ideal beam with phase errors across the wavefront may result in non-$TEM_{00}$ mode profiles. (Adapted from CVI Laser, LLC.)

Wavefront errors (WFEs) across the beam reduce the beam quality, creating a $TEM_{pq}$ beam that is not diffraction limited and, as illustrated in Fig. 3.7, cause the beam to either:

- Diverge more than a diffraction-limited ($TEM_{00}$) beam by a factor $M^2 > 1$, or
- Focus to a spot size $B$ that is larger than a diffraction-limited beam by a factor of $M^2 > 1$.

These consequences of a non-ideal beam depend on how the laser is being used. Specifically, if the laser is used to illuminate the far field with the same waist $w_o$ [Fig. 3.8(a)], then the far-field divergence angle of the non-diffraction-limited beam is larger by $M^2$ (Fig. 3.7). If, on the other hand, the beam is being focused with the same convergence angle $\theta_o$ [Fig. 3.8(b)], then the focused spot is larger by $M^2$ but diverges in the far field at the same angle $\theta_o$ as the diffraction-limited beam.

Phase errors across the beam are the dominant cause of the difference between the ideal irradiance and the actual irradiance. For example, a $TEM_{00}$

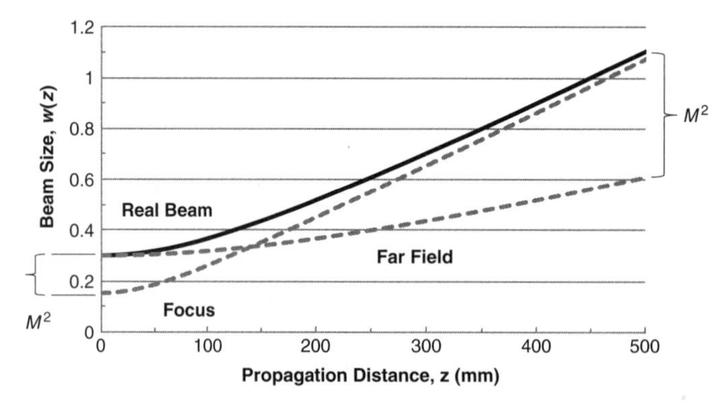


**Figure 3.7** Depending on the reference beam, a non-ideal ("real") beam will either diverge faster or focus to a spot that is larger than a diffraction-limited ($TEM_{00}$) beam by a factor $M^2 > 1$.

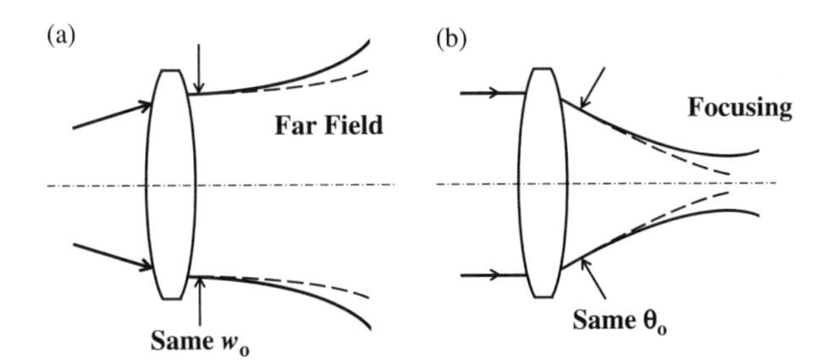


**Figure 3.8** (a) With the same spot size $w_o$ incident on the lens, the far-field divergence angle increases by $M^2$. (b) With the same far-field angle $\theta_o$ propagating away from the waist, the focused spot size is larger than a $TEM_{00}$ diffraction-limited beam by $M^2$.

beam has no phase variations across it in comparison with an ideal parabolic profile (Fig. 3.6); higher-order $TEM_{pq}$ ($p$, $q \neq 0$) spatial modes, on the other hand, have phase errors across the beam that may be large enough to cause the ideal Gaussian irradiance profile to split (as in Fig. 3.9).

In practice, many beams do not have the correct phase variation or profile for a $TEM_{pq}$ mode and can be modeled as aberrated Gaussians (see Section 4.2.4). In addition, beams can be a combination of $TEM_{pq}$ modes, and the phase errors of individual modes combine to produce a beam that is not a specific $TEM_{pq}$ profile. An example is the "donut" mode—a combination of $TEM_{01}$ and $TEM_{10}$ phase and irradiance profiles, giving a circular transverse irradiance with a "donut" hole in the center.

Sources of WFE are many and include the laser modes themselves, optical fabrication WFE, alignment WFE, thermal lensing in the optics, and so on. The $M^2$ beam-quality factor for the laser modes is illustrated in Fig. 3.10, where the rectangular Hermite–Gaussian profile can result in an $M^2$ value that is different in the $x$ and $y$ coordinates.[3]

For a pure $TEM_{pq}$ mode, the beam quality factors are given by[4]

$$M_x^2 = 2p + 1 \tag{3.5}$$

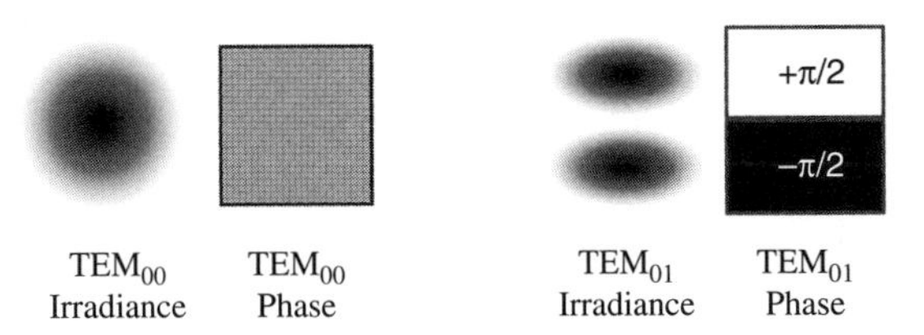


**Figure 3.9** Phase variations of $TEM_{pq}$ modes result in irradiance profiles that are quantified by the product of the ideal Gaussian field and a Hermite polynomial $H(x,y)$.[1] In practice, a superposition of transverse modes can be expected.

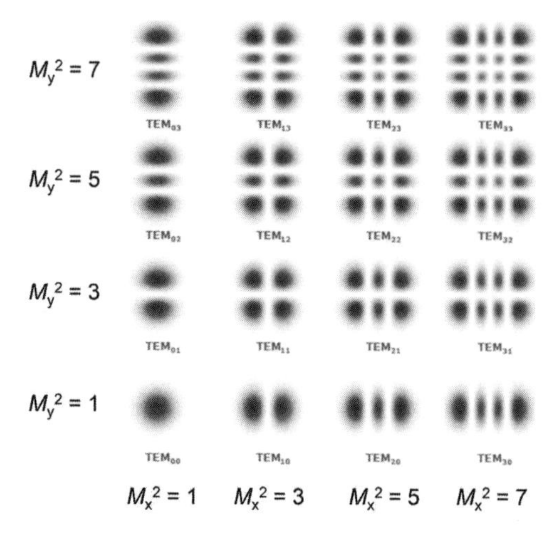


**Figure 3.10** Hermite–Gaussian modes exhibit a rectangular irradiance profile with a beam quality $M_x$ and $M_y$. [Adapted from R. Paschotta, *Field Guide to Lasers*, SPIE Press, Bellingham, Washington (2008)].

$$M_y^2 = 2q + 1 \tag{3.6}$$

and the overall beam quality is given by the product of the individual factors:

$$M^2 = M_x M_y \tag{3.7}$$

For example, the $TEM_{32}$ mode shown in Fig. 3.10 has $M_x = (7)^{1/2}$ and $M_y = (5)^{1/2}$, giving $M^2 = M_x M_y = (35)^{1/2} = 5.9$, a fairly large value that indicates a poor quality beam with a large beam divergence or focused spot size.

To quantify the divergence $\theta_o$ or focused spot size $B$ for an aberrated or higher-order-mode laser, the individual $M_x$ and $M_y$ components can be used, but they are often sufficiently similar in magnitude that the overall $M^2$ value is commonly used for first-order estimates:[5]

$$\theta_o = \frac{\lambda}{\pi w_o} M^2 \qquad [\text{rad}] \tag{3.8}$$

$$B \approx \frac{4}{\pi} \frac{\lambda f}{D_{1/e^2}} M^2 \qquad [\mu\text{m}] \tag{3.9}$$

where $f$ is the focal length of the focusing lens, $D_{1/e^2}$ is the collimated beam diameter incident on the lens, and the $4/\pi$ factor applies to an untruncated beam (see Section 4.2.2). To obtain the same spot size as a $TEM_{00}$ mode, a smaller $f$ or larger $D_{1/e^2}$ must therefore be used when $M^2 > 1$. Also note that the far-field angle $\theta_i$ of an incoherent source—with $\theta_i \approx s/f$ for a collimated beam—can be reduced to that of a diffraction-limited laser with waist $w_o$ for a source size $s \leq \lambda f/\pi w_o$.

The beam-quality factor can also be incorporated into the equations for the propagating beam size $w(z)$ and the wavefront radius of curvature $R(z)$:

$$w(z) = w_o \left[ 1 + \left( \frac{\lambda M^2 z}{\pi w_o^2} \right)^2 \right]^{1/2} \qquad \text{[mm]} \tag{3.10}$$

$$R(z) = z \left[ 1 + \left( \frac{\pi w_o^2}{\lambda M^2 z} \right)^2 \right] \qquad \text{[mm]} \tag{3.11}$$

where we can also define a modified Rayleigh range as[6]

$$z_R = \frac{\pi w_o^2}{\lambda M^2} \qquad \text{[mm]} \tag{3.12}$$

as long as we are careful to use the waist size $w_o$ of the real beam where $R(0)$ is infinite (planar). For example, if the far-field beam with $M^2 = 1$ and the real beam with $M^2 > 1$ are compared in Fig. 3.7 at $z = 0$ where they have the same waist $w_o = 0.3$ mm, then the divergence is larger [Eq. (3.8)] and the Rayleigh range is smaller [Eq. (3.12)] for $M^2 > 1$. If, on the other hand, we compare the focused beams in Fig. 3.7 at $z = 0$ where the waist $w_o$ is larger by $M^2$, then the far-field divergence angle of both beams is the same [as seen in Eq. (3.8) where the $M^2$ terms cancel, and graphically in Fig. 3.7 for $z \gg 0$], and the Rayleigh range of the non-ideal beam *increases* by $M^2$ [since the terms in Eq. (3.12) have $\pi w_o^2 \sim (M^2)^2$ in the numerator and $M^2$ in the denominator].

In addition to the $M^2$ metric for beam quality, a different metric known as the beam-parameter product (BPP) is often used for multimode semiconductor or fiber lasers with large $M^2$:

$$BPP = w_o \theta_o \approx \frac{\lambda}{\pi} M^2 \qquad \text{[mm-mrad]} \tag{3.13}$$

which can be obtained from Eq. (3.8) and where the second-moment waist size $w_o$ and far-field angle $\theta_o$ are combined to characterize the beam quality.[7] Units are millimeters for the waist and milliradians for the angle, for which the wavelength $\lambda$ must then be measured in microns. For example, for $\lambda = 1$ μm and $M^2 = 1$, we obtain $BPP = \lambda/\pi = 0.32$ mm-mrad for the best possible beam quality; typical numbers for high-power commercial products are 3–10 mm-mrad.

The use of either $M^2$ or the BPP has many details and subtleties that are beyond the scope of this book—see Ref. 8 for a highly detailed discussion of the many aspects of measuring beam quality. As we have seen for the first-order use of $M^2$ for either far-field propagation or focusing applications—and as Siegman once observed—"The $M^2$ value...although a useful parameter for characterizing a laser beam, is best viewed as providing only a 'propagation factor' for a laser beam, rather than a unique or universal measure of beam quality, *since the 'quality' of a laser beam depends on the application for which it was intended.*"[9]

---

**Example 3.1**

What is the $M^2$ of the laser used to obtain the curves in Fig. 3.7? If we are fortunate enough to have the data shown in the figure, we can estimate the beam quality from the ratio of waist sizes at $z = 0$ for the real and ideal beams at focus. This gives us $M^2 = w_{or}/w_{oi} = 0.3$ mm/0.15 mm $= 2$. Alternatively, we can also compare the ideal and real beams at $z = 500$ mm, giving $M^2 = w_{or}/w_{oi} = 1.1$ mm/0.6 mm $= 1.83$, with the discrepancy from the focus data indicating that this measurement might not be in the far field. Estimating the Rayleigh range, we see that $z_R = \pi w_o^2/\lambda = \pi(0.3 \text{ mm})^2/0.001 \text{ mm} = 283$ mm for $\lambda = 1$ μm; the distance $z = 500$ mm is thus much less than the rule-of-thumb estimate that defines the far field, namely, $z \geq 5z_R$.

In practice, we do not have a real and an ideal beam to compare, and the $M^2$ must be extracted from the real beam by itself. This is done using a series of measurements of the second-moment (ISO-11146 D4σ) beam size $\sigma_o$ along the propagation direction out to the far field, and fitting to Siegman's quadratic propagation equation.[6] The net result of this measurement—applicable to multimode beams, flat tops, etc., with small error in the conversion of second-moment beam size to $1/e^2$ beam size $w_o \approx 2\sigma_o$ for aberrated Gaussians with $M^2 \leq 2$ or so (see Section 4.2.4)—is that for either the far-field diffraction angle [Fig. 3.8(a)] or focused spot size [Fig. 3.8(b)], "...the $M^2$ value can serve as a rigorous definition of the times-diffraction-limited (TDL) value for an arbitrary real beam compared to a $TEM_{00}$ Gaussian beam."[6]

---

## 3.3 Beam Imaging

As we have seen, a Gaussian, fiber, or semiconductor-laser beam can be focused with a lens or mirror to a spot whose size depends on the beam quality. With the assumptions that: (1) a planar, single-transverse-mode ($M^2 = 1$) wavefront is incident on the lens; (2) the depth of focus (DOF) is $\ll f$ (focal length), and (3) the lens diameter $D \geq 2D_{1/e^2}$, Eq. (3.9) shows that the focused spot size $B = (4/\pi) \times \lambda f / D_{1/e^2}$. This is illustrated in Fig. 3.11, where for $f \ll \pi D_{1/e^2}^2 / 4\lambda$ there is also a planar wavefront at the focal length of the lens that acts as a new waist for beam propagation to the next lens or the far

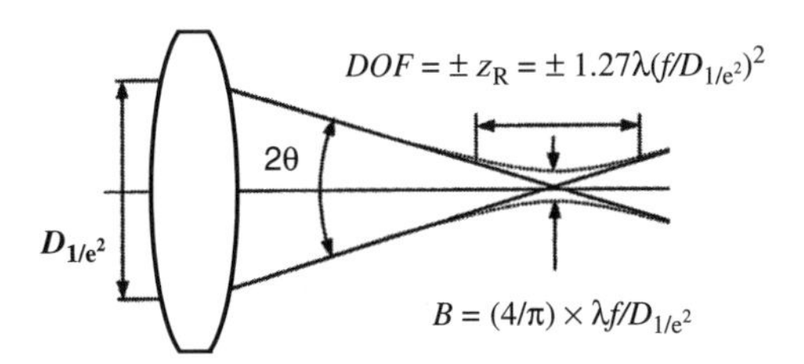


**Figure 3.11** An untruncated Gaussian beam incident on the lens from the left is focused to a spot with a $1/e^2$ blur diameter $B = 4\lambda f/\pi D_{1/e^2}$ and a Rayleigh range $z_R = \pi B^2/4\lambda$.

field.[10] The usual propagation equations for $w(z)$ and $R(z)$ thus apply based on the new beam size $B$.

The focused spot size is similar to the well-known $2.44\lambda \times f/D$ size for diffraction-limited imaging of a conventional point source,[11] with two important differences. The first is that pre-factor is now $4/\pi$, or about one-half the 2.44 pre-factor that applies to a uniform plane wave. The second is that the $4/\pi$ pre-factor applies only if the beam is not truncated; i.e., the lens diameter $D$ is sufficiently larger than the incident beam diameter $D_{1/e^2}$. If there is significant truncation, then the spot size will be bigger, a topic we look at in detail in Chapter 4.

The imaging properties of Gaussian beams are a bit unusual in comparison with those of incoherent sources, and as we will also see in more detail in Chapter 4, the focused spot for a laser may or may not be at the focal length of the lens. In addition to spatial coherence, laser beams are different from incoherent objects because the wavefront curvature $C(z) = 1/R(z)$ of a Gaussian beam varies in a unique way with propagation distance $z$ [see Fig. 3.5 and Eq. (3.3)]. The physical trends of Gaussian-beam imaging are straightforward to understand, however, if we look at the curvature of the wavefront incident on the lens.

Specifically, the equation describing incoherent imaging for a thin lens is given by[11]

$$\frac{1}{f} = \frac{1}{s_o} + \frac{1}{s_i} = C_o + C_i \qquad [1/\text{m}] \tag{3.14}$$

where the object distance $s_o$ determines the wavefront curvature $C_o = 1/s_o$ incident on the lens, and the image distance $s_i$ is determined by the wavefront curvature $C_i = 1/s_i$ exiting the lens. The degree to which the wavefront curvature is changed by the lens thus depends on the lens refractive power $\Phi_L \equiv 1/f$. A lens can therefore be viewed as a converter of wavefront curvature, and this is the case for incoherent objects, Gaussian beams, non-Gaussian beams, etc.

In contrast, the equation describing Gaussian-beam imaging for a thin lens is given by[12]

$$\frac{1}{f} = \frac{1}{z_1 + \frac{z_R^2}{z_1 - f}} + \frac{1}{z_2} \qquad [1/\text{m}] \tag{3.15}$$

where the first term on the RHS now depends on the distance $z_1$ of the object waist to the lens (as with incoherent objects), but also on the focal length and Rayleigh range. The dependence of image distance—i.e., the new waist location $z_2$ after propagating through the lens—on the object distance is plotted in Fig. 3.12 for an $M^2 = 1$ beam and a range of values for $z_R/f$. Note the critical importance of the laser's Rayleigh range: if $z_R = 0$, then Eq. (3.15) reduces to the incoherent imaging equation. Also note that once the wavefront curvature $C_o$ incident on the lens is known from Eq. (3.3), the physical interpretation of the lens as a wavefront converter allows us to use the RHS of Eq. (3.14) to find the wavefront curvature $C_i$ exiting the lens which, when combined with $z_2$ from Eq. (3.15), determines the image waist size [see Eq. (3.3) and Example 4.1].

As an example of the use of Eq. (3.15), a laser's waist is placed one focal length away from a focusing lens; where is the image for an $M^2 = 1$ ($TEM_{00}$) beam? The "object" is the waist at a distance $z_1 = f$ from the lens; the "image" is the waist at a distance $z_2$ from the lens. From the plot in Fig. 3.12, we obtain an image waist at $z_2 = f$ for an object waist at $z_1 = f$. So the focused spot in this example is at the focal length $f$ of the lens—a result that is quite a bit different from incoherent imaging ($z_R = 0$), where the image is at infinity. The physical significance of this unusual result—and its explicit dependence

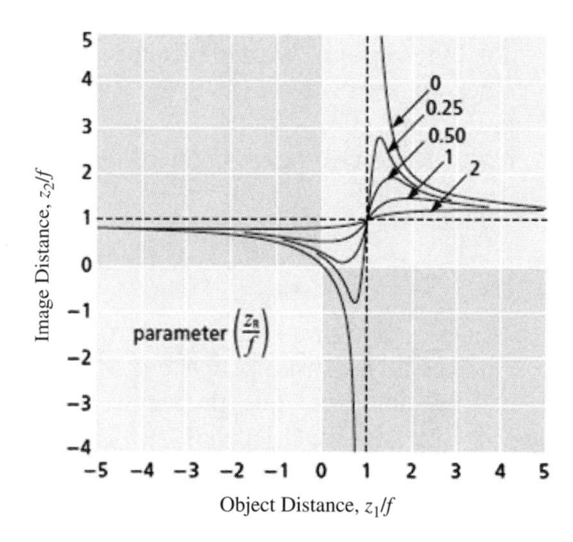


**Figure 3.12** The image distance for a Gaussian beam shows unusual properties in comparison with the incoherent imaging that occurs for the parameter $z_R/f = 0$. (Credit: CVI Laser, LLC.)

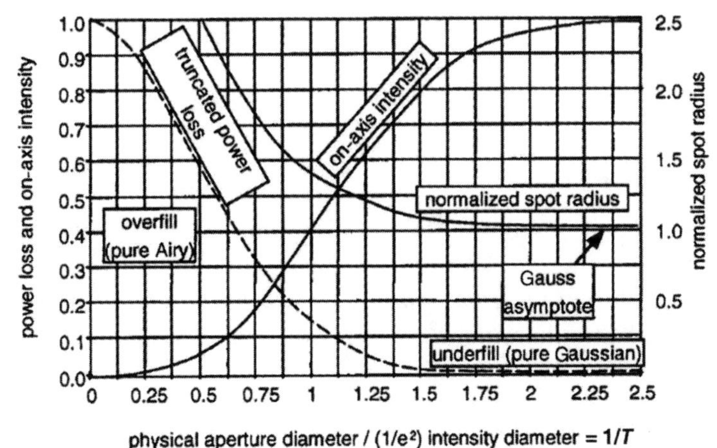


**Figure 3.13** Focused spot size, power loss, and on-axis irradiance ("intensity") depend on the truncation ratio $T = D_{1/e^2}/D$. (Credit: R. E. Fischer, "Practical Optical System Design," SPIE Short Course SC003.)

on incident wavefront curvature—will be explored in more detail in Chapter 4.

In addition to image location, Gaussian beam propagation has a number of additional differences compared to conventional imaging. For example, it is sometimes thought that the $1/e^2$ beam diameter is also an acceptable lens size (clear aperture diameter) for beam propagation and imaging. Figure 3.13, however, shows that using a $1/e^2$ lens diameter:

- Results in a spot size ≈ 40% larger than ideal ($1.83\lambda f/D_{1/e^2}$ versus $1.27\lambda f/D_{1/e^2}$),
- Blocks (truncates) ≈ 13.5% of the power in the beam (86.5% transmitted), and
- Reduces the on-axis irradiance by a factor of 2.5.

These consequences of beam truncation are not acceptable for many applications, and an aperture $D \geq 1.5 \times$ the $1/e^2$ diameter is often recommended. These topics will also be explored in more detail in Chapters 4 and 6.

## 3.4 Problems

**3.1** Is there an optimum waist size $w_o$ to obtain a given beam size $w(z)$ in the far field? That is, a smaller waist results in a larger beam size due to its diffraction-limited far-field angle (Fig. 3.2). A larger waist, on the other hand, expands at a smaller angle but propagates from a larger initial aperture. Is there an optimum waist that balances these two competing effects on far-field beam size? Does it depend on the far-field distance $z_{FF}$ that you assume? What about the wavelength?

**3.2** By what ratio does the Gaussian-beam wavefront radius of curvature $R(z)$ given by Eq. (3.3) differ from each point of an incoherent source? At what distance is the ratio the same to within 10%? Does your answer depend on the Rayleigh range $z_R$?

**3.3** Using Eq. (3.11), plot $R(z)$ versus $z$ for $M^2 = 1$ and $M^2 = 2$. Does the plot depend on what assumption you make as to application (i.e., far-field propagation or focusing)?

**3.4** Does the Rayleigh range at focus increase or decrease for a beam with $M^2 > 1$? Hint: What is the waist size $w_o$ in Eq. (3.12), and how does it relate to $M^2$ for a focused beam?

**3.5** Convert the $M^2$ data given in Table 2.4 into BPP values in units of mm-mrad.

**3.6** A semiconductor-laser manufacturer is measuring the far-field divergence angles of their new high-power diodes. It is found that, with the same waist size at the output facet, the far-field angle for their new laser is twice as large as their diffraction-limited legacy design. What is $M^2$ for the new laser?

**3.7** A laser manufacturer specifies the waist size $w_o = 1$ mm and the far-field half-divergence angle $\theta_o = 1$ mrad. The wavelength of the laser is 1.064 μm. What is the beam quality measured as an $M^2$ value?

**3.8** Given that $BPP = \lambda M^2/\pi$, does it logically follow that different lasers with the same BPP have the same $M^2$?

**3.9** A key difference between Gaussian beams and incoherent sources is that the waist does not necessarily image planar wavefronts at the same location as the focal length of the lens, as seen in the figure. What is the significance of the fact that the ideal lens focus $f$ and the beam-waist focus $f_w$ are not at the same axial location? Does the difference $\Delta f$ between the two foci depend on what the focal length is?

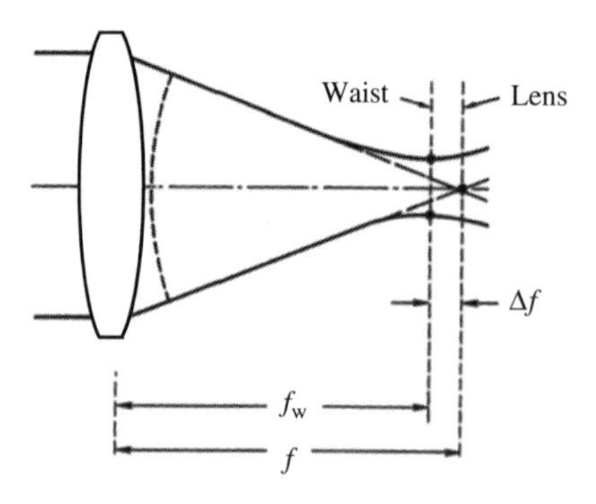


**3.10** In Section 3.3, it is stated that the focal length $f \gg DOF$ and $f \ll \pi D^2_{1/e^2}/4\lambda$ for the spot size to be given by $B = (4/\pi) \times \lambda f/D_{1/e^2}$. Why does the focal length need to be much greater than the DOF? And are these two restrictions on focal length consistent? Hint: see Note 5.

**3.11** Plot Eq. (3.15) for $M^2 = 1$ and for $M^2 = 2$; use $z_R/f = 0.25$ for both plots. Do both plots show the same image distance for $z_1 = f$? Are there any differences of importance?

**3.12** What Rayleigh range is needed to produce an image waist size $w_{02}$ equal to the object waist size $w_{01}$ at the focal length of the lens? Use $f = 100$ mm and $\lambda = 1$ μm. Hint: An algebraic solution is possible but not necessary.

## Notes and References

1. See, for example, A. E. Siegman, *Lasers*, University Science Books, Sausalito, California (1986) and A. E. Siegman, "How to (maybe) measure beam quality," *Diode-Pumped Solid-State Lasers: Applications and Issues*, OSA Annual Meeting (Oct. 1997).

2. The 1/e radius is often selected for the Gaussian electric field distribution, but the irradiance depends on the square of the field, so this is equivalent to using the $1/e^2$ radius for the irradiance distribution.

3. While Hermite–Gaussian $TEM_{pq}$ modes are the most common for free-space lasers—a result of asymmetric pumping, thermal distortions, or misalignments between cavity mirrors—circularly symmetric Laguerre–Gaussian modes are also possible; see Ref. 1 for more details.

4. W. H. Carter, "Spot size and divergence for Hermite–Gaussian beams of any order," *Applied Optics* **19**(4), 1027–1029 (1980).

5. Equation (3.9) can be derived by noting that the far-field divergence angle $\theta$ of the focused spot in Fig. 3.11 is determined from Eq. (3.8) as $2\theta = 2\lambda M^2/\pi w_f$. In addition, with a beam diameter $D_{1/e^2}$ on the lens located a focal length $f$ away, we also see that the convergence angle $\theta \approx D_{1/e^2}/2f$. Equating these two expressions and re-arranging, we find that $B \equiv 2w_f = 4\lambda f M^2/\pi D_{1/e^2}$.

6. See A. E. Siegman, "Defining, measuring and optimizing laser beam quality," *Proc. SPIE* **1868**, 2–12 (1993) and A. E. Siegman, "How to (maybe) measure beam quality", *Diode-Pumped Solid-State Lasers: Applications and Issues*, OSA Annual Meeting (Oct. 1997).

7. The BPP is usually measured using the physical size of the emitting aperture, but this is an approximation that is valid only when the semiconductor or fiber mode is "strongly guided" (i.e., tightly contained in the waveguide or fiber) and the second-moment waist size does not extend far beyond the aperture dimensions.

8. T. S. Ross, *Laser Beam Quality Metrics*, SPIE Press, Bellingham, Washington (2013) [doi: 10.1117/3.1000595].

9. A. E. Siegman, "Laser beams and resonators beyond the 1960s," *IEEE J. Selected Topics in Quantum Electronics* **6**(6), 1389–1399 (2000).

10. Through focus, the converging beam has a wavefront curvature opposite that of the diverging beam. Therefore, the curvature must "flip" at (or near) focus—and be zero at some point, where it acts as a waist.

11. K. J. Kasunic, *Optical Systems Engineering*, McGraw-Hill, New York, Chapter 2 (2011).

12. S. A. Self, "Focusing of spherical Gaussian beams," *Applied Optics* **22**(5), 658–661 (1983).

# Chapter 4
# Laser System Optics

It is surprising how easy it is to damage a lens or other optical component with a laser. A typical occurrence is during the alignment of lab optics, where the slightest tweak results in the sound of a cracked coating, broken glass, or worse. This is not due to any inherent weakness of laser system optics, but of the tight focus to which coherent beams can be imaged, resulting in unintended consequences when re-imaged back-reflections are focused to a high power density.

Laser system optics are also susceptible to—and will contribute to—system wavefront error. As we have seen in Chapter 3, one source of WFE in a laser system is the laser modes themselves, for which the beam-quality factor $M^2$ is used to estimate the focused spot size and far-field divergence angle. In this chapter, we will see that there are other sources as well: thermal lensing, optical fabrication WFE, aberration WFE, and so on.

In addition to damage and WFE, laser-grade optics—including windows, focusing lenses, beam expanders, mirrors, beamsplitters, polarizers, etc.—have some of the most challenging performance requirements:

- Material absorption – Extremely low to reduce heating and thermal lensing
- Surface figure – Minimal WFE to maintain good beam quality ($M^2$)
- Surface roughness – Minimal scattering (forward and back) to reduce background glare
- Surface quality – Low scratch-dig to prevent scattering or fracture

Table 4.1 summarizes how the requirements on laser-grade optics differ in cost and performance from those needed for less-demanding applications such as imaging.

The meaning of the terms in Table 4.1 will be reviewed throughout this chapter. They apply to laser-system components such as windows and filters (Section 4.1), focusing lenses (Section 4.2), beam expanders and collimators (Section 4.3), and homogenizers and beam shapers (Section 4.4). In addition, a number of other requirements on the optical components must be taken

**Table 4.1** Comparison of laser-grade performance specifications with commercial and precision-grade optics.

| Specification | Commercial | Precision | Laser Grade |
|---|---|---|---|
| Surface Power | 10 fringes | 5 fringes | 3 fringes |
| Surface Figure | λ/10 RMS | λ/40 RMS | λ/100 RMS |
| Surface Finish | 50 Å RMS | 20 Å RMS | 10 Å RMS |
| Surface Quality | 60–40 | 40–20 | 10–5 |
| Absorption | 2–5% | < 0.5% | < 0.1% |
| Cost | Low | Moderate | High |

into account, including materials selection, optical coatings, laser damage threshold, and polarization (Section 4.5).

## 4.1 Windows and Filters

It would seem that windows and filters—i.e., plane parallel plates—are the simplest of optical components used in laser systems. Yet their use can be surprisingly difficult due to back-reflections, which can cause interference fringes; material absorption, which can result in thermal lensing and distortion; surface roughness, which scatters light both forward and backward; and poor surface quality, which can reduce the laser damage threshold (LDT) and result in catastrophic failure of the window or its coating.

A typical laser window spec is shown in Fig. 4.1; the figure shows that a wedged window is common. Back-reflections and forward-reflections can interfere to create fringes if the laser's coherence length $d_c > 2nd$ for a window index $n$ and thickness $d$ (Fig. 4.2); in that case, the wedge forces the reflections off of the front and back surfaces in different directions, where they cannot interfere if the beams do not overlap. The wedge can also prevent back-surface

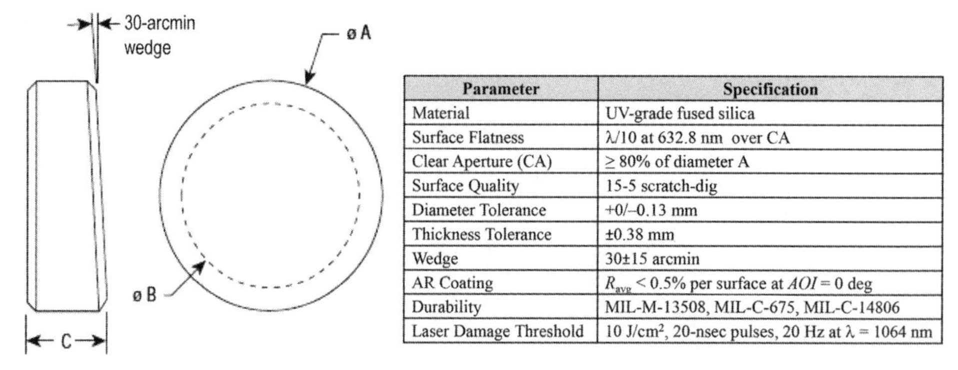


| Parameter | Specification |
|---|---|
| Material | UV-grade fused silica |
| Surface Flatness | λ/10 at 632.8 nm over CA |
| Clear Aperture (CA) | ≥ 80% of diameter A |
| Surface Quality | 15-5 scratch-dig |
| Diameter Tolerance | +0/–0.13 mm |
| Thickness Tolerance | ±0.38 mm |
| Wedge | 30±15 arcmin |
| AR Coating | $R_{avg} < 0.5\%$ per surface at $AOI = 0$ deg |
| Durability | MIL-M-13508, MIL-C-675, MIL-C-14806 |
| Laser Damage Threshold | 10 J/cm$^2$, 20-nsec pulses, 20 Hz at $\lambda = 1064$ nm |

**Figure 4.1** Typical laser-grade specs for a commercial window. (Reprinted with permission from Newport Corp., all rights reserved.)

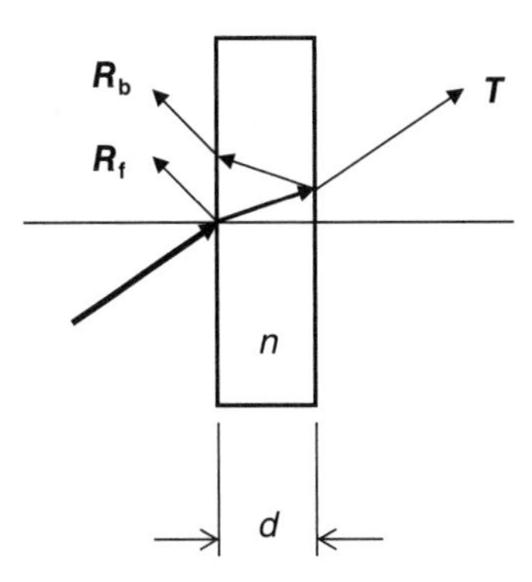


**Figure 4.2** The front and back surface reflections ($R_f$ and $R_b$) of a window or lens can coherently combine (interfere) to create fringes in an image.

reflections from propagating back towards the laser cavity as detrimental optical feedback. In addition to wedge, antireflection (AR) coatings are essential to reducing the magnitude of these effects (Section 4.5.3).

Material absorption will heat the window and cause changes in the refractive index $n(T)$ via the thermo-optic effect ($\mathrm{d}n/\mathrm{d}T$). That is, the refractive index depends on temperature $T$, such that $n(T) \approx n_o + (\mathrm{d}n/\mathrm{d}T)\Delta T$ over a limited temperature range $\Delta T$. For example, thermal lensing from the Gaussian irradiance distribution of the high-power pump shown in Fig. 4.3 creates a positive lens out of the window (higher index at the beam center), slightly focusing the IR beam and also introducing optical aberrations due to the non-uniform temperature and index profile.

Predicting the focus shift and induced aberrations for a Gaussian irradiance distribution is not straightforward, but to first order the focal shift for a radial thermal gradient created by a uniform ("flat-top") beam depends on $\mathrm{d}n/\mathrm{d}T$, the thermal conductivity $k$ of the window material, the absorbed power $Q$, and the area $A$ of the beam:[1]

$$\frac{1}{f_t} = \frac{\mathrm{d}n/\mathrm{d}T}{2k}\frac{Q}{A} \qquad [1/\mathrm{m}] \tag{4.1}$$

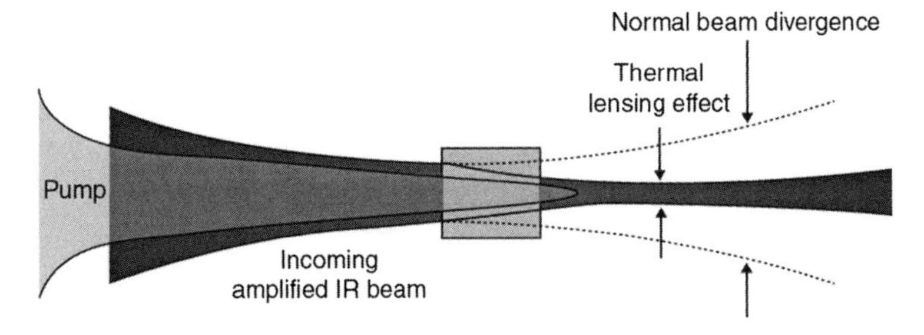


**Figure 4.3** Thermal lensing from non-uniform heating and temperature distributions in a laser window creates a positive lens, slightly focusing the beam. (Credit: Coherent, Inc.)

**Table 4.2** Comparison of thermal lensing of sapphire and fused silica, including material absorption. The incident power $P_{inc} = 1$ W, and the uniform beam diameter $D_b = 1$ mm.

| Parameter | Sapphire | Fused Silica | Units |
|---|---|---|---|
| Heat Absorbed, $Q$ | $6.00 \times 10^{-5}$ | $2.00 \times 10^{-6}$ | W |
| d$n$/d$T$ | 13.1 | 11.9 | ppm/K |
| Conductivity, $k$ | 27.2 | 1.3 | W/m-K |
| Beam Area, $A$ | $7.85 \times 10^{-5}$ | $7.85 \times 10^{-5}$ | m$^2$ |
| Thermal Lensing, $f_t$ | 5.4 | 8.6 | m |

Minimizing the thermal lensing—i.e., keeping the nominally infinite focal length of the window as large as possible—thus requires a window with a small d$n$/d$T$, a small power density $Q/A$ (units of W/m$^2$), and a large thermal conductivity. A comparison of sapphire and fused silica as potential window materials is given in Table 4.2 for an incident power $P_{inc} = 1$ W, a flat-top beam diameter $D_b = 1$ mm, and a window thickness $d = 2$ mm; the comparison shows that even though fused silica has a very poor thermal conductivity, it also absorbs less than sapphire at a wavelength $\lambda = 1.5$ μm, thus giving silica less of a tendency to thermal lensing (i.e., a larger $f_t$).

In addition to changes in index, increases in window temperature also cause the window to expand in thickness by an amount $\Delta d = \alpha_t \cdot d \cdot \Delta T$ for a coefficient of thermal expansion (CTE) $\alpha_t$ measured in units of parts per million (ppm) per degree K.[2] If there is also a radial thermal gradient $\Delta T_r$ (as in Fig. 4.4), then the defocus WFE due to thermal lensing is given by[3]

$$WFE = d\left[\alpha_t(n-1) + \frac{dn}{dT}\right]\Delta T_r \tag{4.2}$$

Even with perfectly uniform heating of a lens, mirror, or window, the transfer of heat to or from the optic can lead to these gradients. In Eq. (4.2), we make no assumptions as to the uniformity of the beam profile; the material-dependent terms in the square brackets, however, lead to the

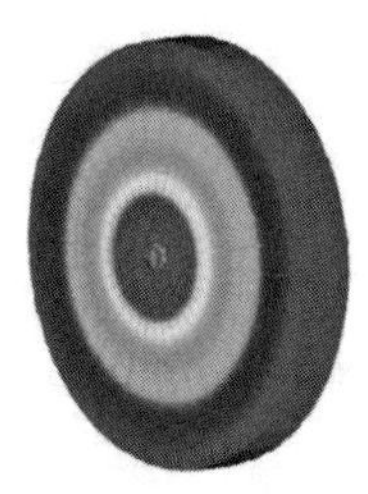

| Material | Index | CTE (ppm/K) | d$n$/d$T$ (ppm/K) | Wavelength | $G$ (ppm/K) |
|---|---|---|---|---|---|
| N-BK7 | 1.52 | 7.1 | 3.0 | 541.6 nm | 6.7 |
| Fused Silica | 1.46 | 0.5 | 10.2 | 541.6 nm | 10.4 |
| Sapphire | 1.77 | 5.3 | 13.1 | 541.6 nm | 17.2 |
| Silicon | 3.40 | 2.6 | 162 | 3-5 μm | 168 |
| Germanium | 4.00 | 6.1 | 385 | 8-12 μm | 403 |

**Figure 4.4** The thermo-optic constant $G$ shows that N-BK7 is less sensitive to radial thermal gradients compared to fused silica.[4] [Image reprinted from K. B. Doyle, V. L. Genberg, and G. J. Michels, *Integrated Optomechanical Analysis*, Second Edition, SPIE Press, Bellingham, Washington (2012).] (See color plate.)

definition of the thermo-optic constant $G = \alpha_t(n - 1) + dn/dT$, used as a metric for material sensitivity to radial gradients (where smaller $G$ is better—see Fig. 4.4 for typical values at room temperature). This does not mean that the least-sensitive material is the best option, as other factors such as material absorption and thermal resistance to the heat sink determine the radial temperature gradient $\Delta T_r$ itself.[2]

More generally, the thermal-lensing focus shift and optical aberrations are predictable and can be partially compensated for if the mode irradiance is well behaved ($TEM_{00}$, e.g.). In practice, many laser beams are not a pure $TEM_{mn}$ mode, but an aberrated Gaussian or a combination of modes (which may also change with time). The resulting wavefront phase error after the beam propagates through an optical component is then not well-defined and results instead in an increase in divergence angle and focused spot size (Figs. 4.5 and 2.24).

Specific techniques may therefore be required to reduce thermal lensing. For example, if the mode is well behaved, then warm-up time should be allowed for temperature stabilization, with accommodations made to adjust (or compensate with a negative lens) the thermal focus shift and optical aberrations. In addition, a heater may be used around the circumference of the window to compensate for radial thermal gradients. For high-power (directed-energy) systems, more advanced techniques such as water cooling of the window may even be necessary.[5] Finally, low-absorption materials are critical, as is reducing the radial thermal gradient $\Delta T_r$ (which depends on the diameter $D$, thickness $d$, and thermal conductivity $k$ of the window). Laser-grade fused silica (Suprasil or equivalent) and low-absorption N-BK7HT are likely the best options for UV-to-SWIR wavelengths (see Section 4.5.1).

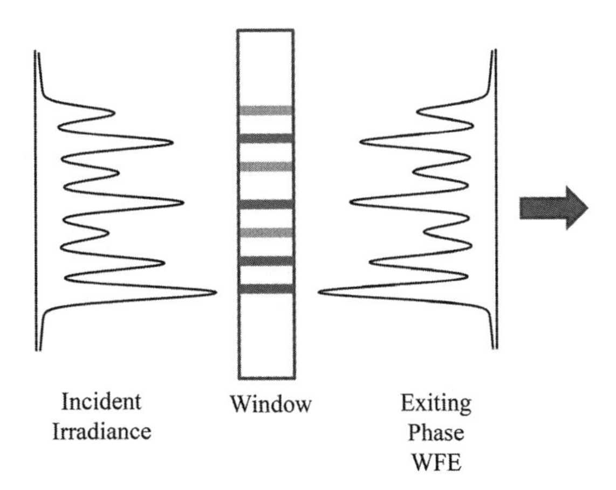


**Figure 4.5** Through absorption, thermo-optic, and thermal expansion effects, a non-uniform irradiance profile results in non-uniform phase shifts after propagation through a window.

## 4.2 Lenses

The back-reflections and thermal lensing that can cause problems with laser-system windows can also be a concern for lenses. The applications for these lenses include beam shaping (elliptical to circular, e.g.), uniformity control ("top hat"), beam divergence (collimation), photon collection, specialized focusing lenses for scanning, and many others. Depending on the application, the design issues that might be considered include focusing (Section 4.2.1), beam truncation (Section 4.2.2), aberrations (Section 4.2.3), surface figure (Section 4.2.4), surface ripple (Section 4.2.5), surface finish (Section 4.2.6), and surface quality (Section 4.2.7).

### 4.2.1 Focusing

We briefly looked at focusing in Section 3.3, where we saw that the diffraction-limited blur size depends on the wavelength $\lambda$, focal length $f$, and $1/e^2$-beam diameter $D_{1/e^2}$ [Eq. (3.9)]. Table 4.3 summarizes how Gaussian-beam focusing differs from the imaging of incoherent sources; key differences include the smaller spot size and depth of focus (DOF) of the $TEM_{00}$ beam, the dependence of the spot size on the $1/e^2$ diameter of the beam (and not the lens diameter $D$ for an untruncated beam), and the unusual $1f$:$1f$ conjugate distances. In this section, we look in more detail at the reasons for (and consequences of) these differences.

In general, the image location and spot size of a Gaussian beam will depend on both the laser *and* the lens. This is not the case for incoherent sources where the $f/\#$ ($\equiv f/D$) determines the blur size; instead, a laser also has a Rayleigh range $z_R$ that must be taken into account. And while the spot size $B = 2w_{02} = 4\lambda f/\pi D_{1/e^2}$ under certain conditions, there are other spot sizes that the focusing optics may give. For example, what is the spot size in Fig. 4.6 if the focus distance is not $f$, but $z_2$? And under what conditions will the focus distance equal $z_2$?

We start by considering the situation shown in Fig. 4.7, where the focal length $f \ll z_R$. This is a common situation, as a typical $f = 100$ mm will be much smaller than $z_R = \pi w_{01}{}^2/\lambda = 1000$ mm for an object waist $w_{01} = 0.564$ mm at a laser wavelength $\lambda = 1$ μm.

Using Eq. (3.15), Fig. 4.8 plots the image waist location $z_2$ as the object waist position $z_1$ is varied. This simple plot has a couple of interesting features.

**Table 4.3** Comparison of imaging properties of incoherent and Gaussian beams.

| Property | Incoherent Imaging | $TEM_{00}$ Gaussian |
|---|---|---|
| Spot Size | $B = 2.44 \times \lambda f/D$ | $B \approx (4/\pi) \times \lambda f/D_{1/e^2}$ |
| Depth of Focus | $DOF = \pm 2\lambda \times (f/D)^2$ | $DOF \approx \pm(4\lambda/\pi) \times (f/D_{1/e^2})^2$ |
| Conjugates | $2f$:$2f$ | $1f$:$1f$ |

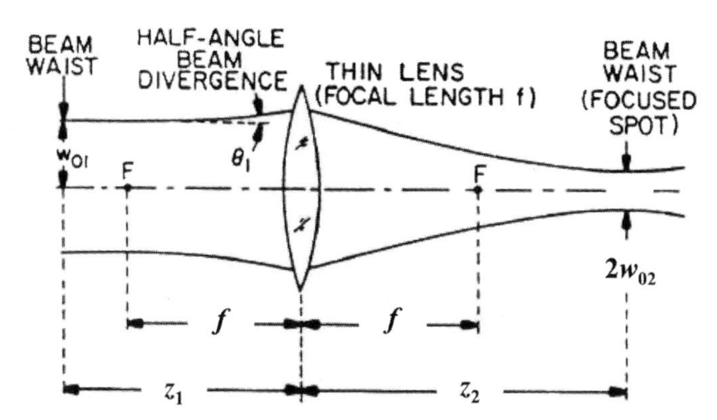


**Figure 4.6** The object waist (size $w_{01}$) at $z_1$ is focused by the lens to an image waist (size $w_{02}$) at the image location $z_2$. [Credit: H. Weichel and L. S. Pedrotti, "A summary of useful laser equations – an LIA Report," *Electro-Optical Systems Design*, Vol. 8, pp. 22–36 (1976). Reprinted with permission from the 8th edition of *Electro-Optical Systems Design*. ©1976 PennWell.]

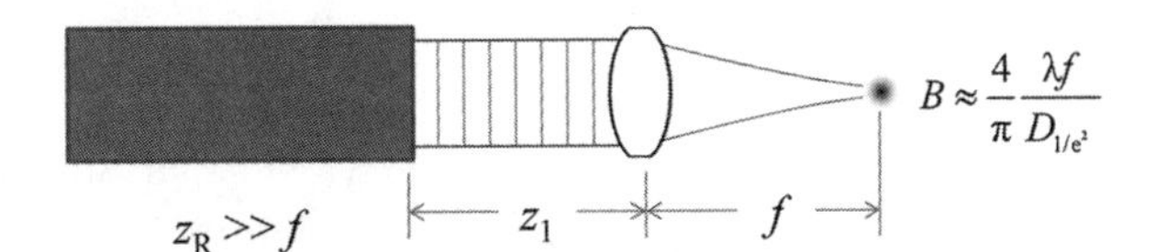


**Figure 4.7** For a Rayleigh range $z_R \gg f$, the wavefronts incident on the lens are planar, and the beam diameter $D_{1/e^2}$ does not change much as the object waist position $z_1$ is varied.

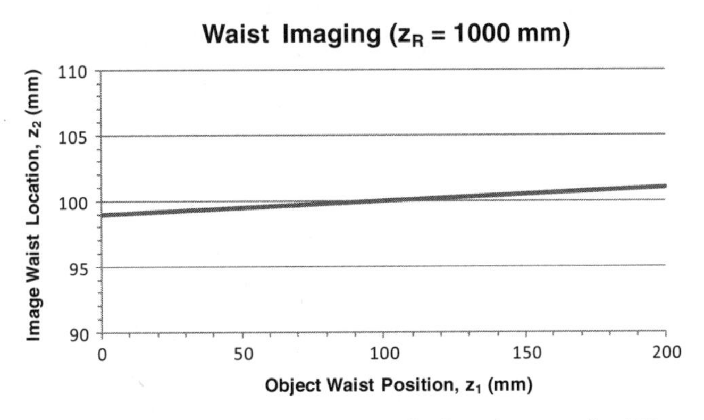


**Figure 4.8** For $z_R \gg f$, the image waist location $z_2 \approx f = 100$ mm.

The first is that $z_2 \approx f$, as expected for planar wavefronts incident on a lens. The second is that $z_2$ is exactly one focal length when $z_1 = f$, illustrating the $1f$:$1f$ object–image conjugates found with Gaussian beams.

The focused spot size depends on the wavefront curvature and beam diameter $D_{1/e^2} \approx 2w_{01}$ incident on the lens, and given that neither changes much when we are near the waist, we expect to see a more-or-less constant

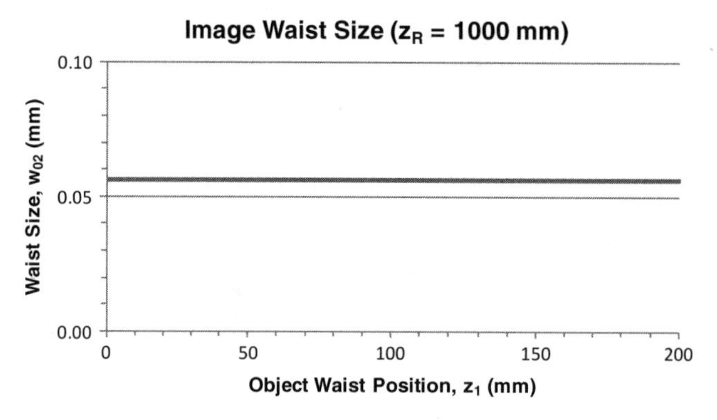


**Figure 4.9** For $z_R \gg f$, the image waist is approximately constant, given by $w_{02} \approx 2\lambda f/\pi D_{1/e^2}$.

blur size as the object distance is varied. This is shown in Fig. 4.9 for a wavelength $\lambda = 1$ μm and a waist size $w_{01} = 0.564$ mm.

To estimate the focused spot size from $B \approx 2w_{02} = 2\lambda/\pi D_{1/e^2}$ for $\theta_{02} \approx D_{1/e^2}/2f$ (see Fig. 3.11), we use the $1/e^2$ diameter $D_{1/e^2} \approx 2w_{01} = 2 \times 0.564$ mm $= 1.128$ mm incident on the lens, giving $w_{02} = 0.056$ mm as shown in Fig. 4.9 across a wide range of object waist positions. The equation given in Table 4.3 for focused spot size $B$—also equal to $2\theta_{01}f$—is thus a commonly used approximation, but as we will soon see, one that is only valid when $z_R \gg f$.

The image waist size $w_{02}$ in Fig. 4.9 and the figures that follow is determined from the distance $z_2$ from the lens to the waist and wavefront radius of curvature $R_i$ converging to that distance.[6] If this were a situation of incoherent imaging, these numbers would be the same; since this is a Gaussian beam, they are related by solving Eq. (3.3) for the Rayleigh range $z_{R2}$ of the focused beam:

$$z_{R2} = \sqrt{z_2 R_i - z_2^2} = \frac{\pi w_{02}^2}{\lambda} \tag{4.3}$$

which in turn determines the waist size $w_{02}$. We thus need to calculate the waist location $z_2$ and the wavefront radius of curvature $R_i$ for any given object position $z_1$.

Equation (3.15) gives us the image distance $z_2$ for a known object distance $z_1$ and Rayleigh range $z_{R1}$ of the beam *incident on* the lens. Fortunately, this is known for Fig. 4.9, as we are given a waist size $w_{01} = 0.564$ mm and wavelength $\lambda = 1$ μm, from which Eq. (3.4) gives us $z_{R1} \equiv z_R = 1000$ mm. We then use a modified form of Eq. (3.15) that avoids division by zero when $z_1 = f$:[7]

$$z_2 = f\left[1 + \frac{\frac{z_1}{f} - 1}{\left(\frac{z_1}{f} - 1\right)^2 + \left(\frac{z_R}{f}\right)^2}\right] \tag{4.4}$$

To calculate the wavefront radius of curvature $R_i$ exiting the lens and converging towards $z_2$, we note from the RHS of Eq. (3.14) that $R_i$ is determined by the incident wavefront radius of curvature $R_o$ and the focal length $f$ of the lens. That is, a lens does not "know" if an incident wavefront is incoherent, coherent, or a combination of the two. Instead, the wavefront-conversion property of the lens simply transforms the wavefront—whatever its type—according to the physical interpretation of the RHS of Eq. (3.14). Since the radius of curvature $R_o$ is known from Eq. (3.3), $R_i$ can easily be found. For the case of $z_{R1} \gg f$, $R_i \approx z_2$, but the errors in the approximation lead to incorrect results when $z_1 \approx f$, and as shown in Example 4.1, the exact values of $R_i$ must be used for the accurate calculation of $w_{02}$.

---

**Example 4.1**

In this example, we illustrate the use of the imaging equations in this section to generate the curves in Figs. 4.8 and 4.9. The method applies to the other curves in this section as well and is easily implemented in a spreadsheet, *Mathcad*, *Mathematica*, etc. Software packages such as Zemax and Code V are also available for propagating Gaussian beams, but an understanding of the imaging equations is necessary for intelligent use of these tools.

Looking first at $1f{:}1f$ imaging for $z_R = 1000$ mm $\gg f = 100$ mm, we know that the incident wavefront is nearly planar and thus focuses to a distance $z_2 \approx f$. Mathematically, the laser waist is located at $z_1 = f$, with Eq. (4.4) giving $z_2 = f$, as expected and as shown in Fig. 4.8.

Choosing $z_1 = 2f$ to calculate a second data point in Fig. 4.8, Eq. (4.4) now gives

$$z_2 = f\left[1 + \frac{\frac{2f}{f} - 1}{\left(\frac{2f}{f} - 1\right)^2 + \left(\frac{10f}{f}\right)^2}\right] = f\left[1 + \frac{1}{1^2 + 10^2}\right] = 1.0099f$$

or very close to $f$, as expected for an incident wavefront that is almost planar. A laser waist placed at $z_1 = 200$ mm thus images to $z_2 = 1.0099 \times 100$ mm $\approx$ 101 mm, as shown in Fig. 4.8. This is, of course, quite a bit different from incoherent imaging with its $2f{:}2f$ conjugates.

With the image location known, we can now estimate the image waist size $w_{02}$. Two approaches are possible; the first approach uses Eq. (4.3) to calculate the $1f{:}1f$ point in Fig. 4.9. To use this equation, we need to know the image distance $z_2$ and the radius of curvature $R_i$ converging to that distance. The radius of curvature is obtained from the wavefront-transformation properties of a thin lens, i.e., the RHS of Eq. (3.14). This depends on the radius of curvature $R_o$ of the wavefront incident on the lens, which we find from Eq. (3.3) for Gaussian propagation as

$$R_o(z_1) = z_1\left[1+\left(\frac{z_R}{z_1}\right)^2\right] = 100\left[1+\left(\frac{1000}{100}\right)^2\right] = 10{,}100\,\text{mm}$$

giving an incident wavefront curvature $C_o = 1/R_o = 0.000099$/mm. From the RHS of Eq. (3.14), we find that $C_i = 1/f - C_o = 0.01$/mm – 0.000099/mm = 0.0099/mm, or $R_i = 1/C_i = 101$ mm. This is nearly identical to the focal length—but not exactly equal—as the radius of the incident wavefront is large but not perfectly planar.

We can now find the image waist size $w_{02}$. Substituting $z_2$ and $R_i$ in Eq. (4.3), we find that the Rayleigh range of the focused spot is $z_{R2} = [z_2R_i - z_2^2]^{1/2} = [100 \times 101 - (100)^2]^{1/2} = 10$ mm. The waist size is then obtained from Eq. (3.4), giving $w_{02} = [z_{R2}\lambda/\pi]^{1/2} = [10\text{ mm} \times 0.001\text{ mm}/\pi]^{1/2} = 0.0564$ mm, as shown in Fig. 4.9 for $1f{:}1f$ imaging and $\lambda = 1$ μm.

The second approach to finding $w_{02}$—simpler mathematically, but without the physical insight that wavefront transformation gives us in the first approach —is to use Eq. (4.5). For the $1f{:}1f$ case, this gives a waist magnification $m = w_{02}/w_{01} = 1/[(1 - f/f)^2 + (10f/f)^2]^{1/2} = 0.1\times$, or $w_{02} = w_{01}/10 = 0.0564$ mm, consistent with the first approach.

Finally, we finish this example by illustrating the calculation of the $z_1 = 2f$ point in Fig. 4.9. Using the second approach to finding the spot size, we have $m = 1/[(1 - 2f/f)^2 + (10f/f)^2]^{1/2} = 0.0995\times$, or $w_{02} = w_{01}/10.05 = 0.0561$ mm. This is shown in Fig. 4.9 as almost unchanged from $1f{:}1f$ imaging, as expected for a nearly planar wavefront incident on a lens with $z_R \gg f$.

---

As we reduce the Rayleigh range, approximation errors become even larger for the next case we consider, namely, $z_R = f$. Figure 4.10 shows that the beam in this case now has room to expand before being intercepted by the lens; the wavefront radius of curvature incident on the lens is also no longer approximately planar as it was for $z_R \gg f$.

Using Eq. (4.4), Figure 4.11 plots the image waist location $z_2$ as the object waist position $z_1$ is varied. As with $z_R \gg f$, the $1f{:}1f$ Gaussian conjugates are clear; physically, the object location at $z_1 = z_R = f$ results in a wavefront radius of curvature incident on the lens $R(z_1) \equiv R_o = 2z_R = 200$ mm. The

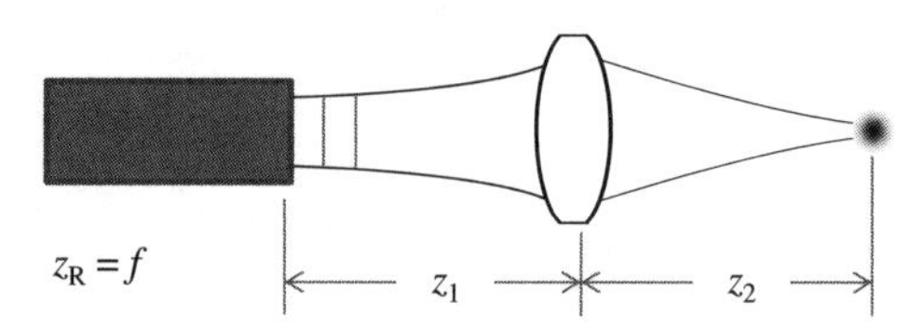


**Figure 4.10** For a Rayleigh range $z_R = f$, the wavefront radii incident on the lens are given by Eq. (3.3), increasing (as illustrated in Fig. 3.5) as the lens is moved away from the laser.

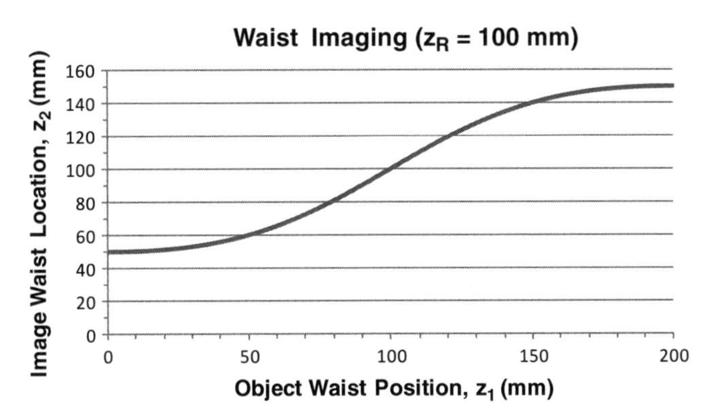


**Figure 4.11** For $z_R = f$, the image waist location is determined by Eq. (4.4) and is now more sensitive to changes from $z_1 = f$ as the incident wavefront curvature changes quickly near $z_R$.

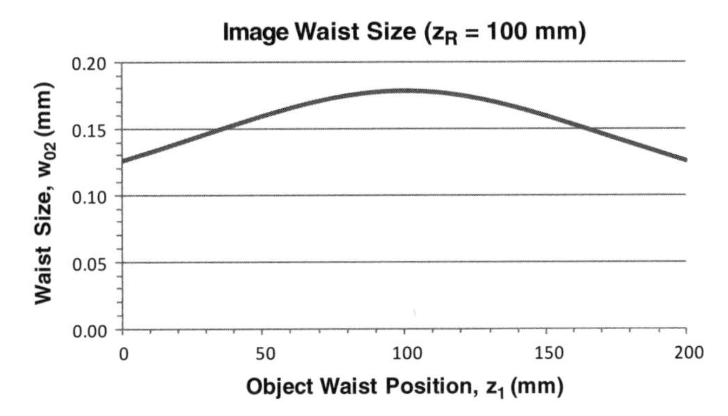


**Figure 4.12** For $z_R = f$, the image waist gets smaller as the lens is moved away from the object waist position at $z_1 = f = 100$ mm, a result of the changes in wavefront curvature and beam size incident on the lens.

wavefront-transformation properties of a lens [Eq. (3.14)] then require that $R_i = 2z_2 = 200$ mm, placing the image waist at the back focal length [i.e., $z_{R2} = f = 100$ mm from Eq. (4.3)].

The image waist size $w_{02}$ for $z_R = f$ is plotted in Fig. 4.12. The image waist is now *largest* at the conjugates, where the focused spot $B \approx 2\theta_{01} f$ and peak magnification $m_p = w_{02}/w_{01} = f/z_R = 1\times$, and the lens can be thought of as relaying or re-imaging the waist, rather than focusing. As the waist is moved away from the lens, however, focusing to a smaller spot occurs—a result of the incident beam diameter $D_{1/e^2}$ increasing faster than the image position $z_2$ for $z_1 \geq 1.5(f + z_R)$ or so.

Quantitatively, we can calculate the image waist using the same methods described in Example 4.1; here we use the waist magnification $m$ for a given $z_R$ and object position $z_1$:[7]

$$m = \frac{w_{02}}{w_{01}} = \frac{1}{\sqrt{\left(1 - \frac{z_1}{f}\right)^2 + \left(\frac{z_R}{f}\right)^2}} \tag{4.5}$$

Note that we cannot in general estimate the blur size from $B = 2w_{02} \approx 4\lambda z_2/\pi D_{1/e^2}$, as the distance $z_2$ varies quickly near the $1f$:$1f$ conjugates (Fig. 4.11); away from the conjugates, however, the approximation is good for $z_1 \geq 1.5(f + z_R)$ or so. For example, using the blur-size estimate $B = 2w_{02} \approx 4\lambda f/\pi D_{1/e^2}$ for $z_2 = f$, the $1/e^2$ diameter incident on the lens $D_{1/e^2} \approx 2w_{01} = 2 \times 0.2523$ mm $= 0.5046$ mm [from Eq. (3.2)], giving $w_{02} = 0.126$ mm. This is only 70% of the actual waist size $w_{02} = 0.178$ mm for $z_1 = f$ in Fig. 4.12, clearly illustrating the inaccuracy of the commonly used approximation for blur size.

Finally, when we shorten the Rayleigh range even further such that $z_R \ll f$, even more dramatic changes in image position are found. Figure 4.13 shows that the beam in this case now has a large distance to expand before being intercepted by the lens; since the lens is well outside the Rayleigh range, the wavefront radii incident on the lens nearly equal the distance $z_1$ [i.e., $R(z_1) \approx z_1$, as shown in Fig. 3.5]. This situation is typical of semiconductor or fiber lasers, or a tightly focused waist before the lens giving a small $w_{01} \approx 10$–$100$ μm.

Figure 4.14 shows that the image waist location $z_2$ now changes quickly as the lens is moved away from the $1f$:$1f$ conjugates. In addition, the image waist has the very unusual property of first moving away from the lens as the lens is moved away from the laser—and then coming back *towards* the laser as the lens is moved even farther away.

This unusual property of Gaussian-beam imaging can best be understood by remembering that the image position depends on both the wavefront curvature and the beam size exiting the lens. When $z_1 \approx f$, the incident curvature is very close in value to $1/f$, given that $R_o = R(z_1) \approx z_1 \approx f$ for $z_R \ll f$. The wavefront transformation properties of a thin lens then show that

$$\frac{1}{f} = \frac{1}{R_o} + \frac{1}{R_i} = \frac{1}{f + \delta} + \frac{1}{R_i} \tag{4.6}$$

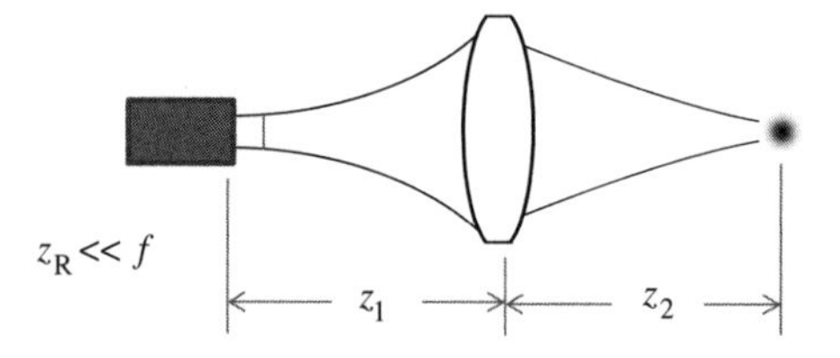


**Figure 4.13** For a Rayleigh range $z_R \ll f$, the size $w(z)$ and radius of curvature $R(z)$ of the wavefronts incident on the lens change approximately linearly with $z_1$ as the lens is moved.

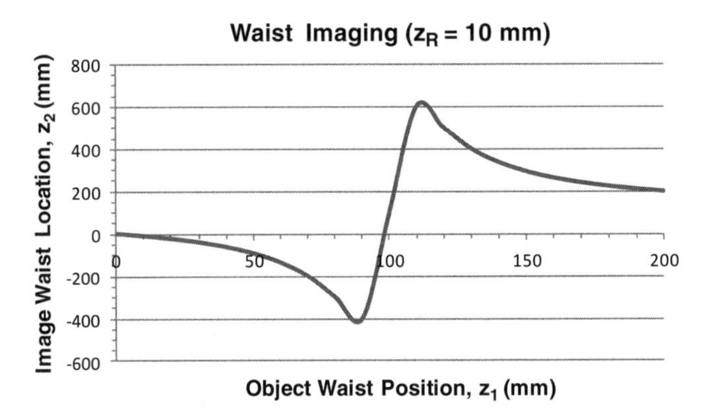


**Figure 4.14** For $z_R \ll f$, the image waist location is extremely sensitive to changes in object position due to the wavefront transformation becoming highly dependent on changes from $z_1 = f$.

for which the exiting curvature $C_i = 1/R_i$ is very sensitive to variations δ from $f$. The exiting curvature thus dominates over the beam size in determining the image distance for $z_1 \approx f$.

As $z_1$ increases, however, the incident radius of curvature increases approximately proportionally to $z_1$, thus reducing the sensitivity of $z_2$ to $R_i$. As this occurs, the beam size $w(z_1)$ starts to play a larger role in the image location, and the balance between these two competing effects determines the maximum in Fig. 4.14.

The imaged waist size also depends on the wavefront curvature and beam diameter incident on the lens. This is plotted in Fig. 4.15, where we see a large change in size near $z_1 \approx f$, also a result of the sensitivity of the exiting curvature to lens position. The image waist is again largest at the conjugates, where the peak magnification $m_p = w_{02}/w_{01} = f/z_R = 10\times$, and the lens can now

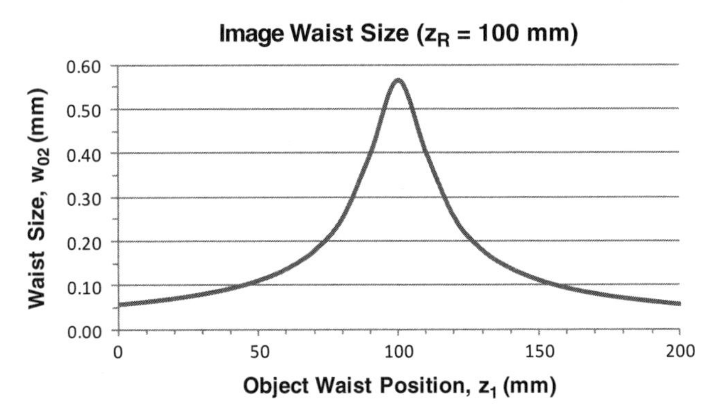


**Figure 4.15** For $z_R \ll f$, the image waist size drops quickly for $z_1 \neq f$ as the exiting wavefront curvature $1/R_i$ is highly sensitive to these changes in object waist position.

be thought of as a beam expander. As the waist is moved away from the lens, however, focusing to a smaller spot occurs—a result of the incident beam diameter $D_{1/e^2} = 2w(z_1)$ increasing faster than the image position $z_2$ for $z_1 \geq 1.5(f + z_R)$ or so.[8] For large $z_1$ where the wavefronts incident on the lens are close to planar, the blur size can be approximated by $B = 2w_{02} \approx 4\lambda z_2/\pi D_{1/e^2}$.

Summarizing, Gaussian beam imaging is unique in that the wavefront curvature exiting a thin lens does not converge to the geometrical focus for an incident plane wave. Instead, propagation through the lens starts from a known waist size $w_{01}$ and its distance $z_1$ to the lens; the beam size $w(z_1)$ and wavefront radius of curvature $R(z_1) \equiv R_o$ incident on the lens are then known from Eqs. (3.2) and (3.3), respectively. In propagating through the lens, the beam size does not change, and the wavefront radius of curvature $R_i$ exiting the lens is determined from the wavefront transformation properties of the lens [RHS of Eq. (3.14)]. Physically, this is sufficient to determine the image waist location $z_2$ and waist size $w_{02}$; mathematically, they are calculated from the simultaneous solution of Eqs. (3.2) and (3.3), as given by Eqs. (4.4) and (4.5), respectively. Useful approximations and rules of thumb obtained from these equations include:

- The imaging properties of a Gaussian beam depend on both the laser *and* the lens, where we have looked at the use of a lens for focusing ($z_R \gg f$), conjugate relay ($z_R = f$), or beam expansion ($z_R \ll f$).
- Independent of Rayleigh range and focal length, a laser waist placed at the front focal length of a thin lens will image to the back focal length (i.e., the object–image conjugates are at the $1f$:$1f$ locations).
- An often-used approximation for focused spot size is that $w_{02} = \theta_{01} f$, such that a small beam divergence $\theta_{01}$ incident on the lens results in a small spot. This equation is valid only for the $1f$:$1f$ conjugates, but is also useful away from the conjugates for $z_R \gg f$.
- The peak magnification $m_p = f/z_R$ at the $1f$:$1f$ conjugates, so a conjugate spot size smaller than the incident waist can be obtained with a lens with $z_R \gg f$ (as in Fig. 4.9).
- For $z_R \gg f$, we see from Fig. 4.9 that $B \approx 4\lambda f/\pi D_{1/e^2} = 2\theta_{01} f$ is valid for a wide range of near-field ($z_1 \ll z_R$) waist positions.
- Another often-used approximation for focused spot size is $B = 4\lambda z_2/\pi D_{1/e^2}$; we have seen that this approximation is only valid for $z_1 \geq 1.5(f + z_R)$ or so (Fig. 4.15). For $z_R \ll f$, diffraction-limited spot sizes are obtained at the focal length for the classic far-field object-at-infinity scenario with the wavefront radius of curvature $R(z_1)$ incident on the lens close to infinite and $z_2 \rightarrow f$ for $z_1 \gg f + z_R$.

A key assumption in the estimate of spot sizes in this section is that the lens is large enough to not truncate the beam to any significant degree. How to include this complication is addressed in the next section.

### 4.2.2 Beam truncation

Truncation—also known as beam clipping—can increase the focused spot size well beyond that given by the analysis in Section 4.2.1. The concept is illustrated in Fig. 4.16, where the $1/e^2$ beam diameter $D_{1/e^2}$ in comparison with the lens, mirror, or window aperture $D$ determines the truncation ratio $T \equiv D_{1/e^2}/D$. Given that a Gaussian beam is infinite in radial extent, any optical aperture will truncate some portion of the beam, but large truncation values have the biggest effect on increasing focused spot size and reducing power transmission.

One approach to quantifying the effect on spot size uses the truncation factor $K_T$:[9]

$$B \approx K_T \frac{\lambda f}{D_{1/e^2}} \qquad [\mu m] \tag{4.7}$$

where it is understood that this equation applies to the focusing of planar wavefronts. In this scenario, the truncation factor applies, as illustrated in Fig. 4.16 and tabulated in Table 4.4. In this table, an ideal untruncated beam has $K_T = 4/\pi = 1.27$ for a $TEM_{00}$ beam—the same prefactor we have been

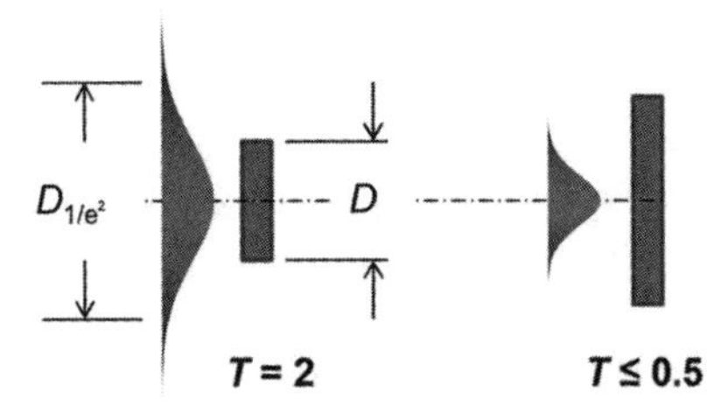


**Figure 4.16** The truncation ratio $T \equiv D_{1/e^2}/D$ of a Gaussian beam affects the focused spot size.

**Table 4.4** The truncation factor $K_T$ results in smaller $1/e^2$ spot sizes for a smaller truncation ratio $T$. (Data courtesy of Sill Optics GmbH.[9])

| Truncation Ratio, $T$ | Truncation Factor, $K_T$ |
|---|---|
| ≤ 0.50 | 1.27 (Gaussian) |
| 0.67 | 1.41 |
| 0.80 | 1.56 |
| 1.00 | 1.83 |
| 1.11 | 1.99 |
| 1.33 | 2.32 |
| ≥ 2.00 | 2.44 (Airy disk) |

using in all previous spot-size equations in this book. As the truncation increases, diffraction from the aperture beam clipping increases the spot size until we reach a point where the Gaussian profile is lost and an approximately uniform distribution is focused by the lens; in this case $K_T = 2.44$, the same as that for the Airy disk resulting from the focusing of a uniform, incoherent plane wave. Note that in this case—and in all cases for which $T > 1$—it is the lens diameter $D$ that is used in Eq. (4.7) when $D_{1/e^2} > D$.

In addition to the effects on focused spot size and power transmission—as well as spot-size-dependent parameters such as Rayleigh range and depth of focus—truncation of a spatially coherent beam also results in near-field diffraction ripple across the beam (Fig. 4.17).

As shown in Fig. 4.17, diffraction ripple $R$ is defined as a percentage of the on-axis irradiance:

$$R = \frac{\Delta E}{E} = \frac{E_{\text{peak}} - E_{\text{Gaussian}}}{E_{\text{Gaussian}}} \tag{4.8}$$

One consequence of such near-field ripple is that propagation to the far field reduces the on-axis irradiance. For example, a relatively good truncation ratio $T = 2/\pi = 0.64$ gives a near-field ripple of $\pm 17\%$; this also gives a 16% reduction in focused or far-field on-axis irradiance.[10]

In general, a truncation that blocks $R^2$ of the Gaussian power gives a near-field ripple of $\pm 2R$ and a reduction in peak far-field irradiance by a factor of $(1 - R)^2$.[10] For example, a $1/e^2$ truncation ($T = 1$) blocks 13.5% of the Gaussian power (Fig. 3.4), giving a near-field ripple of $\pm 2(0.135)^{1/2} = \pm 73.5\%$. The peak irradiance is then reduced by a factor of $(1 - 0.367)^2 = 0.4$ due to truncation, or a factor of 2.5× smaller than if there were no truncation—a significant drop for applications such as manufacturing, microscopy, or directed energy that may be

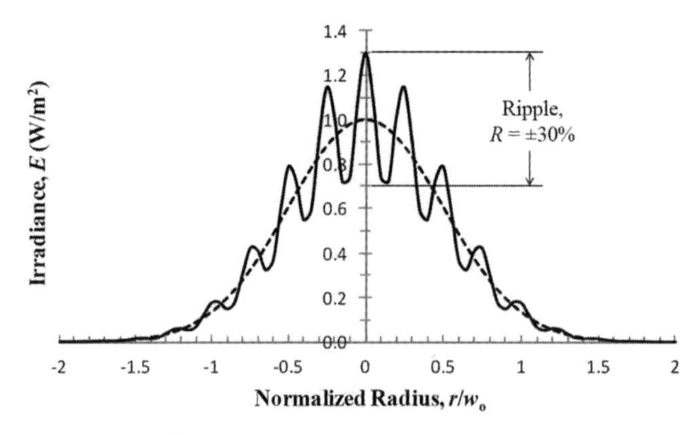


**Figure 4.17** Truncation creates near-field diffraction ripple that propagates to a far-field reduction in the peak irradiance.

relying on the larger peak irradiance for material removal, nonlinear excitation, or heating (see Chapter 6).

---

**Example 4.2**

Combining the effects of truncation and laser beam quality, what is the focused spot size for a $\lambda = 1$-μm laser with $M^2 = 1.5$, $z_R \gg f = z_1 = 100$ mm, and a lens diameter $D = 1.5D_{1/e^2} = 50$ mm?

Using a truncation ratio $T = D_{1/e^2}/D = 1/1.5$, we find from Table 4.4 that $K_T = 1.41$. Combining Eqs. (4.7) and (3.9), the spot size $B = K_T \lambda f M^2 / D_{1/e^2} = 1.41 \times 1\ \mu\text{m} \times 100\ \text{mm} \times 1.5/33.3\ \text{mm} = 6.35\ \mu\text{m}$.

---

### 4.2.3 Aberrations

The equations for focused blur size in the previous sections imply that increasing the $1/e^2$ beam diameter decreases the spot size without limit. This is shown in Fig. 4.18 where, based solely on untruncated Gaussian-beam diffraction, the blur size decreases linearly with the ratio $f/D_{1/e^2}$.

In practice, lens aberrations limit the blur size for many applications; this is also shown in Fig. 4.18, where a lens limitation known as *spherical aberration* controls the blur size for $f/D_{1/e^2} < 10.1$. While this value is specific to the parameters assumed for the plot, other values (and other aberrations) can dominate the division between beam diffraction and aberrations. The purpose of this section is to provide an overview of the aberrations typically found in laser systems. As this is not intended to be a book on lens design—there are many excellent books available for that[11,12]—we cover here the important problems the lens designers are concerned with, and the COTS lenses available to solve them.

The laser system requirements that affect aberrations may include:

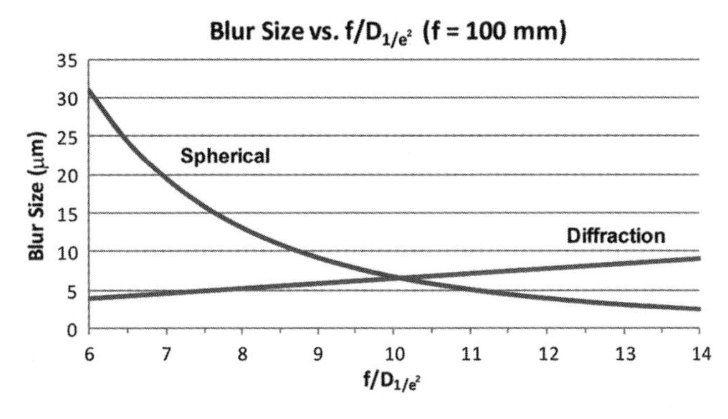


**Figure 4.18** Depending on the ratio $f/D_{1/e^2}$, untruncated blur size may be limited by Gaussian-beam diffraction or lens aberrations such as spherical aberration.

- Small field-of-illumination (FOI) beam delivery such as manufacturing and biomedical microscopy
- Larger FOI and field-of-view (FOV) imaging of reflected laser light such as laser radar or active imaging
- Collimation or astigmatism correction for fiber and diode lasers with large far-field angles resulting from their small emission apertures
- Chromatic correction for multiwavelength laser systems

In this section, then, we briefly review the aberrations associated with each of these requirements, namely: spherical aberration, coma, astigmatism, and wavelength-dependent aberrations.

**Spherical Aberration.** While it is sometimes incorrectly thought that third-order spherical aberration (SA) is the dominant spot-size limitation in laser systems, SA *can* be important for small FOV systems where beam diameter controls the amount of SA. In particular, Fig. 4.19 shows an on-axis beam with planar wavefronts incident on a lens; for a lens (or mirror) with spherical surfaces, the outer (or *marginal*) zones of the wavefront are incident on the lens at a larger Snell's law refraction angle θ than the inner (or *paraxial*) zones near the optical axis. The larger angle causes the rays to bend more at the outer zones of the lens, resulting in a blur that has no clearly defined focus and in increase in laser-plus-lens $M^2$.[13]

An incident plane wave will converge to a "best-focus" position very close to the focal length $f$ of the lens. Ignoring truncation, the blur size $B_{SA}$ for a singlet is given by[11]

$$B_{SA} = \beta_{SA} f = \frac{K_{SA} f}{(f/D_{1/e^2})^3} = \frac{K_{SA} D^3_{1/e^2}}{f^2} \qquad [\mu\text{m}] \tag{4.9}$$

where the size of the blur depends on the $1/e^2$ diameter because the refraction angle increases with diameter. In addition, $K_{SA}$ is a unitless constant that depends on the lens index and shape, and the physical blur size $B_{SA} = \beta_{SA} f = K_{SA} D^3/f^2$. For an index $n = 1.5$, Table 4.5 shows that $K_{SA} = 0.067$; the angular blur for an $f/2$ lens is thus $\beta_{SA} = K_{SA}/(f/\#)^3 = 0.067/2^3 =$

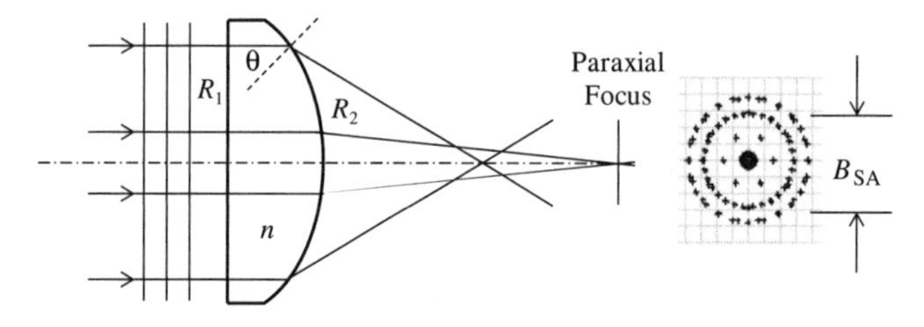


**Figure 4.19** Spherical aberration (SA) is a result of a different refraction angle θ across a spherical surface.

**Table 4.5** The spherical aberration coefficient $K_{SA}$ and associated best-form shape factor $q$ for minimum SA varies with lens index $n$.[11]

| Index, $n$ | $K_{SA}$ | Shape Factor, $q$ |
|---|---|---|
| 1.5 | 0.0670 | 0.714 |
| 2.0 | 0.0273 | 1.50 |
| 2.5 | 0.0174 | 2.33 |
| 3.0 | 0.0129 | 3.20 |
| 3.5 | 0.0103 | 4.09 |
| 4.0 | 0.0087 | 5.00 |

8.375 mrad, a relatively large blur. The physical blur for the same *f*/2 lens with a 100-mm focal length is $B_{SA} = \beta_{SA} f = 8.375$ mrad × 100 mm = 837.5 μm, confirming our guess that the blur due to SA is large for this lens. Reducing the SA thus requires using a slower beam (larger $f/D_{1/e^2}$), which Eq. (4.9) implies can yield an arbitrarily small SA. This is true up to the point where diffraction begins to dominate (as in Fig. 4.18).

Table 4.5 also shows that the lens index affects SA. Mathematically, the parameter $K_{SA}$ in Eq. (4.9) becomes smaller as the index increases.[11] Physically, a larger index allows a smaller surface curvature to obtain the same focal length; smaller curvature in turn implies smaller incident angles and thus a smaller difference between marginal and paraxial rays. Unfortunately, this index cannot be chosen arbitrarily as $n \approx 1.5$ happens to be a common index for materials (e.g., N-BK7) that transmit well in the visible spectrum. In contrast, infrared materials (e.g., silicon and germanium) typically have $n \approx 3$ to 4, values for which a low-SA design can be readily obtained using a shape that's a meniscus rather than plano-convex.

The $K_{SA}$ factors in Table 4.5 apply only if the shape (or *bending*) of the lens is that of the "best-form" singlet associated with its index. That is, a shape factor $q$ of a lens can be defined as

$$q = \frac{R_2 + R_1}{R_2 - R_1} = \frac{C_1 + C_2}{C_1 - C_2} \tag{4.10}$$

where $R_n = 1/C_n$ is the radius of curvature of each surface of the lens (Fig. 4.19). For example, a plano-convex lens facing towards the object waist with $R_1 = \infty$ ($C_1 = 0$) and any value of $R_2$ gives $q = C_2/(-C_2) = -1$, while a convex-plano lens with $R_2 = \infty$ ($C_2 = 0$) gives $q = +1$ (Fig. 4.20).

When SA is the dominant aberration, the smallest spot size obtained with a singlet is when the best-form shape is used. The minimum-SA shape thus depends on the index, and COTS convex-plano lenses with $n \approx 1.5$ to 1.7 are thus commonly used for visible-wavelength lasers, while IR materials with high indices ($n \approx 3$ to 4) use a meniscus shape ($q > +1$) such as that shown in Fig. 4.20 for $q = +3.2$.

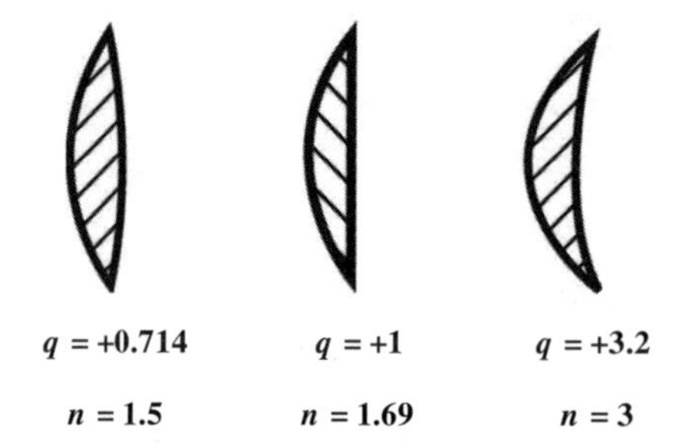


**Figure 4.20** Best-form shape factor $q$ for minimum SA is determined by the index $n$. Key assumptions are that the object waist is to the left of the lens and the incident wavefronts are planar.

From the perspective of using low-cost off-the-shelf lenses, then, vendors offer convex-plano lenses as a close approximation to the $q = +0.714$ shape for UV, visible, and near-IR wavelengths, as well as a variety of meniscus lenses for IR wavelengths. Alternatively, a larger spot size is sometimes necessary—to increase manufacturing throughput, for example—and in this case a high-index convex-plano lens is used for IR wavelengths (such as $CO_2$ lasers with $\lambda = 10.6$ μm). Lower SA (and higher cost) can be obtained by using two-component (doublet) or three-component (triplet) lenses; with these lenses an off-axis aberration known as coma can be reduced as well.

**Coma.** When going beyond small-FOV systems where aperture size controls the amount of SA, an off-axis aberration known as coma may dominate. Typical examples are active illumination or laser radar systems that collect reflected light over a large FOV; what is seen in these cases is that a focused spot no longer has the symmetric shape of the diffraction- or spherical-limited blur; instead, it has the asymmetric shape of a comet and its tail (Fig. 4.21).

The design of a lens with neither SA nor coma—i.e., an *aplanat*—is beyond the scope of this text. However, a best-form singlet for minimum SA will also have reduced coma.[11] In addition, the use of a doublet allows the

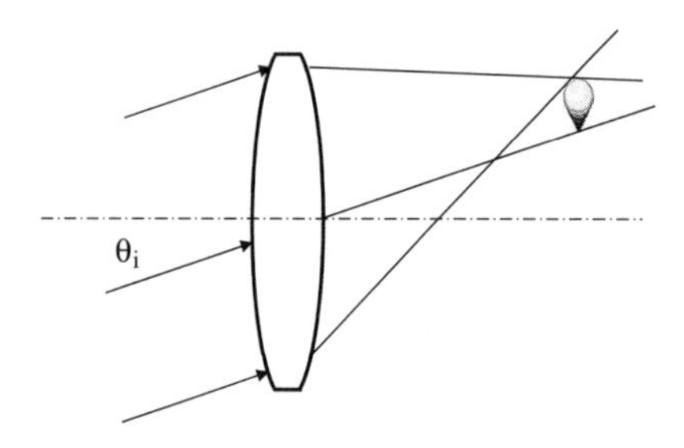


**Figure 4.21** The asymmetric blur of an off-axis beam is a result of the asymmetry of the Snell's law refraction determined by the angled wavefront incident on the lens with an $\text{FOV} = 2\theta_i$.

removal of both of these aberrations. For critical applications where the smallest-possible spot size is necessary, aplanatic doublets are available from a number of vendors; triplets are also available to reduce the focal length of the doublet by the index *n* of the third lens.

**Astigmatism.** At the other extreme, the small emission apertures of fiber and semiconductor lasers result in a large far-field angle; the optics used with these lasers require sophisticated designs to turn these laser beams into something useful for the laser systems engineer.

As shown in Fig. 4.22, the first problem encountered with edge-emitting semiconductor lasers is that the waist for the quickly diverging angle (or "fast axis" associated with the smaller waveguide dimension and waist size) is at the facet of the laser, while the larger waist of the slowly diverging angle $\theta_{slow}$ (or "slow axis") is behind the facet by approximately 10 μm for a conventional edge emitter. When focused, the different waist locations result in different focus positions—an effect known as astigmatism.

Also shown in Fig. 4.22 is that a lens placed at a given distance from the laser intercepts different beam sizes from the different beam divergences—i.e., the power profile is also elliptical. The use of an edge-emitting semiconductor laser thus requires correction of astigmatism and circularization of the beam ellipticity; VCSELs and single-mode fiber lasers with circularly symmetric single-mode beams do not have either issue associated with their use.

A traditional approach to solving the astigmatism problem has entailed the use of an aspheric collimating lens [which creates planar wavefronts expanding at a diffraction-limited angle $\theta_{slow}$ from Eq. (3.8) for only the slow

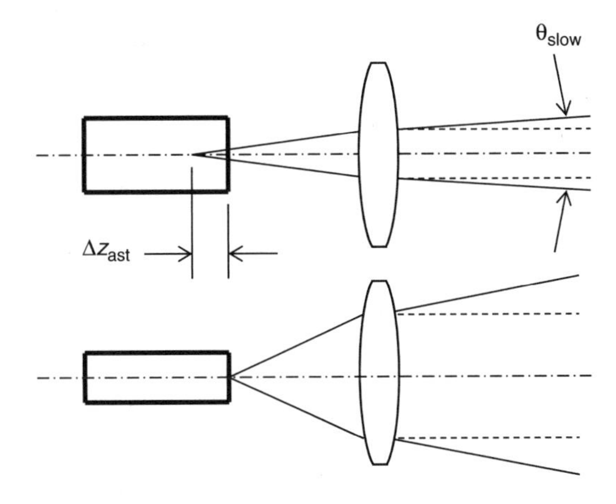


**Figure 4.22** The top view of a single-mode, edge-emitting semiconductor laser shows a waist location for the slowly diverging dimension that is offset by an amount $\Delta z_{ast} \approx 10$ μm from the waist location on the facet for the quickly diverging dimension.

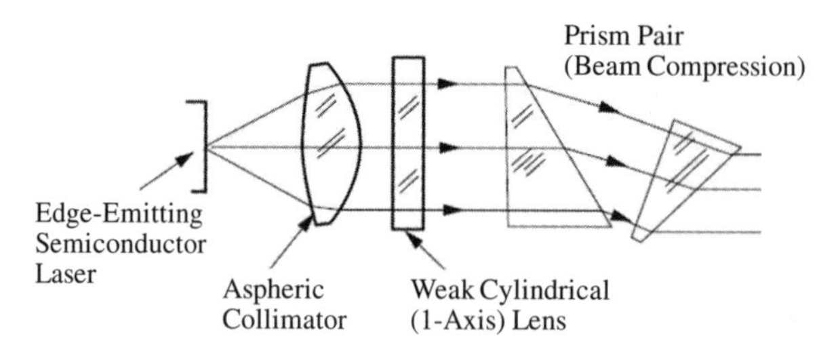


**Figure 4.23** The diameter of the fast-axis beam is compressed by the prism pair to match that of the slow axis and maintain the same direction of propagation as the laser. [Adapted from Warren Smith, *Modern Optical Engineering*, Fourth Edition, McGraw-Hill, New York (2008).]

axis] and a cylindrical lens (with refractive power in one dimension to finish the collimation in the fast axis); Fig. 4.23 shows that the circularization then requires a single-axis (anamorphic) beam expander, typically implemented as a prism pair to also maintain the same direction of propagation as the laser.

However, the prisms are relatively large and expensive, so some semiconductor laser manufacturers place an aspheric lens at the position where the fast and slow beams have the same diameter, thus circularizing without a prism pair. The astigmatism—and thus difference in wavefront radius of curvature—is still present, and this is corrected by using an asphere with more curvature in the fast direction than the slow. Alternatively, a cylindrical lens is used for circularization, followed by an asphere for collimation and astigmatism correction.[14]

**Chromatic Aberrations**. Finally, there are laser systems where a lens must be corrected for wavelength-dependent (chromatic) refractive-index aberrations—a strange thought given the narrow linewidth of most lasers. However, it is sometimes necessary for a single lens to focus two different lasers; for example, an infrared Nd:YAG laser emitting at $\lambda = 1064$ nm is difficult to align, so a co-aligned "pilot" beam of a visible HeNe wavelength of 633 nm is used instead. A typical example of a commercial two-wavelength (or multiline) lens is shown in Fig. 4.24; note the air spacing between lenses—a necessary design

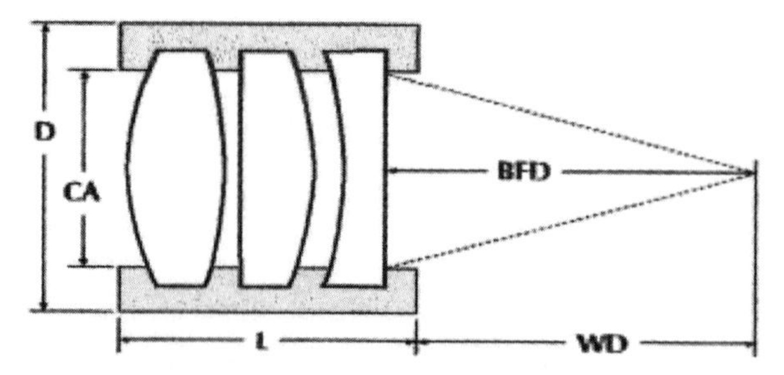


**Figure 4.24** An air-spaced achromat is corrected for chromatic aberrations to give the same focal length at $\lambda = 1064$ nm and 633 nm. (Credit: CVI Laser, LLC.)

detail that distinguishes laser achromats from cemented doublets to avoid the laser-induced damage of the epoxy used in doublets.

### 4.2.4 Surface figure (irregularity)

In the fabrication of a lens, the form of each surface—spherical, cylindrical, aspheric, or free-form—will not exactly match the ideal, and the deviation from this ideal is known as the surface figure or irregularity. The surface-figure errors (SFEs) result in WFE, which affects beam quality and therefore also affects focused spot size and far-field divergence angle.

A simple example of SFE for a mirror and a window and its effect on WFE are shown in Fig. 4.25. The SFE is the height (or depth) $\Delta d$ of the irregularity; the resulting peak-to-valley (PV) $WFE = 2\Delta d$ for a mirror (with which the wavefront interacts twice), and $WFE = (n - 1)\Delta d$ for a lens or window in air.

WFE can be measured as either a PV or a root-mean-square (RMS) quantity. The RMS WFE is an averaged WFE over the area of the optic[15]—a better measure of surface figure, as it removes the effects of $6\sigma$ outliers that do not affect optical performance.[2] For example, the PV geography of the state of California includes Mt. Whitney at an elevation of 4420 m (14,494 feet) and Death Valley at –86 m (–282 feet), but an RMS elevation over the area of California that is much smaller. For optical components, a factor of 5 is used in practice for random fabrication errors (i.e., $WFE_{PV} = 5WFE_{RMS}$), although a factor of $(12)^{1/2} \approx 3.5$ based on defocused wavefronts is also commonly used.

As measured by the Strehl ratio, lens WFE reduces the peak power of a focused spot. As shown in Fig. 4.26, the Strehl ratio $S$ is the peak power of the blur with $WFE > 0$ in comparison with the peak power for a blur with $WFE = 0$. Physically, the lens WFE redistributes power into the outer regions of the spot, thus reducing the peak value from its ideal diffraction limit.

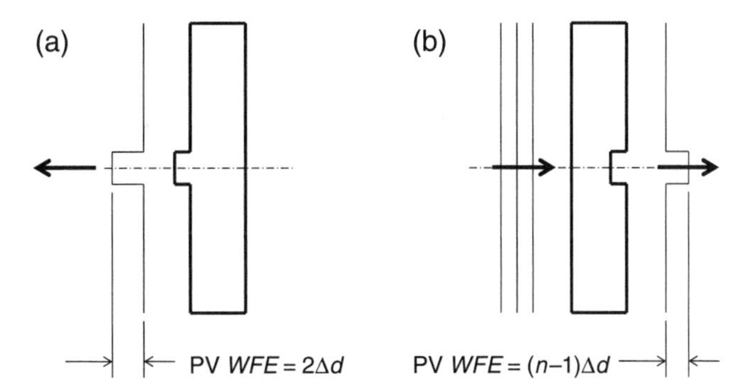


**Figure 4.25** Wavefront error is created by surface irregularities in (a) reflection from a mirror or (b) transmission through a lens or window with refractive index *n*.

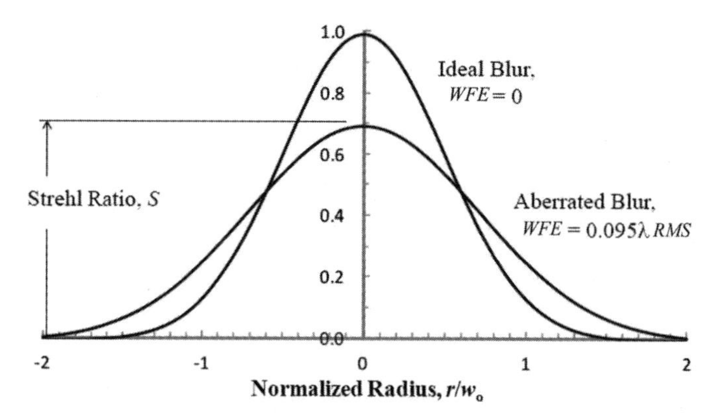


**Figure 4.26** Strehl ratio $S \equiv E_{WFE}/E_o$ with the ideal $E_o$ for WFE = 0 typically normalized to 1. From Eq. (4.11), $S = 0.7$ for an aberrated Gaussian implies that WFE = 0.095λ RMS, as shown in the plot.

This is similar to what we have seen for laser WFE, where $M^2 > 1$ reduces the peak power of a focused spot, as well as increases the spot size. To combine the effects of the laser and the optics, we first note that the Strehl ratio $S$ is related to the $\mathrm{WFE_{RMS}}$ of a lens or mirror by[11]

$$S = \exp[-(2\pi \cdot WFE_{\mathrm{RMS}})^2] \tag{4.11}$$

which is valid for $WFE_{\mathrm{RMS}} \leq \lambda/5$ or so for the wavefront errors such as spherical aberration or surface-figure errors typically found in laser systems, and $\mathrm{WFE_{RMS}}$ is measured in units of λ.

For a Gaussian or aberrated-Gaussian beam,[16] we can define a Strehl-equivalent $M^2$ for the WFE of the lens or mirror as[17]

$$M^2 \approx \frac{1}{\sqrt{S}} \tag{4.12}$$

As a result, we can think of a lens as having an $M^2$ value associated with its WFE, but how do we combine the $M^2$ values of the optical subsystem with the $M^2$ of the laser? The next step down that trail is to notice that if the wavefront errors of the optics and the laser are uncorrelated and independent of each other over the aperture, then the errors add as a root sum square (RSS):

$$WFE^2_{\mathrm{sys}} = WFE^2_{\mathrm{laser}} + WFE^2_{\mathrm{optics}} \tag{4.13}$$

where the WFE is understood to be an RMS value. An example of a situation where the errors *are* correlated is when the laser is of high enough power to induce thermal-distortion wavefront errors of the type we have seen in Section 4.1. In that case, Eq. (4.13) does not apply.

When Eq. (4.13) does apply, the exponential dependence of the Strehl ratio on WFE shows that the WFE RSS leads to a multiplicative dependence for combining $M^2$:

$$M^2_{\text{sys}} = M^2_{\text{laser}} \cdot M^2_{\text{optics}} \tag{4.14}$$

For a laser with less-than-perfect beam quality—a high-power semiconductor laser, for example—it thus may not be necessary to put a lot of effort into designing diffraction-limited optics. The laser beam quality is already much worse than diffraction limited, and Eq. (4.14) shows that the addition of small amounts of lens WFE will not significantly affect the beam divergence or image size.

---

**Example 4.3**

A lens that has manufacturing wavefront errors of 0.1 waves (λ/10) RMS is used to focus a Gaussian beam. If the laser does not induce any additional WFE in the optics, what is the total $M^2$ for the system if the laser's $M^2 = 1.4$?

From Eq. (4.11), the Strehl ratio for the lens is $S = \exp[-(2\pi \text{WFE})^2_{\text{optics}}] = \exp[-(2\pi \times 0.1)^2] = 0.67$. Using Eq. (4.12), the $M^2$ associated with the Strehl ratio is $M^2 = 1/S^{1/2} = 1.218$. From Eq. (4.14), the system $M^2$ is then $M^2_{\text{sys}} = M^2_{\text{laser}} \times M^2_{\text{optics}} = 1.218 \times 1.4 = 1.71$, within the bounds of the $M^2 \leq 2$ assumption for which these equations are valid. This value of $M^2_{\text{sys}}$—not just that of the laser itself—is what is used in the equations for the propagation of the beam to determine the far-field angle [Eq. (3.8)] or focused spot size [Eq. (3.9)].

---

### 4.2.5 Surface ripple ("quilting")

Robert Parks relates the story of the fabrication of a very expensive laser-system mirror that "... met both the RMS figure error spec and the RMS finish spec, but was going to be useless for its intended purpose,"[18] apparently a directed-energy application that required large amounts of power in a small area. While the mirror did have low irregularity, its fabrication unfortunately did not include another critical spec, namely, that of surface ripple or quilting.

Surface ripple—distinct from the irradiance ripple we saw in Section 4.2.2—is a mid-spatial-frequency (MSF) surface "waviness" resulting from substructural print-through patterns or "quilting" errors from stitching of subaperture fabrication zones.[19] Fabrication processes such as single-point diamond turning (SPDT) or magnetorheological finishing (MRF), for example, can create surface features with a smaller spatial separation $\Delta x$—or a higher spatial frequency $f_s = 1/\Delta x$—than that found for figure errors (Fig. 4.27).

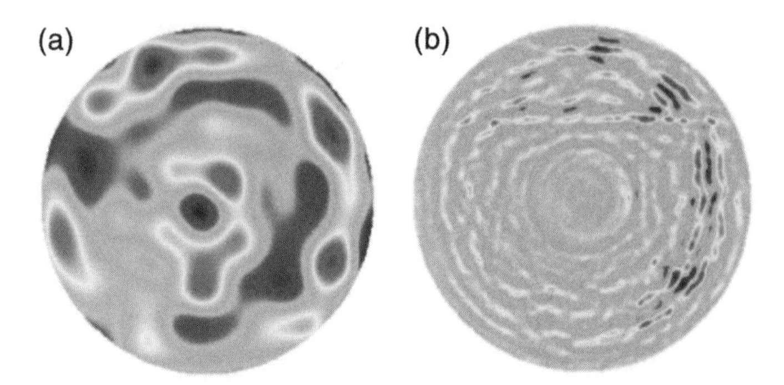


**Figure 4.27** (a) Low-spatial-frequency figure errors and (b) mid-spatial-frequency ripple errors from the fabrication process. (Reprinted from Ref. 19.) (See color plate.)

**Figure 4.28** MSF surface errors diffract light into a larger angle (right) than surface figure errors (left). (Reprinted from Ref. 19.)

The consequence of such MSF errors is that some light is diffracted off of the mirror into larger angles than predicted by the figure errors (Fig. 4.28). Thus, a high-power laser will have its energy spread into a larger angle than expected, reducing the irradiance ($W/m^2$) on the target and the energy over a specified area. Alternatively, the designer of a confocal microscope may be surprised to find that there is not enough power on the specimen to create the nonlinear two-photon effects required, even with a high-peak-power femtosecond laser.

Using the small-angle paraxial grating equation, the angle $\theta_d$ into which light is diffracted depends on the wavelength and spatial separation $\Delta x$ of the surface features:

$$\theta_d \approx \frac{\lambda}{\Delta x} = \lambda f_s \qquad [\text{rad}] \tag{4.15}$$

where the spatial frequency $f_s = 1/\Delta x$. For example, the spacing $\Delta x$ between peaks for low-spatial-frequency aberrations and surface figure errors is relatively large (≤ 5 cycles over an aperture), while that for MSF errors is on the order of 5–1000 cycles. That is, each cycle of MSF error takes up from $1/5^{th}$ to $1/1000^{th}$ of the aperture, thus diffracting light from a smaller $\Delta x$ into a larger range of angles than the blur determined by the aberrations and surface figure.

It is sometimes said that MSF errors do not increase the blur size or the far-field angle, but only add to the glare surrounding the beam. However, this statement depends on how the blur is defined—and the use of a second-moment (rather than a $1/e^2$) criterion that includes the power in the outer regions clearly indicates a larger blur, as the second-moment diameter emphasizes the power in the larger radii ($\sim r^2$). How much larger also depends on the amount of light diffracted by the MSF errors, indicating the need to understand and control this surface spec.

Allowable MSF surface errors are often specified using a power spectral density (PSD) plot (Fig. 4.29). Here, the term *spectral density* implies a measurement as a function of spectrum—in this case, a spatial frequency spectrum measured in units of $1/\Delta x$ (such as cycles/m, for example). This is shown as the horizontal axis of the PSD plot in Fig. 4.29.

The vertical axis then has the physical interpretation of surface "power" per unit spatial frequency. That is, the surface power—or more accurately, the elastic energy associated with the surface distortion[20]—varies with the square of the depth of the surface error, giving units of $y^2$ (such as nm$^2$). The division by the spatial frequency to make the vertical axis a spectral power density thus gives the vertical axis units of $L^3$ (such as nm$^2$-m).

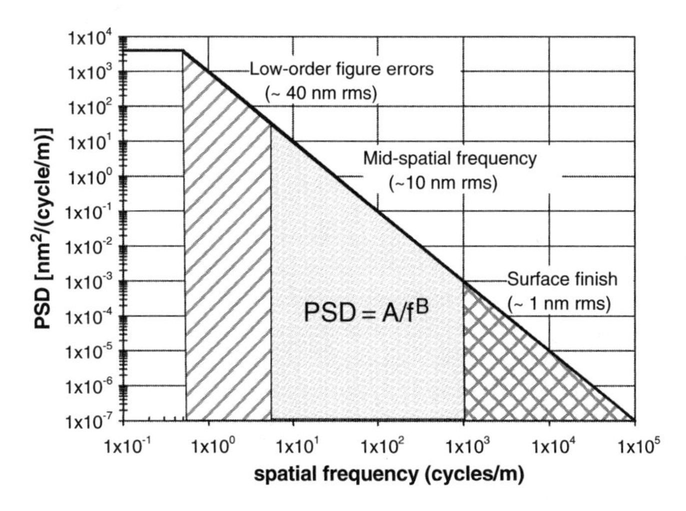


**Figure 4.29** Ideal one-dimensional PSD plot illustrating the relative PSD of surface figure errors, MSF errors, and surface finish. For this ideal plot, the RMS MSF error $y_{RMS} = 10$ nm, or one-fourth of the surface figure WFE. (Reprinted with permission from Prof. Jim Burge, Univ. of Arizona.)

The ideal PSD plot shows that the surface distortion drops off with spatial frequency. For example, the low-spatial-frequency figure errors shown in Fig. 4.29 have a spatial frequency on the order of 0.5–5 cycles/m and a surface distortion of $\leq \lambda/20$ RMS at $\lambda = 800$ nm. The MSF errors, on the other hand, encompass $f_s \approx 5$–1000 cycles/m and have an RMS surface distortion ranging from $\lambda/20$ to $\lambda/1000$. The dividing line between surface figure errors and MSF errors depends on the size of the aperture, with 0.5–5 cycles per lens or mirror diameter $D$ being a more general specification range for figure errors over a diameter $D \geq 10$ mm or so.

While the MSF error may be measured as the amount of power diffracted out of a given measurement diameter—thus determining the *encircled energy*—it is useful from a design standpoint to understand its dependencies on physical parameters. Specifically, using the PSD curves to obtain an estimate of the RMS MSF error requires integrating the PSD over the spatial frequency range $\Delta f_{\mathrm{MSF}}$ (giving units of $y^2$), and taking the square root to obtain the RMS MSF surface error $y_{\mathrm{MSF}}$,

$$y_{\mathrm{MSF}} = \sqrt{\int PSD \cdot df_s} \qquad [\mathrm{nm}] \tag{4.16}$$

If $y_{\mathrm{MSF}}$ is on the order of the surface figure WFE, then the effects on the Strehl ratio will be approximately comparable [Eq. (4.11)], and the PSD spec must be changed to reduce the MSF errors. For example, if $y_{\mathrm{MSF}} = \lambda/5$, then the MSF-induced Strehl ratio $S \approx 0.2$ and significant amounts of incident power will be scattered away from the central core of the blur or propagating beam—to the point where the blur size is indeed increased, even using a $1/e^2$ criterion.

If specified properly, then, the MSF errors will not significantly affect the Strehl ratio or optical $M^2$, indicating a relatively small diffraction of power into the diffraction angle $\theta_d$ for each spatial separation $\Delta x$. If left to chance, however, it is entirely possible that the MSF error can be larger than the surface figure WFE, and the effects on Strehl and optical $M^2$ can be dominated by the ripple or waviness. This leads to situations where the figure spec may be perfectly acceptable, yet the performance of the laser system is not because the allowable MSF errors have not been specified.[18]

Summarizing: to ensure that MSF surface errors do not diffract a significant amount of power away from the focused blur or propagating beam, the RMS MSF error $y_{\mathrm{MSF}}$ must be much smaller than the surface figure WFE. Since a good spec for surface figure WFE is $\lambda/20$ RMS, a first-order design goal for $y_{\mathrm{MSF}}$ is $\lambda/80$ (or less) based on the integrated PSD given by Eq. (4.16). An additional complication is that a poor MSF PSD can also result from environmental conditions—see Ref. 19 for more details.

### 4.2.6 Surface finish (roughness)

In addition to figure errors and MSF errors, Fig. 4.30 shows that there are high-spatial-frequency (HSF) errors associated with the fabrication of an optical surface. These errors are more commonly known as surface finish or surface roughness. With a large spatial frequency and scatter angle [Eq. (4.15)], and a percentage of scattered power that is typically very low, the surface finish does not increase the blur size, which is instead surrounded by a "veil" of background glare when the surface finish is relatively rough.

As the final polishing of a lens or mirror reduces the surface figure and ripple to acceptable levels, surface finish must simultaneously be maintained; it is measured as the RMS height variations across the surface with a spacing $\Delta x \approx 1$ μm to 1 mm (Fig. 4.29). State-of-the-art fabrication and characterization methods are able to provide extremely fine, molecular-level finishes as smooth as 2 Å (angstroms). Surface finish thus occurs on a nanometer scale much smaller than surface irregularities or MSF errors, and has no effect on WFE or Strehl ratio.

However, poor surface finish increases the scattering off of a surface, which is measured as angular scattering (bidirectional scatter distribution function, or BSDF) or as the nonspecular power $P_{\text{nsp}} \equiv P_{\text{o}} - P_{\text{sp}}$ over nonspecular angles (i.e., the total integrated scatter, or TIS) for a specular power $P_{\text{sp}}$. As a fraction of the total reflected power $P_{\text{o}}$, the TIS depends on the RMS roughness $\delta_{\text{RMS}}$ compared with the laser wavelength $\lambda$:

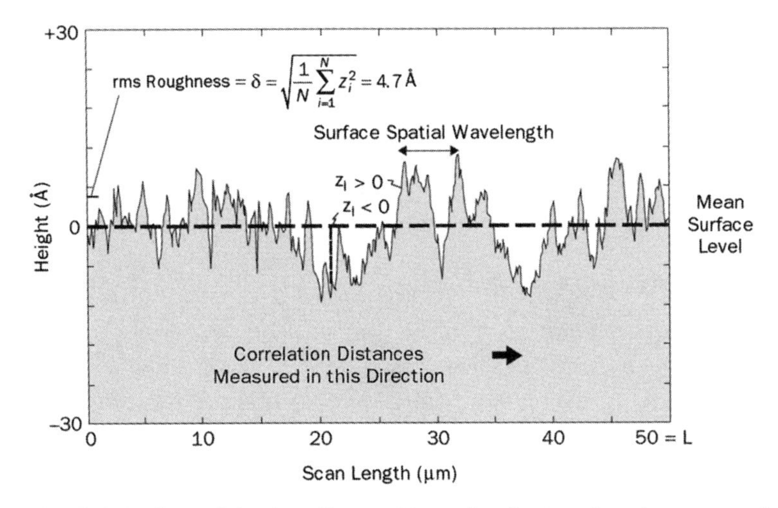


**Figure 4.30** Finish of a polished or diamond-turned optical surface is measured as RMS surface roughness. [Reprinted with permission from J. M. Bennett and L. Mattsson, *Introduction to Surface Roughness and Scattering*, Optical Society of America, Washington, D.C. (1989).]

$$TIS = \frac{P_o - P_{sp}}{P_o} \approx \left(\frac{2\pi \cdot \Delta n \cdot \delta_{RMS}}{\lambda}\right)^2 \quad (4.17)$$

where $\Delta n$ is the index difference across the optical surface ($\Delta n = -2$ for mirrors), and even a smoothly polished mirror scatters some light into large angles based on the HSF of the surface finish. For example, a mirror polished to a surface finish $\delta_{RMS} = \lambda/1000$ (or 10 Å at $\lambda = 1$ μm) scatters 0.016% of the incident light into nonspecular angles. While this may seem like a small quantity, a small fraction of a large number—kilowatts of laser power, for example—can be significant, even if the beam is no longer spatially coherent. In addition, note that a short-wavelength laser scatters significantly more than a longer-wavelength laser for the same roughness.

Most applications do not require a superpolished surface with only 2-Å microroughness; more typical specs that are uniquely determined by the stray-light requirements for each system are 5 to 10 Å for high-performance laser systems. Metals such as beryllium and aluminum are "sticky" and typically cannot be polished to better than about 50 Å, so they are coated with electroless nickel when used as mirror substrates requiring better surface finish. In contrast, fused silica and ultralow expansion (ULE) glass can be polished to very fine finishes—down to 5 Å if required—but cannot be diamond turned, as the glass breaks from the diamond tool in a brittle manner, resulting in excessive surface roughness and poor surface quality.

Along with surface figure, surface finish can be a major cost component, as meeting the finish specs involves a time-consuming process of fine polishing. It is expensive to simultaneously obtain high-precision figure and finish, since the additional polishing required to give good finish often affects the figure. A recent fabrication method that avoids this trade is MRF, which uses a magnetic material (iron) in the polishing fluid to control figure and finish (although it also introduces MSF stitching errors). The method is useful for surface figures down to $\lambda/20$ as well as surface finishes down to about 10 Å RMS.[21]

### 4.2.7 Surface quality (scratch-dig)

The polishing process can leave marks on surfaces that are too large for the finishing process to remove. These are the types of scratches often seen on a windshield or pair of eyeglasses, but they also include larger pits and divots known as "digs." They are mostly cosmetic defects for imaging systems but can be seen as shadows when found on lens surfaces—for example, field flatteners and field lenses—that are located near the image. They can also be important in systems where scattered light and interference fringes are a concern, as well as in high-power laser systems where the enhanced electric field strength at these small-area imperfections can shatter the optic.

Scratches and digs are specified in terms of allowable sizes, spacings, and densities. In its simplest form, the scratch is measured in units of length and specified as 10× larger than the scratch width in microns. A scratch specification of 60, for example, corresponds to surface scratches that are no more than 6 μm in width.

The dig spec is also in units of length but is given as 10× smaller than the actual diameter in microns; a dig spec of 40 thus refers to a dig with a 400-μm diameter. Both scratch and dig are usually evaluated visually by an experienced inspector; a typical scratch-dig spec for laser systems is 20-10 or 10-5, with smaller values not currently specified. Smaller apertures are less expensive to use with a tighter (10-5) spec, as there is less of a chance that a scratch or dig exceeding the spec occurs over a smaller area.

Applying the concepts in this section to the evaluation of optical components, we next look in more detail at beam expanders and collimators (Section 4.3), homogenizers (Section 4.4), and miscellaneous topics such as absorption and laser damage threshold (Section 4.5).

## 4.3 Beam Expanders and Collimators

A beam expander is a common optical component that increases the diameter of a laser beam; once increased, the beam can be focused to a smaller spot [Eq. (3.9)] or propagate with a smaller divergence angle [Eq. (3.8)].

Two architectures are possible for laser beam expanders—the same architectures as are commonly used for afocal telescopes.[22] These are the Keplerian and Galilean designs (Fig. 4.31) with a $1/e^2$ beam expansion $m = D_f/D_i = f_2/|f_1| = \theta_i/\theta_f$, which depends on the ratio of the focal lengths of the lenses if the input beam is collimated (i.e., has planar wavefronts).

In comparing architectures, most of the advantages go to the Galilean. Specifically, the negative lens results in a shorter overall ("track") length and is thus a lighter design as well. More importantly for many applications, the Keplerian design has an intermediate focus where the power density ($W/m^2$) in the small spot can be large enough to ionize air, causing "crackling" discharge noise and changes in beam pointing.[23] While it is possible to use an evacuated chamber at the location of the spot, a better answer is often the Galilean beam expander. On the other hand, if the power density at the intermediate focus is low enough, an advantage of the Keplerian design is that it is possible to use a pinhole for spatial filtering of any scattered light.

Beam expanders can also be used to increase the working distance between a lens and the image plane—often useful in manufacturing where clearance is required between the lens and workpiece. For example, if the spot size is fixed, then a longer focal length lens is possible with an expanded beam. This is illustrated by Eq. (3.9), where an expanded $D_{1/e^2}$ can be used

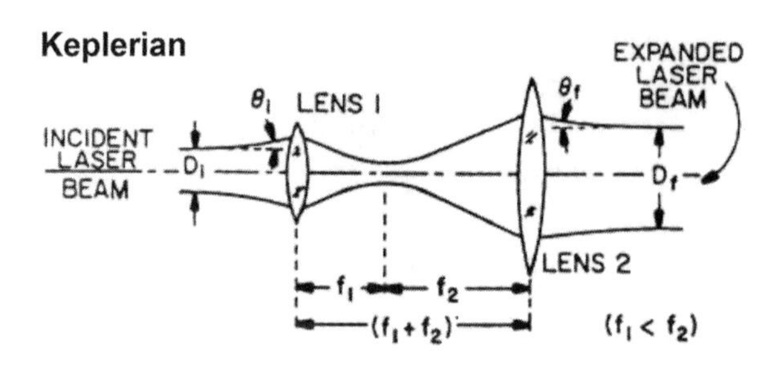


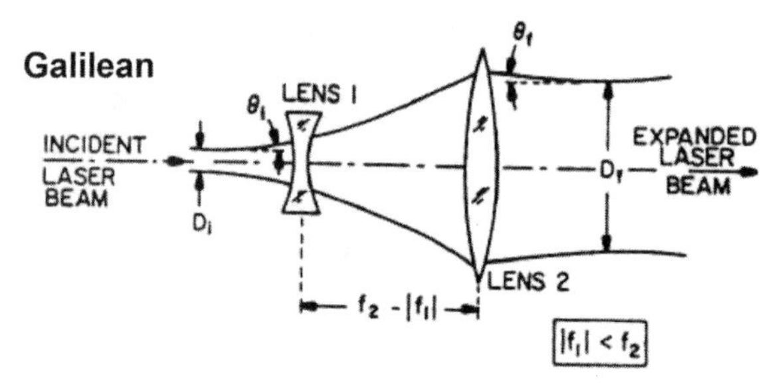


**Figure 4.31** Laser beam expanders use one of two afocal architectures for increasing the beam diameter. [Credit: H. Weichel and L. S. Pedrotti, "A summary of useful laser equations – an LIA Report," *Electro-Optical Systems Design*, Vol. 8, pp. 22–36 (1976). Reprinted from the 8th edition of *Electro-Optical Systems Design*. © 1976 by PennWell.]

to produce a smaller spot, or it can also be used to produce the same spot size if the focal length is increased in the same proportion to increase the working distance.

Commercial beam expanders can have a fixed or variable magnification $m = f_2/|f_1| = D_f/D_i$ from 1.5× → 15×. A larger magnification will have more internal optics to compensate for aberrations; high-power beam expanders may also be water cooled. Typical specs to consider when purchasing or developing an expander include:

- Input beam diameter $D_i$
- Magnification $m$—fixed or variable
- Transmitted wavefront error
- Optical transmission (insertion) losses
- Optical power limits
- Beam deviation
- Size, weight, cooling, etc.

The wavefronts leaving a laser beam expander may or may not be collimated (i.e., planar and expanding at the diffraction limit), though expanders often combine the features of both. If the input wavefront is planar, for example, then the ideal output beam will be as well, although in practice, the lenses will introduce some degree of transmitted WFE.

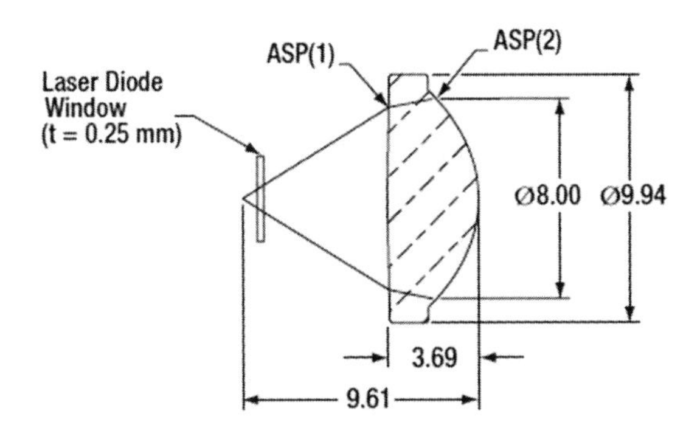


**Figure 4.32** A collimator converts diverging wavefronts into planar wavefronts (all dimensions are in millimeters). (Reprinted with permission from LightPath Technologies.)

If the input wavefront is not planar, however, then a typical optical component that makes it so is known as a collimator. As we have seen in Section 4.2.3, for example, collimators are used with lasers with very small areas and therefore highly diverging beams—typically semiconductor and fiber lasers. They range from single injection-molded aspheres for diode lasers to water-cooled multi-element lenses for high-power fiber lasers. Figure 4.32 shows a typical aspheric collimator used with edge-emitting semiconductor lasers; many other COTS parts are also available from vendors such as Thorlabs, IPG Photonics, etc.

It is also important with the use of these lenses to remember what collimation is not. Specifically, even though the wavefronts coming from the collimator are planar in any direction, they are also expanding in diameter. If the lens is diffraction limited with low WFE, the beam divergence will be that given by Eq. (3.8), as diffraction ensures that there will always be some divergence and, as with Keplerian or Galilean expanders, the larger the collimated beam diameter the smaller the angle.

## 4.4 Homogenizers

Another common off-the-shelf component used in laser systems is a homogenizer. As shown in Fig. 4.33, homogenizers convert a Gaussian irradiance profile into something more uniform (or *homogeneous*) and are thus

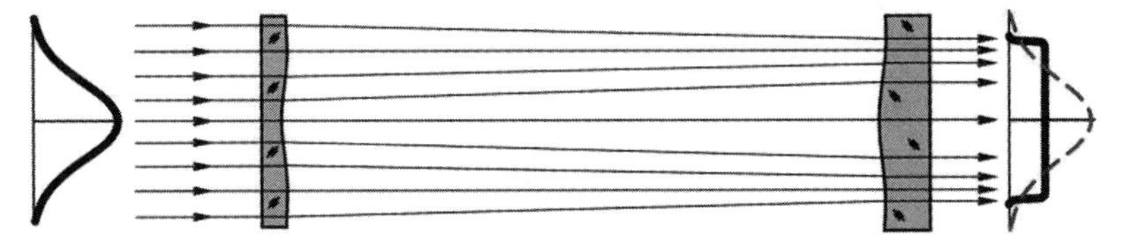

**Figure 4.33** A homogenizer converts a near-Gaussian power profile into a homogeneous (or "top-hat") profile. (Reprinted from Ref. 25.)

also known as "Gaussian to top-hat" converters or beam shapers. The motivation for using such components is that many laser-based processes require uniform illumination—photolithography exposure or materials processing tasks such as the machining of tight-tolerance holes,[24] for example.

Two architectures are available for homogenizers: refractive and microlens. The refractive architecture is shown in Fig. 4.33; it uses aspheric lenses to redirect power from the central core of the Gaussian into the edges.[25] Limitations on the use of refractive homogenizers are that the input beam be near-Gaussian ($M^2 \leq 1.4$, for example) and have a divergence less than some critical value (5 mrad, e.g.).

The microlens architecture uses a microlens array to sample an inhomogeneous profile such as a Gaussian beam (Fig. 4.34). The samples (of spacing $P_{LA1}$) are then recombined with diameter $D_{FT}$ at the focal plane (FP) of a focusing lens (FL), where their overlap reduces the inhomogeneity in a way that is less sensitive to the value of $M^2$ for the input beam. Disadvantages of the microlens homogenizers include higher optical loss and output divergence angle, and the potential for coherence effects (interference fringes and speckle) affecting uniformity due to the overlap of spatially coherent samples.[26]

For either refractive or microlens homogenizers, typical specs to consider include:

- Top-hat shape and homogeneity (%)
- Input beam $M^2$
- Alignment sensitivities and transmitted wavefront error
- Optical transmission (insertion) losses
- Optical power limits
- Output beam diameter $D$ or field size
- Output beam divergence $2\theta$
- Flat-top length (working distance) $L \sim \lambda D^2$
- Size, weight, cooling, etc.

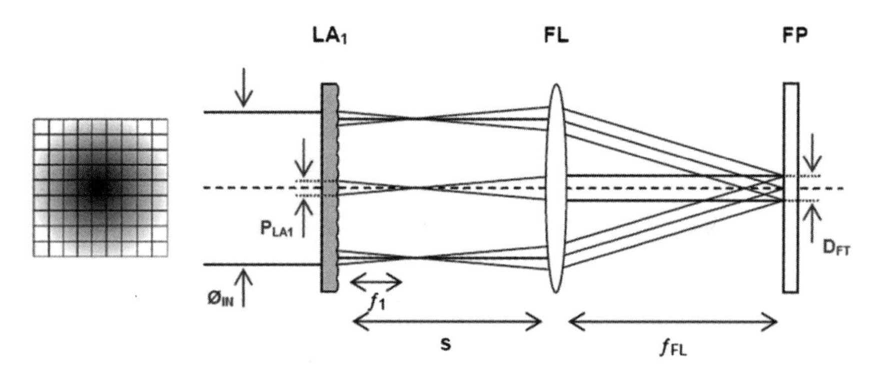


**Figure 4.34** A non-imaging homogenizer uses a microlens array ($LA_1$) to sample and recombine an inhomogeneous profile. (Reprinted from Ref. 26.)

## 4.5 Miscellaneous

Whether using focusing lenses, mirrors, beam expanders, collimators, homogenizers, and so on, a number of issues common to all laser system optics must be addressed. In this section, we review five of these issues in more detail, namely, material absorption, back-reflections, optical coatings, laser damage threshold, and polarization.

### 4.5.1 Material absorption

As we have seen in Section 4.1, low material absorption is required to reduce thermal lensing in windows; in addition, the optical power limits for beam expanders, homogenizers, and other optical components are determined in part by the absorption of the lenses used. The attenuation of light as it propagates through a material is determined by Beer's law:

$$P_{\mathrm{t}} = P_{\mathrm{i}} e^{-\alpha_{\mathrm{m}}(\lambda) d} \tag{4.18}$$

where the transmitted power $P_{\mathrm{t}}$ is smaller than the incident power $P_{\mathrm{i}}$ by an exponential factor that depends on the propagation distance $d$ and the material's attenuation coefficient $\alpha_{\mathrm{m}}(\lambda)$. The attenuation coefficient depends on wavelength $\lambda$ and consists of optical loss due to both absorption and scattering, but not that due to Fresnel surface reflections.[27]

If all of the attenuation is due to material absorption, then the absorbed power leads to a thermal heat load $P_{\mathrm{th}} = P_{\mathrm{i}} - P_{\mathrm{t}} = P_{\mathrm{i}}[1 - \exp(-\alpha_{\mathrm{m}} d)]$ on the optic. In general, it is not known from vendor data whether the attenuation is due to absorption or scattering, and a conservative assumption is that the attenuation is entirely due to absorption. High-power laser mirrors also have requirements on low absorption, and in this case the assumption is that any power that is not reflected is absorbed, giving $P_{\mathrm{th}} = P_{\mathrm{i}} - P_{\mathrm{r}}$ for a reflected power $P_{\mathrm{r}}$.

Some optical materials—silica optical fibers for long-haul telecommunications, for example—are extremely pure and have the lowest available attenuation coefficients ($\alpha_{\mathrm{m}} = 0.2$ dB/km $= 4.6 \times 10^{-7}$/cm at $\lambda = 1.55$ μm). Unfortunately, the selection of optical materials for the lens design of components such as beam expanders and homogenizers is limited. For example, it was not until relatively recently that low-absorption materials for high-power visible-wavelength laser systems were available, when laser-grade low-impurity ($<1$ part per million) and low-water-content fused silica (Suprasil or equivalent) was developed to replace conventional fused silica. Typical internal transmittance $T_{\mathrm{int}}$ for laser-grade fused silica is shown in Fig. 4.35. Note the logarithmic scale used to illustrate the extremely high transmittance—and thus low absorptance $A = 1 - T_{\mathrm{int}}$ of these materials for UV, visible, and NIR wavelengths.

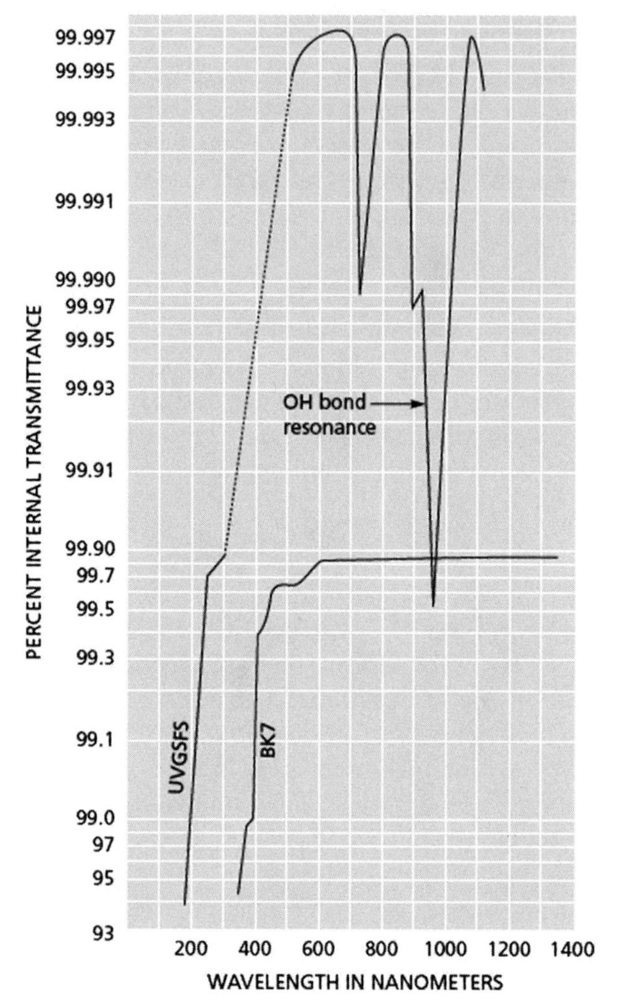


**Figure 4.35** Internal transmittance $T(\lambda) = P_t/P_i$ for UV-grade synthetic fused silica (UVGSFS) in comparison with BK7; sample thickness $d = 10$ mm. (Credit: CVI Laser, LLC.)

The availability of only one type of low-absorption material leads to lens-design challenges; however, new materials have recently been introduced to give lens designers more refractive-index options. These include a high-transmission (HT) version of a common crown material (SCHOTT's N-BK7) known as N-BK7HT, as well as high-index flints such as N-SF6HT. Fig. 4.36 compares the transmission of N-BK7 with its HT variant.

While N-BK7HT has somewhat better transmission in the UV, some applications—photolithography with ArF excimer lasers, for example—require much better transmission in the $\lambda = 200$- to 300-nm range. Materials developed for such applications include excimer-grade fused silica (such as HPFS 8650 from Corning) and calcium fluoride ($CaF_2$). An additional

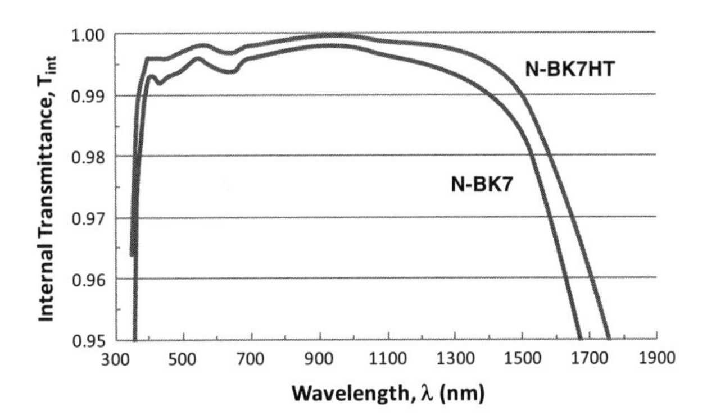


**Figure 4.36** Comparison of the internal transmittance of N-BK7 with N-BK7HT for a sample thickness $d = 25$ mm. (Data courtesy of SCHOTT.)

complication in materials selection for UV optics is the possibility of material fluorescence induced by high-energy UV photons, which the UV-grades typically reduce to near zero. Photodarkening due to impurity absorption from long-term exposure to UV light can also be an issue; see the manufacturers' literature for more details.

In addition to VIS- and UV-optimized materials, a number of laser systems use IR wavelengths; for these systems, HT IR-grade fused silica, germanium, sapphire, multispectral zinc sulfide (aka CLEARTRAN™), and zinc selenide (ZnSe) are available.

## 4.5.2 Back-reflections

In addition to excess absorption, unwanted reflections can also cause problems in laser systems; the most common of these is unintentional focusing of back-reflections from a lens surface. Shown in Fig. 4.37, for example, are the focused back-reflections of surfaces 6 and 8 to a location

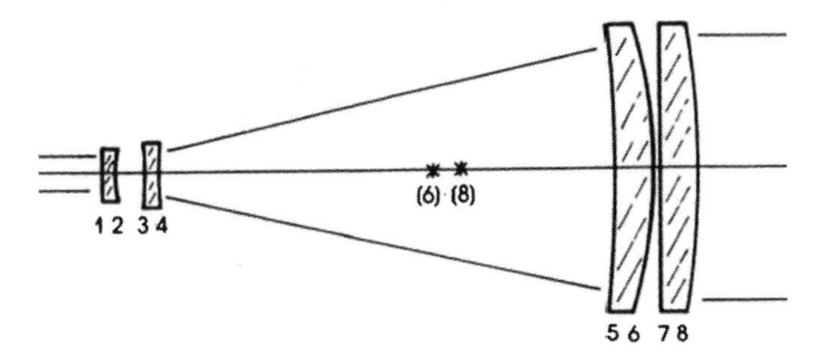


**Figure 4.37** Back-reflections from individual lens surfaces may focus on or near another lens with high power density. [Reprinted with permission from D. A. Roberts, "Laser Optics: Design Considerations," in *The Photonics Design and Applications Handbook*, Laurin Publishing, Pittsfield, Massachusetts (1988).]

between surfaces 4 and 5—exactly where they should be to avoid re-focusing of the beam onto (or near) a lens where it can do significant damage.

Based on the radius of curvature and the reflected beam diameter of surface 5, however, it turns out that the reflected wavefront focuses onto surface 4 and must therefore be changed. In contrast with incoherent systems where reflections image to an area, coherent reflections from a laser may re-image to a small, near-diffraction-limited waist with a potentially damaging power density ($W/m^2$), even with low-reflectivity coatings (Section 4.5.3).

### 4.5.3 Optical coatings

If the refractive index $n$ of a lens is relatively large, a high internal transmittance $T_{int}$ does not guarantee a large net (or external) transmittance. The reason is that the inherent Fresnel reflection loss $R_f$ from each surface of the lens reduces the amount of light transmitted:

$$R_f = \left[\frac{n(\lambda) - 1}{n(\lambda) + 1}\right]^2 \tag{4.19}$$

where this equation applies only at normal incidence [a 0-deg angle of incidence (AOI)] for a surface in air (with $n_{air} = 1$). For example, if $n = 1.5$, then $R_f = 0.04$ per surface, and the external transmittance $T_{ext} = T_{int} \times T_{refl} \approx T_{int}(1 - R_f)^2$ for two surfaces.

A common method for reducing surface reflections from their inherent Fresnel value is a single-layer antireflection (AR) coating. That is, a "thin," quarter-wave ($= \lambda/4n_f$) film of dielectric material—whose index $n_f$ is between that of the lens and the surrounding medium (typically air)—can be deposited on the surface of a lens; destructive interference between the reflections at each interface reduces the Fresnel surface-reflection loss to something much smaller (Fig. 4.38). The use of such coatings is clearly essential for reducing the effects of back-reflections. Magnesium fluoride ($MgF_2$) is the most common single-layer AR coating due to its low cost and near-optimal index ($n_f = 1.38$) for many lens materials with high transmission in the visible and NIR wavelengths.

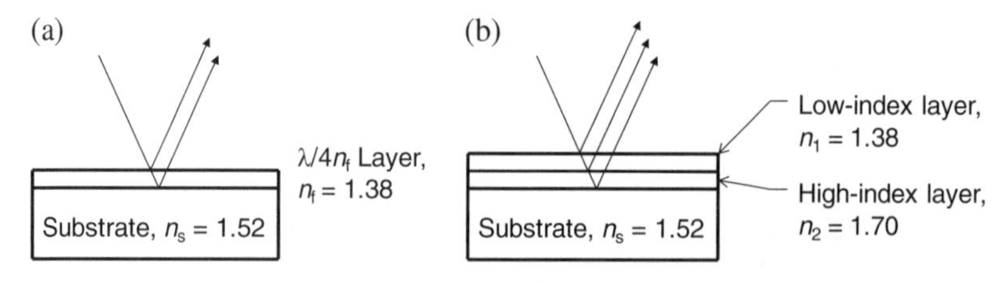


**Figure 4.38** (a) Single-layer and (b) two-layer dielectric coatings are commonly used to reduce the inherent Fresnel reflectivity of an optical surface.

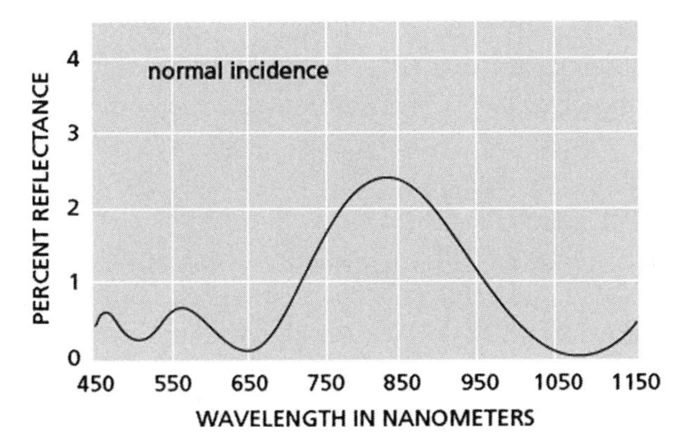


**Figure 4.39** A two-layer AR coating shows < 1% reflectivity at both the fundamental Nd:YAG wavelength (1064 nm) and the second harmonic (532 nm). (Credit: CVI Laser, LLC.)

Because the refractive index of $MgF_2$ does not exactly match the ideal index for zero reflectivity of a single-layer coating at all wavelengths for common visible-transmission glasses, more complex multilayer coatings to further reduce the surface reflection are also used [Fig. 4.38(b)]. A two-layer coating known as a V-coating, for example, has near-zero reflectivity at a specific laser wavelength; other types of coatings are designed for near-zero reflectivity at two wavelengths, with a varying reflectivity over the range between them (Fig. 4.39).

In addition to reflectivity, a number of additional specifications must be met for dielectric coatings; these are summarized in Table 4.6 and illustrate the complexity of thin-film coating design. Items unique to laser systems include:

- These coatings can be single or dual wavelength, as shown in Fig. 4.39.
- Coating performance is never perfect, so "leakage" will occur in either transmission or reflection. That is, a high-reflectivity (HR) dielectric

**Table 4.6** Typical specifications required for optical coatings used with laser system optics.

| Specification | Comments |
|---|---|
| Filter Type | Broadband, notch, two-color, etc. |
| Bandwidth, $\Delta\lambda$ (nm) | Specify value from peak (FWHM, 0.1%, etc.) |
| Wavefront Error (RMS) | Affected by coating stresses, substrate stiffness |
| Transmission or Reflection (%) | Over $\lambda$ at 0-deg AOI and operating temperature |
| Angle of Incidence, AOI (rad) | "Blue" shift with angle |
| Beam Convergence (rad) | "Blue" shift with numerical aperture |
| Temperature Range, $\Delta T$ (K) | "Red" shift with temperature |
| Leakage (%) | Residual transmission of reflective coatings, e.g. |
| Scattering (dB) | Increases with number of layers |
| Polarization | Polarization reflectivity and splitting with AOI |
| Durability | Scratch-dig, peel, salt spray, etc. |
| Laser Damage Threshold | Depends on coating deposition technology |

mirror coating will transmit a small amount of light, while an AR coating will reflect a small amount (Fig. 4.39). These residual transmissions and reflections may lead to problems if not quenched elsewhere in the system. Leakage of other wavelengths may also occur, and the unwanted transmission of 1064-nm light is the reason that frequency-doubled green (532 nm) laser pointers can be hazardous to the eye.

- Harsh environments such as manufacturing applications with evaporated or ablated material can result in splatter on a window or lens. Diamond-like carbon (DLC) coatings are sometimes used in such cases; alternatively, regular replacement of a damaged window is also an option.
- The surface finish at each coating interface results in scattering, so multilayer coatings with more interfaces generally scatter more light than single-layer coatings.
- The coating-deposition technology affects a number of important parameters. For example, high-energy ion-beam sputtering (IBS) results in compacted coatings with fewer adsorption sites and voids of a different character than e-beam coating technology. The choice of coating technology also affects coating adhesion and its susceptibility to laser-induced damage (Section 4.5.4).

In short, coating design should not be underestimated in the development of laser systems, for as Koechner has mentioned: "Multilayer films are often the weakest elements of any laser system."[1] The meaning of coating "weakness" is reviewed in the next section.

### 4.5.4 Laser damage threshold

As mentioned in Section 4.5.2, a large energy density (aka fluence, units of $J/cm^2$) or power density (irradiance, units of $W/cm^2$) can damage an optic or its coating. It's not necessary that the beam be tightly focused—an unfocused beam may be perfectly capable of damaging a material or coating if the incident fluence or irradiance exceeds a measured value known as either the laser damage threshold (LDT) or the laser-induced damage threshold (LIDT).

The material damage that occurs can range from melting to evaporation to cold ablation to fracture. For CW and QCW lasers with an average power $P_{avg}$, material absorption and the resulting heating is a key factor in determining damage; the LDT in this case is measured as a power density, as the incident power distributed over a small area has little area for heat transfer and thus causes a large temperature increase. A typical dielectric (nonmetallic) surface-damage LDT for Nd:YAG wavelengths ($\lambda = 1064$ nm) is $\approx$ 1–10 $MW/cm^2$ based on a CW or QCW $P_{avg}$, where the macroscopic mechanisms of heat transfer and energy balance—absorption coefficient, thermal mass, thermal conductivity, and so on[2]—affect the LDT.

With pulsed lasers, on the other hand, the LDT is measured as the energy density deposited by the pulse. Depending on the thermal diffusivity of the material, pulses with $\Delta t \geq 100$ psec or so cause thermal damage by absorption and thus increase the local temperature,[1] resulting in dielectric melting or boiling at a fluence on the order of 10–20 J/cm$^2$ for 20-nsec Nd:YAG pulses. For $\Delta t < 100$ psec, electron ionization and two-photon absorption resulting from the high peak power—and the resulting material breakdown and ablation without thermal damage—is the damage mechanism (which is also used to advantage with USP machining).

In all cases, material defects or imperfections that enhance the local electric field strength reduce the LDT.[28] Laser-induced damage usually occurs at a surface where scratches, digs, cracks, contamination (dust, polishing compound, condensates), and so on can reduce the LDT. Bulk damage can also occur if a beam is focused inside the material, where the heating of trapped air, water, impurities, metallic inclusions, defect sites, excess material absorption, or USP ablation can shatter the material; the LDT for bulk damage, however, will typically be higher than that for surface damage. Materials with a large bulk LDT include laser-grade fused silica, sapphire, and N-BK7.

In addition to (difficult to quantify) surface conditions, the LDT depends on a number of variables. If the pulse energy is constant, then the peak power is larger as the pulse width $\Delta t_p$ is reduced, with less time for heat transfer via thermal diffusion lowering the pulsed LDT:[29]

$$LDT \propto \lambda^m \sqrt{\Delta t_p} \qquad [\text{J/cm}^2] \tag{4.20}$$

thus placing an emphasis on using longer pulses to increase (improve) the LDT when thermal damage dominates ($\Delta t_p \geq 100$ psec). Equation (4.20) also shows that a shorter wavelength—for which each photon has higher energy [Eq. (1.2)], thus requiring fewer photons per pulse—also reduces the LDT, even if the material absorption is the same.[30] Also note that Eq. (4.20) is a proportionality, illustrating the scaling laws if the LDT is already known for a given $\Delta t_p$ and $\lambda$. For example, if the LDT = 10 J/cm$^2$ for a 20-nsec pulse, then a 10-nsec pulse with twice the peak power will reduce the damage threshold to 10 J/cm$^2$ $\times$ $(10/20)^{1/2} = 7.1$ J/cm$^2$.

If the peak power $P_{peak} = Q_p/\Delta t_p$ is constant and the pulse energy $Q_p$ varies, then the trend with pulse width goes in the opposite direction. That is, shorter pulses—with their lower pulse energy deposited on the material—have a larger LDT than longer pulses. For either constant pulse energy or peak power, the thermal damage predicted by Eq. (4.20) is valid for a pulse width $\Delta t_p \geq 0.1$ nsec and $\leq 0.1$ μsec; shorter pulses result in nonthermal (cold ablation) damage, whereas longer pulses are considered to be QCW. The measured damage may also depend on the number of pulses incident on a site, as the initial pulse may create nanoscopic damage that is then expanded to micro- or macroscopic damage by subsequent pulses; as a result, the number of pulses (or the PRF and exposure time) should also be specified for pulsed damage.

In addition to pulse width, wavelength, and number of pulses, the LDT also depends on the surface finish, where a smoother finish with a smaller $\delta_{RMS}$ has a higher LDT:

$$LDT \propto \frac{1}{\sqrt{\delta_{RMS}}} \tag{4.21}$$

illustrating that a smooth surface that has less enhancement of the local electric field strength increases the LDT. Extremely critical applications such as directed energy may thus require superpolished surfaces with $\delta_{RMS} \approx 2$ Å or less, reducing the surface scattering as well.

The method by which the surface is polished also affects the LDT. For example, subsurface damage results from conventional polishing techniques, where the use of an abrasive polishing compound leaves scratches, digs, and particulates *below* the surface after multiple passes of the polishing tool. Damage can then occur due to excess absorption (by the particulates) or electric field enhancement (by the scratches and digs). The use of an MRF polishing method is thought to reduce this damage,[31] although as we have seen in Section 4.2.5, this is at the expense of a possible increase in MSF surface errors.

There are, then, a large number of parameters that affect laser-induced damage. Summarizing the primary methods from this section (and elsewhere) for reducing laser damage:

- If possible, use a large beam area to reduce the incident irradiance, longer pulses (for a given pulse energy or fluence), and longer wavelengths.
- A smaller-diameter beam will likely irradiate fewer critical-defect sites than a larger-diameter beam, *increasing* the LDT if the incident irradiance is the same.
- Surface quality (scratch-dig) defect spec should be 20-10 or 10-5.
- Surface finish spec $\delta_{RMS} \leq 10$ Å.
- Use ion-assisted deposition (IAD) or ion-beam sputtering (IBS), which produces denser coatings with lower porosity, giving better environmental stability in a humid environment and fewer defect sites where damage can initiate; one disadvantage is greater sensitivity to coating stresses.
- Cleanliness: Dust, dirt, and residual polishing compound can ignite and cause damage at low fluence and should be removed.
- Surface polishing: Use MRF polishing to reduce subsurface damage.

- Use single-layer or rugate-based dielectric coatings whenever possible to avoid the electric-field enhancements that can occur at large-$\Delta n$ interfaces.
- Similarly, use AR subwavelength microstructures that increase the LDT with a slowly varying axial $\Delta n$ gradient, as has been reported by TelAztec LLC[32] and others.

This is an ongoing area of research, focusing on the surface and material imperfections that allow laser damage to initiate, and reminiscent of the improvements that were made in material quality in the early days of semiconductor lasers—improvements that allowed huge reductions in threshold current and increases in output power. It is expected that LDT research will continue to show similar improvements in material quality and LDT for both coatings and bulk materials.

### 4.5.5 Polarization

We have seen in Section 2.1.12 how a laser beam can be linearly or randomly polarized; to take advantage of—or at least not be penalized by—this laser property, the laser-system optics and their coatings must be able to accommodate or modify the polarization.

The effects of using a polarized laser are seen when the beam is incident on the optics at a non-normal angle, with an angle of incidence $\theta_i > 0$. In that case, the Fresnel reflectivity given by Eq. (4.19) now depends on $\theta_i$, incident refractive index $n_i$, and incident polarization:[33]

$$R_s = \left[\frac{\cos\theta_i - \sqrt{(n/n_i)^2 - \sin^2\theta_i}}{\cos\theta_i + \sqrt{(n/n_i)^2 - \sin^2\theta_i}}\right]^2 \tag{4.22}$$

$$R_p = \left[\frac{-(n/n_i)^2\cos\theta_i + \sqrt{(n/n_i)^2 - \sin^2\theta_i}}{(n/n_i)^2\cos\theta_i + \sqrt{(n/n_i)^2 - \sin^2\theta_i}}\right]^2 \tag{4.23}$$

which both reduce to Eq. (4.19) when $\theta_i = 0$ and $n_i = 1$. The equations assume that the beam reflections are governed by external reflection, i.e., a beam propagating in a low-index medium (air, e.g., with $n_i = 1$) incident on an optical component whose index $n > n_i$; the equations for internal reflection ($n < n_i$) are well known and available in the literature.[33]

The "s" and "p" subscripts in Eq. (4.22) and (4.23) refer to the incident polarization. This is shown in Fig. 4.40(a), where the horizontal and vertical components—as measured with respect to the laser—are now measured with respect to the optical component on which the beam is incident. Specifically, the plane of incidence and reflection—i.e., the plane of the page in Fig. 4.40(a), as determined by the propagation direction and the normal to the surface—is used as the reference.[34]

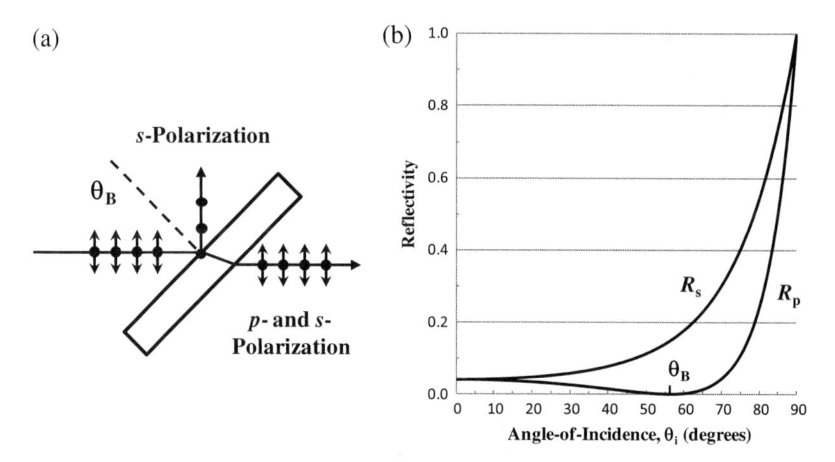


**Figure 4.40** External reflectance $R_s$ and $R_p$ for the *s*- and *p*-polarized components of the incident beam varies with incident angle $\theta_i$, with $R_p = 0$ for $\theta_i = \theta_B$ [given by Eq. (4.24)].

This change in reference also changes the vocabulary used to describe the incident polarization, with a horizontally polarized laser becoming an *s*-polarized beam [because it is perpendicular (*senkrecht* in German) to the plane of incidence] when incident on a window, lens, mirror, etc., as shown in Fig. 4.40(a) at an angle $\theta_i$. Similarly, the vertically polarized laser becomes a *p*-polarized beam when it is parallel to the plane of incidence.

The *s*- and *p*-polarized beams have a different reflectivity, and one that varies with incident angle. This is shown in Fig. 4.40(b), where Eqs. (4.22) and (4.23) are plotted versus incident angle $\theta_i$. An interesting (and useful) feature of the plots is the initial drop in the *p*-polarized reflectivity $R_p$, which reaches zero at an angle known as Brewster's angle $\theta_B$:

$$\theta_B = \tan^{-1}\frac{n}{n_i} \tag{4.24}$$

where Fig. 4.40(b) shows a Brewster's angle $\theta_B = \tan^{-1}(1.5/1) = 56.3$ deg for external reflection from a window with index $n = 1.5$ used in air. Physically, $\theta_B$ is the angle at which the radiating dipole excited by the incident electromagnetic field has no component in the direction of the reflected beam, hence giving zero reflectivity for *p*-polarized light.

A Brewster window—i.e., a plane-parallel plate placed at Brewster's angle (see Figs. 2.34 and 2.35)—is commonly used in free-space (solid-state or gas) lasers to insure linearly polarized output. To understand why, the lack of reflection at Brewster's angle for *p*-polarized light in Fig. 4.40(b) implies nearly 100% transmission for a low-absorption window. This contrasts with *s*-polarized light, which has 15% reflection loss at Brewster's angle and therefore only 85% transmission at best. Assuming that the window or gain-medium absorption does not change the dominant loss, the lower-loss polarization will be the first to lase, thus ensuring laser output of *p*-polarized light. The laser can then be specified as being either vertically or horizontally polarized, depending on how the mounting surface is oriented with respect to this output (see Problem 4.14).

Once outside the laser, however, a Brewster window is not a particularly efficient way of modifying the polarization. This is shown in Fig. 4.40(b), where the reflected beam at Brewster's angle is *s*-polarized with a high polarization extinction ratio (PER), but only 15% of the incident power is reflected.

A lower-loss method of polarization splitting—used to separate *s*- and *p*-polarized beams for power measurement with different detectors, for example—is a polarizing beamsplitter (PBS), where two prisms are bonded together to send *p*-polarized light in a direction that is perpendicular to the *s*-polarized light.[35] These are based on a multilayer thin-film optical coating on the surface of one of the prisms to create a succession ("pile of plates") of Brewster polarizers. Small-aperture ($\leq$ 20 mm) PBS cubes are available with a loss of $\leq$ 5% for each polarization, and a $PER_R \equiv R_s/R_p = 10{:}1$ to 50:1 for the reflected (*s*-polarized) component and $PER_T \equiv T_p/T_s = 200{:}1$ to 1000:1 for the transmitted (*p*-polarized) component.

Because of the AOI dependence of $R_s$ and $R_p$, the dominant errors in the use of these devices for narrow-band laser systems are most often due to angular misalignments between the laser and the PBS. The LDT can also be an issue when the two prisms in a PBS are bonded using optical cement; however, adhesive-free (optical contact) bonding or thin-film plate beamsplitters are available with a CW LDT up to 1 MW/cm$^2$ at $\lambda = 1064$ nm.

A number of other polarization-splitting options using two birefringent crystals such as calcite or $MgF_2$ are also available. With different refraction angles for the *s*- and *p*-polarizations, these don't rely on Brewster's angle and as a result have a much larger $PER_T$ and acceptance angle than a thin-film PBS. Sold commercially as Glan–Thompson, Rochon, and Wollaston prisms, they are available as either polarizers or polarization splitters, with $PER_T \geq 10^5{:}1$, $T_s \geq 95\%$, and $T_p \geq 90\%$ for the splitters, but a CW LDT of only 10 W/cm$^2$ or so at $\lambda = 1064$ nm. One difference between these three types of splitters is in the angular deviation—and therefore susceptibility to interference fringing from its own back-reflections—of the output polarizations with respect to the entrance face and each other; another is that the $PER_R$ is not as large for the Glan–Thompson beamsplitter as it is for the Rochon and Wollaston.

In addition to polarizing beamsplitters, there are a number of other components that may be needed in laser systems requiring polarization control, including Glan-laser prism polarizers, sheet polarizers and analyzers, circular polarizers, waveplates and retarders, isolators, and so on; for more details, vendor catalogs and Ref. 35 are excellent resources.

All of these components will use a thin-film AR coating to reduce the Fresnel surface losses; stress birefringence (i.e., the change in coating index $n$ with stress $\sigma$, or $dn/d\sigma$) can change the polarization states, putting requirements on the design of the coating as well as the mechanical stiffness of the component.

The coating specs must also take into account the variation of $R_s$ and $R_p$ with incident angle. This is particularly difficult for optical components with curved surfaces, i.e., lenses and mirrors where the angle of incidence of the beam varies across the diameter of the optic. Quantifying this effect is typically a task for the laser system optical engineer, where the variation of $R_s$ and $R_p$ across a lens diameter may need to be modeled in Zemax, Code V, Polaris, or some other optical design software. As we will see in Chapter 5, this variation in incidence angle—and therefore polarization properties—is also seen when the beam or the optics are scanned.

## 4.6 Problems

**4.1** A window is 2-mm thick and has a refractive index $n = 1.5$. What coherence length is needed from the laser to avoid coherent interference? What lasers meet this requirement?

**4.2** Add to Table 4.2 to include all the materials used in Fig. 4.4. Based on the simple model of Eq. (4.1), which material has the least thermal lensing?

**4.3** Would you expect that a Hermite–Gaussian beam with $M^2 > 1$ has $1f$:$1f$ conjugates? Can you prove it one way or the other, either algebraically or numerically?

**4.4** For an incoherent source, the $2f$:$2f$ object–image conjugates also have an image magnification $m_i = 1$, such that the image size is the same as the object. For a lens with $f = 100$ mm and a Gaussian beam with $M^2 = 1$ and $z_R = 10$ mm, what is the magnification at the $1f$:$1f$ conjugates? What conjugate distances give $m_i = 1$?

**4.5** Looking at Fig. 4.14, we see that there is a maximum image distance $z_2$ for a given ratio of $z_R/f$. What is this image distance, the corresponding object distance $z_1$, and how do they both depend on $z_R$? At what $z_1$ and $z_2$ does the maximum occur?

**4.6** If the curvature of a Gaussian wavefront can be measured, is there a unique distance to the waist? What else do we need to know to find a unique distance?

**4.7** We saw in Section 4.2.2 that a truncation $T = 1$ reduces the peak on-axis irradiance by a factor of 2.5. How much is the peak irradiance reduced if the truncation is changed to $T = 0.658$?

**4.8** If a rectangular focusing mirror is sufficiently large to reflect the $1/e^2$ beam diameter in only one dimension—the beam is truncated in the other dimension—what is the shape of the focused spot?

**4.9** Can a high-order Hermite–Gaussian beam with poor $M^2$ be homogenized to have much better beam quality? If so, what are the disadvantages of doing so?

**4.10** What is the value of the PSD frequency exponent $B$ for the data in Fig. 4.29? Given this value, what is the RMS surface ripple in units of nanometers? Use an integration range of $f_s = 6$ to $10^3$ cycles/m.

**4.11** For a fabrication surface figure WFE $= \lambda/20$ RMS, what is the Strehl ratio? If the MSF error $y_{MSF} = \lambda/100$, what is the Strehl ratio? Which error dominates?

**4.12** Given that the material absorptance $A = 1 - T_{int}$, what is $A$ in terms of the attenuation coefficient $\alpha_m(\lambda)$?

**4.13** If the peak power $P_{peak}$ is constant, does the LDT increase or decrease as the wavelength is reduced from $\lambda = 1$ μm to 0.5 μm? By how much does it change?

**4.14** For the laser shown in Fig. 2.35, is the output beam vertically or horizontally polarized?

## Notes and References

1. W. Koechner, *Solid-State Laser Engineering*, Springer-Verlag, Berlin, Chapter 7 (1996).
2. K. J. Kasunic, *Optomechanical Systems Engineering*, John Wiley & Sons, Hoboken, New Jersey, Chapter 8 (2015). Not included in this equation are thermal expansion and stress-optic effects—see Ref. 1 for more details.
3. N. W. Wallace and M. A. Kahan, "First-order thermo-optical and optomechanical wavefront error analysis," *Proc. SPIE* **3030**, 109–120 (1997) [doi: 10.1117/12.284052]. This analysis does not include stress-optic effects ($dn/d\sigma$), which create an additional (typically small) change in index.
4. Sapphire is birefringent—that is, it has a refractive index that varies with the polarization of the incident electromagnetic field—but the value for $G$ listed here is representative.
5. C. A. Klein, "Materials for high-power laser optics: Figures of merit for thermally induced beam distortions," *Optical Engineering* **36**(6), 1586–1595 (1997) [doi: 10.1117/12/294473].

6. Physically, the wavefront curvature and beam diameter exiting the lens are sufficient to determine the image waist location $z_2$ and size $w_{02}$. This is a key difference between Gaussian and incoherent beams whose wavefront curvature alone determines the geometrical image location. In addition, the beam diameter exiting a thin lens is the same as that incident, and the simultaneous solution of Eqs. (3.2) and (3.3) results in Eq. (4.4), which is used to find $z_2$.

7. S. A. Self, "Focusing of spherical Gaussian beams," *Applied Optics* **22**(5), 658–661 (1983).

8. In Ref. 7, it is shown that the maximum image distance $z_2$ occurs at $z_1 = z_R + f$; the additional factor of 1.5 is included based on this author's numerical simulations.

9. Truncation data was obtained from http://www.silloptics.de/english/printable/products/laser-optics/technical-informations/index.php.

10. A. E. Siegman, *Lasers*, University Science Books, Sausalito, California, Chapter 18 (1986).

11. W. J. Smith, *Modern Optical Engineering*, Fourth Edition, McGraw-Hill, New York (2008).

12. R. R. Shannon, *The Art and Science of Optical Design*, Cambridge University Press, Cambridge (1997).

13. J. A. Ruff and A. E. Siegman, "Measurement of beam quality degradation due to spherical aberration in a simple lens," *Optical and Quantum Electronics* **26**, 629–632 (1994).

14. H. Sun, "Beam circularization and astigmatism-correction," Laser Diode Technical Note 1, Coherent Inc. (1998), http://www.coherent.com/downloads/LaserDiodeTechNote1.pdf.

15. The conversion from PV to RMS depends on the area weighting of the surface errors, such that $SFE_{RMS} = (\sum w_i SFE_i^2)^{1/2}$, where $SFE_i$ is the PV surface error for each area element with area $A_i$, and $w_i = A_i/A_t$ for a total area of the optic $A_t$. In addition, the $SFE_i$ must first be adjusted to give an area-weighted mean $\overline{SFE} = 0$. Also, see Fig. 4.30 for an RMS surface roughness calculation.

16. T. S. Ross, *Laser Beam Quality Metrics*, SPIE Press, Bellingham, Washington (2013) [doi: 10.1117/3.1000595].

17. G. Golnik, "Directed Energy Systems," in *The Infrared and Electro-Optical Systems Handbook* Vol. **8**, S. R. Robinson, Ed., ERIM, Ann Arbor, Michigan and SPIE Press, Bellingham, Washington, Chapter 5 (1993).

18. R. E. Parks, "Specifications: figure and finish are not enough," *Proc. SPIE* **7071**, 70710B (2008) [doi: 10.1117/12.798223].

19. T. Hull, M. J. Riso, J. M. Barentine, and A. Magruder, "Mid-spatial frequency matters: examples of the control of the power spectral density and what that means to the performance of imaging systems," *Proc. SPIE* **8353**, 835329 (2012) [doi: 10.1117/12.921097].

20. The correct units for the vertical axis of the PSD plot are actually energy spectral density (ESD). The reason is that the $L^2$ units are proportional to the strain energy $U = ½ky^2$ of a spring or surface for a distortion $y$. If this energy were a function of time (rather than spatial frequency), the units would be energy per unit time, giving power. Unfortunately, common use has adapted the PSD nomenclature for similarity with other PSD concepts found in detector noise[22] and vibration theory,[2] where the spectrum is temporal, not spatial.

21. A. B. Shorey, D. Golini, and W. Kordonski, "Surface finishing of complex optics," *Optics and Photonic News*, **18**(10), pp. 14–16 (2007).

22. K. J. Kasunic, *Optical Systems Engineering*, McGraw-Hill, New York, Chapter 6 (2011).

23. W. R. Sooy, "Lasers and optics: An overview," *Proc. SPIE* **69**, 3 (1975) [doi: 10.1117/12.954540]. In this reference it is stated that "In clear air the threshold for breakdown at 10 μm wavelength is about $10^9$ W/cm$^2$, and it scales inversely with the square of the wavelength. In ordinary dirty air the threshold at 10 μm reduces to $10^7$ W/cm$^2$ or lower. Once initiated, breakdown can be sustained at much lower irradiances—between $10^4$ and $10^5$ W/cm$^2$ at 10 μm."

24. K. Du, "Thin layer ablation with lasers of different beam profiles—energy efficiency and over-filling factor," *Proc. SPIE* **7202**, 72020Q (2009) [doi: 10.1117/12.810158].

25. A. Laskin and V. Laskin, "Refractive beam shapers for material processing with high power single mode and multimode lasers," *Proc. SPIE* **8600**, 860010 (2013) [doi: 10.1117/12.2001390].

26. R. Voelkel and K. J. Weible, "Laser beam homogenizing: Limitations and constraints," *Proc. SPIE* **7102**, 71020J (2008) [doi: 10.1117/12.799400].

27. In addition, the incident power is that on the surface after Fresnel reflection loss, and the transmitted power is that before Fresnel losses are included.

28. N. Bloembergen, "Role of cracks, pores, and absorbing inclusions on laser induced damage threshold at surfaces of transparent dielectrics," *Applied Optics* **12**(4), 661–664 (1973).

29. It would seem that the constant pulse energy would not change the LDT. However, for pulses in the 0.1-nsec to 0.1-μsec range, thermal diffusion of heat away from the beam affects the LDT. Specifically, we can think of *deposited* energy as a balance between the absorbed pulse energy ($\sim \alpha_m P_{peak}\ \Delta t$ = constant) and the thermally diffused energy, with shorter pulses having less time [$\sim (\Delta t)^{1/2}$] to axially or radially diffuse the same pulse energy.

30. Reference 1 quotes a wavelength exponent $m = 0.43$ for thermal damage, though given the potential for electron ionization and $N$-photon absorption, this will depend on the wavelength range. For nonthermal ablative damage, data from the SCHOTT Laser Grade N-BK7HT data sheet indicates $m \approx 2$ for $\Delta t_p = 74$ psec; also see R. Jedamzik and F. Elsmann, "Recent results on bulk laser damage threshold of optical glasses," *Proc. SPIE* **8603**, 860305 (2013) [doi: 10.1117/12.2000646].

31. R. Williamson, *Field Guide to Optical Fabrication*, SPIE Press, Bellingham, Washington, p. 58 (2011) [doi: 10.1117/3.892101].

32. D. C. Hobbs and B. D. MacLeod, "High laser damage threshold surface relief micro-structures for anti-reflection applications," *Proc. SPIE* **6720**, 672001 (2007) [doi: 10.1117/12.754223]. Note that the pulse-width results reported in this paper do not appear to scale according to Eq. (4.20), possibly due to the extremely high thermal dissipation of the micro-structures. Clearly, Eq. (4.21) is also not valid for these structures.

33. E. Hecht, *Optics*, Fourth Edition, Addison Wesley, Reading, Massachusetts, Chapter 4 (2001).

34. Alternatively, we can think of the plane of the optic as defining the reference plane, with the *s*-polarization shown in Fig. 4.40(a) "sliding" off of the surface and the *p*-polarization "plunging" through it.

35. P. C. D. Hobbs, *Building Electro-Optical Systems*, Second Edition, John Wiley& Sons, Hoboken, New Jersey, Chapter 6 (2009).

# Chapter 5
# Beam Scanning

It is often said that lasers allow directed energy "at the speed of light." While this is true along the direction of beam propagation, it is clearly not the case perpendicular to the beam, where beam scanning, tracking speed, and pointing stability are still (usually) limited by mechanical steering of a two-axis (azimuth-elevation, or "Az-El") gimbal[1,2]—see Fig. 5.1.

While gimbals are useful for scanning through a large field-of-regard (FOR), a typical beam control subsystem for a smaller FOR might look like that shown in Fig. 5.2. The figure shows a two-axis scan system for manufacturing that changes the angle of a beam incident on a focusing lens, rather than changing the pointing of the laser itself. This change in the angle of the beam reflected off of one of the flat mirrors by $\Delta\theta$ results in a scan of the focused spot by $\Delta y = f \times \Delta\theta$.

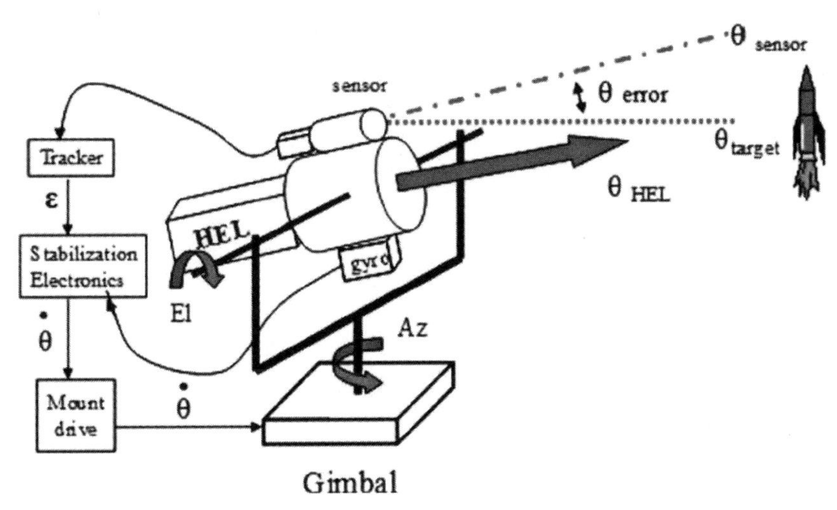


**Figure 5.1** Angular beam scanning over a large field-of-regard requires mechanical steering components such as a gimbal. [Reprinted from P. H. Merritt and J. R. Albertine, "Beam control for high-energy laser devices," *Optical Engineering*, **52**(2), 021005 (2013).]

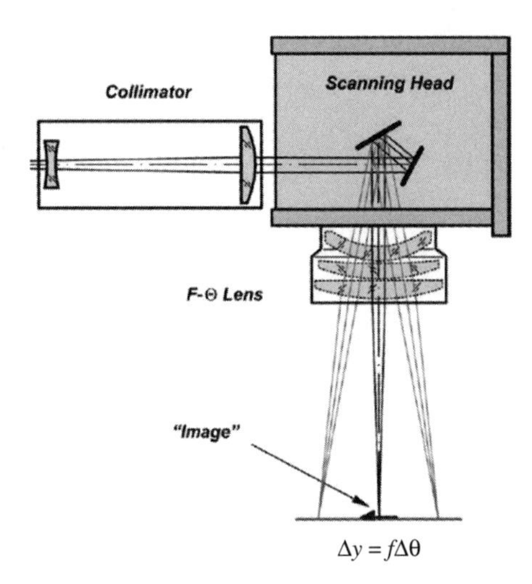


**Figure 5.2** Rotating mirrors in the scanning head change the angle of the beam incident on the focusing lens by $\Delta\theta$, scanning the focused beam through a distance $\Delta y = f \times \Delta\theta$. [Reprinted from A. Laskin and V. Laskin, "Refractive beam shapers for material processing with high power single mode and multimode lasers," *Proc. SPIE* **8600**, 860010 (2013).]

One immediate benefit of rotating a mirror to change the direction of a beam is that the angular deflection of the beam is 2× the mechanical rotation $\Delta\theta_m$ of the mirror. That is,

$$\Delta\theta = 2\Delta\theta_m \qquad [\text{rad}] \tag{5.1}$$

This is a result of the law that the angle of reflection equals the angle of incidence (with both angles measured with respect to the surface normal); consequently, turning a flat mirror by 1 deg deflects the beam reflecting off of it by 2 deg. This simple law is an enormous advantage in favor of the use of mirrors for scanning.

Another advantage is that the mirrors are much smaller and lighter than the laser or any gimbal it may be mounted on. Mirror scanning is thus much easier—in terms of size, speed, precision, etc.—for a smaller FOR than trying to move the platform or the laser itself.

This chapter reviews the scan technologies available for scanning and beam control. Included are a brief discussion of the various types of scanners (Section 5.1) as well as the mirrors and lenses (Section 5.2) and system trades involved with their practical use (Section 5.3). Beam control is an extensive topic, and we only review a small subset of it in this chapter: beam pointing, nongimbaled hardware configurations, and their advantages and errors.

## 5.1 Scan Technologies

The technologies available for scanning are numerous;[3,4] in this section, we review those that will be used 90% of the time in laser system development.

Included are galvanometers, polygon scanners, and MEMS scanners, as well as miscellaneous technologies that have advantages for a narrower range of applications.[5]

### 5.1.1 Galvanometers

A galvanometer—or "galvo" or "paddle," labeled as "X-Axis Scanner" and "Y-Axis Scanner" in Fig. 5.3—oscillates a flat mirror, off which a laser beam is reflected. The single-axis oscillation is driven by a high-torque, low-inertia motor, which is connected to the mirror with a torsionally stiff shaft. As indicated by Eq. (5.1), a mechanical rotation of 1 deg of the motor axis changes the direction of the beam by 2 deg. Either the mechanical or optical scan angle may be specified in vendor catalogs, so caution is advised in reading these

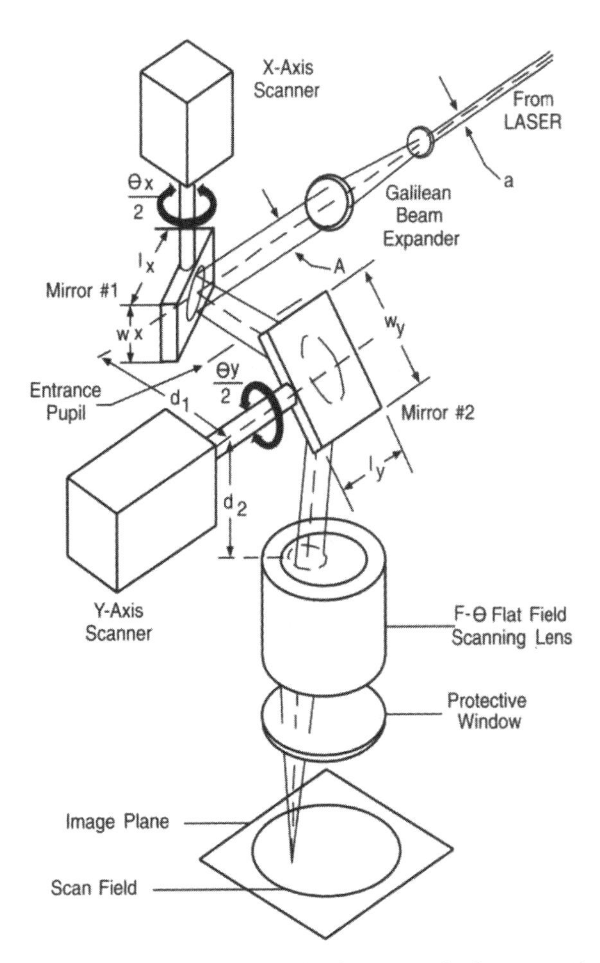


**Figure 5.3** Galvanometers are used in pairs for two-axis ($x$-$y$ or $r$-$\theta$) scanning over a maximum FOR of approximately ±45 deg (optical). (Credit: Special Optics, a Navitar Company; reprinted with permission.)

catalogs. Galvos are used in pairs for two-axis ($x$-$y$ or $r$-$\theta$) scanning; maximum scan angles are on the order of ±45 deg (optical). The mirror flatness can be affected by the scan rate and incident laser irradiance, a topic we look at in more detail in Section 5.2. In addition, for reasons we will explore in Section 5.3.4, the mirrors are placed as close to each other as their geometry allows.

Both closed-loop galvos with position feedback and open-loop resonant galvos are common.[6] The closed-loop response time is limited by the motor torque and mirror inertia, with small-angle response times as small as 0.2 msec and full-angle bandwidths up to 2 kHz (depending on scan angle and mirror inertia); resonant galvos can scan sinusoidal or triangular patterns at oscillation rates up to 18 kHz (also dependent on scan angle and mirror inertia). Closed-loop and resonant scanners are often combined for fast (resonant) raster line scanning in one direction with a slower scan in the other; typical specs for both types of scanners are given in Table 5.1.

In addition to range, resolution, and repeatability, the along-scan jitter and cross-scan wobble can limit the positioning of a galvo. These concepts are illustrated in Fig. 5.4 for an ideal scan that consists of three equally spaced steps. The jitter is the difference in angular position from ideal in the direction of the scan; when used with a focusing lens such as that shown in Fig. 5.2,

**Table 5.1** Typical performance specs for closed-loop galvos and resonant, polygon, and nonresonant 2D MEMS scanners.[7] (RPM is revolutions per minute.)

| Property | Closed-Loop | Resonant | Polygon | 2D MEMS |
|---|---|---|---|---|
| Range, $\theta$ (optical) | ±45 deg | ±8 deg | <720/$n_f$ deg | ±24 deg |
| Resolution | 2–50 μrad | NA | NA | <1 mrad |
| Repeatability | 4–100 μrad | NA | NA | 10 μrad |
| Step Time | 0.2–1 msec | NA | NA | 0.1–1 msec |
| Speed | 2 kHz | 100 Hz–18 kHz | 1–100 kRPM | 1–40 kHz |
| Mirror size, $D$ | 2–100 mm | 3–50 mm | 2–50 mm | 0.8–5 mm |
| Jitter (optical) | 1–50 μrad | <1 μrad[3] | $\Delta v/v \approx$ 0.01–1% | - |
| Wobble (optical) | 2–25 μrad | <1 μrad[3] | 10–200 μrad | - |
| Offset Drift | 1–50 μrad/K | 0.01%/K | NA | - |

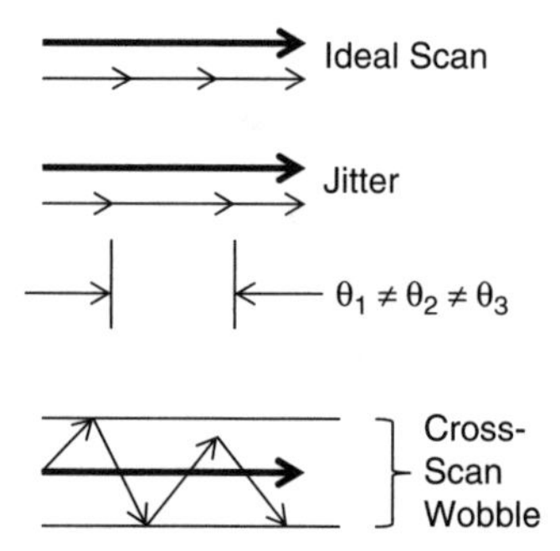


**Figure 5.4** Along-scan jitter and peak-to-peak cross-scan wobble (or "dynamic track").

jitter results in a positional variation $\Delta y = f \times \Delta\theta$ and a velocity variation $\Delta v = \Delta y/\Delta t = f \times \Delta\theta/\Delta t$. Wobble limits the positional resolution perpendicular to the scan and, depending on the blur size from the optics, may therefore may dominate the image resolution in the cross-scan direction.

### 5.1.2 Polygon scanners

The introduction of high-PRF lasers with ultrashort pulses has led to the need for ultrafast scanners. Galvanometers are usually too slow for these lasers, in which case a polygon scanner is used. Polygon scanners consist of a motor that continuously rotates a faceted cylinder—a polygon—about a single axis in the same direction. Each facet is a mirror that scans the beam over a sample, target, or focusing lens (Fig. 5.5); depending on the rotational speed, the polygon is made of aluminum or copper for slow speeds, or a stiffer metal such as beryllium for higher speeds.

The angle over which the polygon scans depends on the number of facets $n_f$. A mechanical rotation $\Delta\theta_m$ of 360 deg ($2\pi$ rad) results in an optical scan angle $\Delta\theta$ of

$$\Delta\theta = \eta \frac{4\pi}{n_f} \qquad \text{[rad]} \tag{5.2}$$

where a geometric efficiency factor $\eta$ has also been included, since the beam cannot be scanned when the beam diameter overlaps the intersections of the facets (Fig. 5.6).

The efficiency factor $\eta$ thus depends on

$$\eta = 1 - \frac{1.5 D_{1/e^2}}{W} \tag{5.3}$$

for a beam diameter $D_{1/e^2}$ and facet width (mirror size) $W$ along the scan direction. The thickness of the facet must also be sufficient to fully reflect the 1%-truncated beam based on $1.5 D_{1/e^2}$.

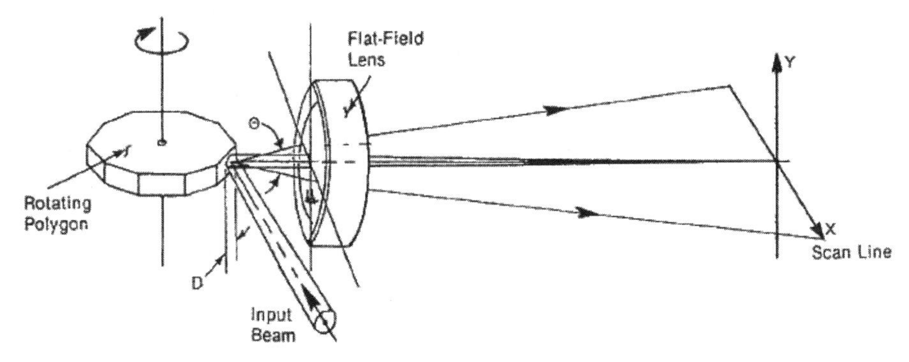


**Figure 5.5** A rotating polygon scanner continuously translates a beam over the surface of a focusing lens and image plane. [Reprinted from L. Beiser, *Laser Scanning Notebook*, SPIE Press, Bellingham, Washington (1992).]

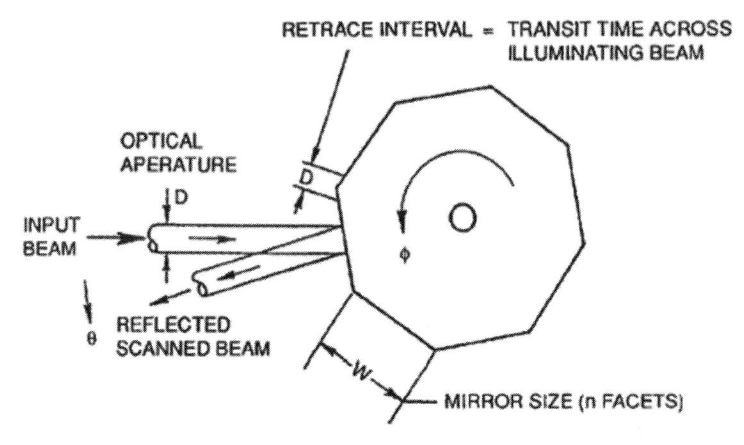


**Figure 5.6** A beam cannot be scanned during the time it takes for a new facet to move into a scan position. This time period is called a "retrace interval" and depends on the beam diameter *D* and mirror size *W*. [Reprinted from L. Beiser, *Laser Scanning Notebook*, SPIE Press, Bellingham, Washington (1992).]

Available scan speeds range from about 500 RPM for barcode scanning to 100K RPM for applications such as laser printers, manufacturing, etc., where a large area must be covered quickly. High-RPM scanners are very expensive, with the polygons mounted in evacuated chambers to reduce air drag. Reducing drag forces is important not because a large acceleration is required; instead, scan-speed stability is a critical specification for polygon scanners, with $\Delta v/v \approx 0.01$–1% being typical stability specs.

Errors in mirror facet angle also affect the scan angle. Random facet-to-facet errors on the order of 5–100 μrad are possible, leading to scan angle errors of 10–200 μrad; additional specs for polygon scanners are shown in Table 5.1.

### 5.1.3 MEMS scanners

Two scan mirrors—either galvanometer, polygon, or a combination—are extremely inconvenient in terms of size, weight, power consumption, and optical design. Miniaturization of a two-axis scan system—along the lines of size reductions of digital SLR cameras into smartphones—is thus an important trend for beam control technologies. The manufacturing process that allows such miniaturization for scanners is known as *micro-electromechanical systems* (MEMS).

Two types of MEMS scanners are available: digital and analog; both use aluminum- or gold-coated silicon mirrors to deflect a beam. The digital MEMS device shown in Fig. 5.7 consists of an array of mirrors that point in one of two directions to reflect light either into or out of a projection lens. When used in desktop or large-scale cinema projectors, the projection lens relays an image of the MEMS array onto a screen, where on-off mirror

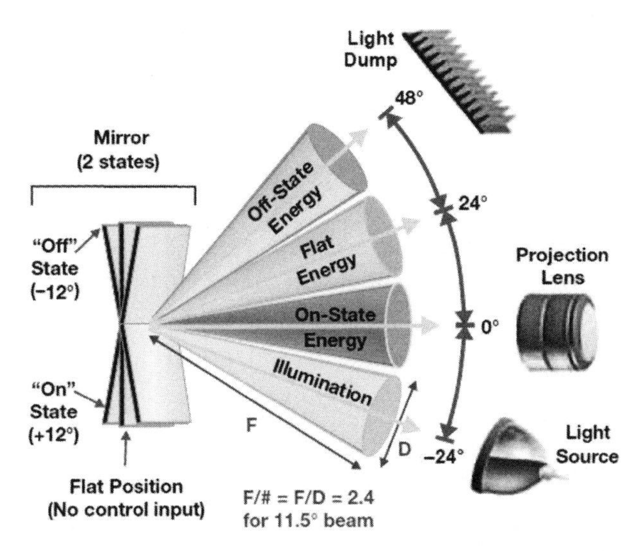


**Figure 5.7** One mirror in an array is shown redirecting light into or out of a video projection lens; each silicon mirror is as small as 10.8 μm × 10.8 μm in size. (Credit: Texas Instruments Inc.; reprinted with permission.)

scanning is synchronized with modulated red, green, and blue lasers (or LEDs) to create a color video image (such as an XGA 1024 × 768 format).

Further miniaturization is possible with the use of analog MEMS mirrors. That is, by using a single, two-axis (tip-tilt) mirror to raster scan a video image onto a wall or screen, an array of on-off mirrors is not required, nor is a projection lens. With MEMS mirror sizes on the order of 1 mm (Fig. 5.8), near-eye wearables, head-up displays, and hand-held pico-projectors have been developed using analog MEMS scanners[8]—miniaturized versions of the fast-steering mirrors (FSMs) used for many years in high-speed optical

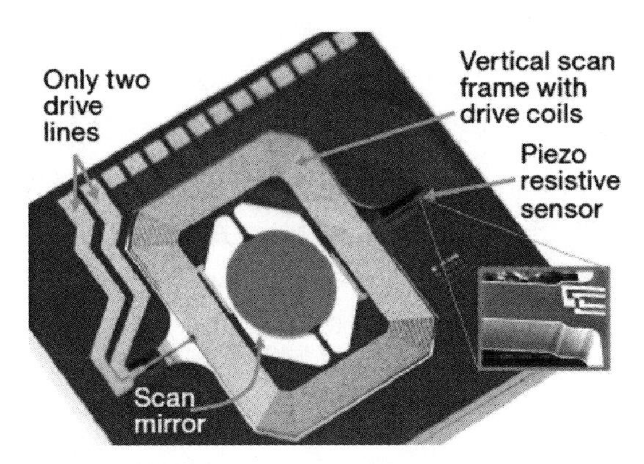


**Figure 5.8** A two-axis (tip-tilt) silicon mirror to raster or vector scan a laser beam is fabricated using MEMS processes. [Reprinted from M. Freeman, M. Champion, and S. Madhavan, "Scanned laser pico-projectors: Seeing the big picture (with a small device)," *Optics and Photonics News* **20**(5), 28–34 (2009).]

systems.[9] Typical specs for 2D analog MEMS scanners are shown in Table 5.1.

In addition to the obvious advantages of reductions in size, weight, and power consumption, analog MEMS scanners have the disadvantage of limited optical resolution. That is, because the mirror sizes are restricted to approximately 1–4 mm, the $1/e^2$ Gaussian beam diameter incident on the mirror cannot be larger than approximately 0.6–2.5 mm (i.e., 1.5× smaller than the mirror size) to avoid truncation and near-field ripple. The far-field divergence angle is therefore fairly large—with $2\theta_o = 4\lambda/\pi D_{1/e^2} \approx 1$ mrad for $D_{1/e^2} = 0.6$ mm and $\lambda = 0.5$ μm—as is the spot size if the scanner is used with a focusing lens.

### 5.1.4 Miscellaneous technologies

In addition to the use of MEMS for miniaturization, there are two additional trends for beam control technologies: nonmechanical scanning[10] and ultrafast devices.

Nonmechanical scanning relies on the concept of "no moving parts" to scan a beam. This has traditionally been done with acousto-optic (AO) scanners (Fig. 5.9); while fast, these scanners are expensive, inefficient, have a limited range and resolution, and can only accept a small input beam—a restriction for use in free-space laser communications and IR countermeasures (IRCM).

An approach to nonmechanical beam steering over a larger aperture is the use of liquid crystal on silicon (LCOS) refractive-index optical phased arrays (OPAs).[11] While these devices have good resolution, their angular range is limited. An increase in range can be obtained with the use of liquid crystal

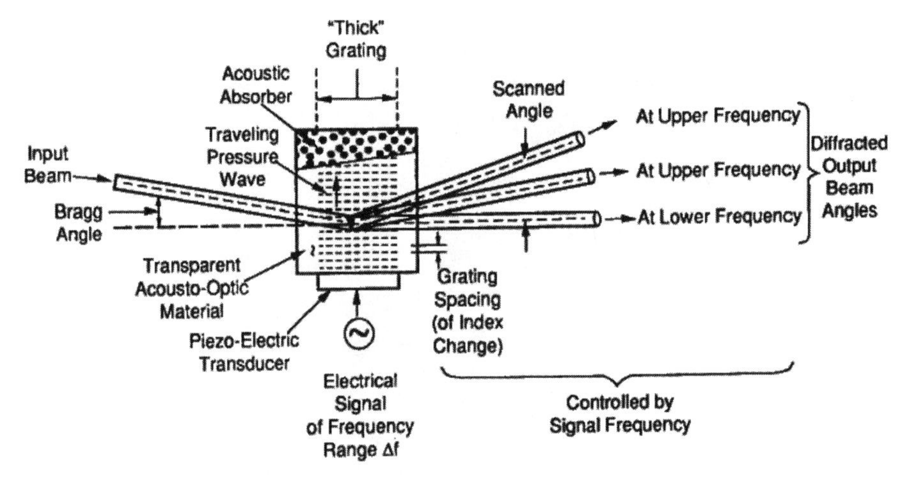


**Figure 5.9** Acousto-optic (AO) scanners use an acoustic wave to create an index grating and therefore control the scan angle to approximately ±3 deg. (Reprinted from Ref. 3.)

polarization gratings (LCPGs) developed by Boulder Nonlinear Systems, a technology that has recently been introduced in commercial products.[12]

Ultrafast scanners are being pushed by the development of ultrafast lasers, high-resolution and high-speed microscopy, and ultrahigh-definition laser-projection systems. A recent innovation is the use of pulse dispersion to control the propagation angle at 90-MHz rates.[13] These and other approaches to nonmechanical beam control will only increase in importance over the years to come.

## 5.2 Scan Optics

We saw in Chapter 4 how a number of requirements—truncation, surface figure, material absorption, and so on—determine the performance of the optical subsystem. In this section, we look in more detail at the optical components unique to scanning and beam control; included are scan mirrors and f-θ focusing lenses.

### 5.2.1 Scan mirrors

While we have used the word "flat" to describe scan mirrors, we have seen in Chapter 4 that nothing is perfectly so, and the deviation from perfection—the surface figure—affects the reflected beam quality. In addition to the manufacturing influences on surface flatness—a MEMS mirror may have a surface radius of about 5 m, for example—even a well-fabricated mirror will suffer from additional surface-figure errors when used in a dynamic and thermal environment.

The dynamic distortions from oscillating a galvo mirror are illustrated in Fig. 5.10. The mirror is being rotated—accelerated and decelerated—about the mechanical axis in-and-out of the page. The angular accelerations create a force that distorts the surface with a dynamic deflection δ that varies with time; the PV value depends on the angular acceleration $\alpha = \ddot{\theta}$, mirror geometry, and material properties.

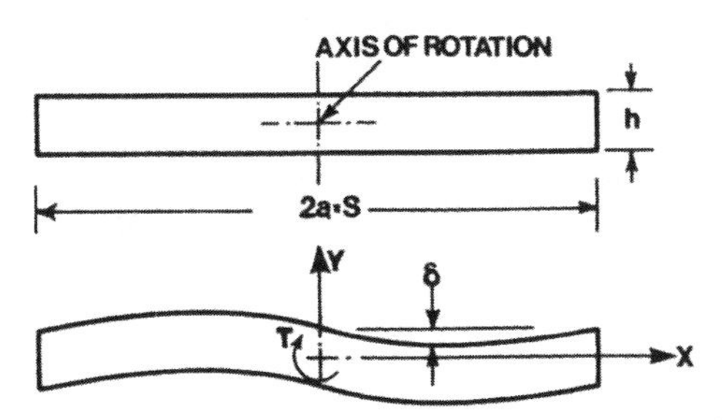


**Figure 5.10** A galvanometric scan mirror distorts as it is rotated about its mounting axis. [Reprinted with permission from P. J. Brosens, "Dynamic mirror distortion in optical scanning," *Applied Optics* **11**(12), pp. 2987–2989 (1972).]

Quantitatively, the dynamic PV deflection δ for a flat glass mirror is given by[14]

$$\delta \approx 0.0055 \frac{\rho}{E} \frac{S^5}{h^2} \ddot{\theta} \qquad [\mu\text{m}] \tag{5.4}$$

for a mirror material with a stiffness $E$ and density ρ, and rectangular width $S$ and thickness $h$ as shown in Fig. 5.10. Minimizing the distortion thus requires a mirror with a large specific stiffness $E/\rho$; material options with high $E/\rho$ include silicon, silicon carbide (SiC), and beryllium (Table 5.2). Aluminum and fused silica are also common for slow-speed, low-cost mirrors when distortion is controllable with mirror geometry or a low angular acceleration.

Minimizing the distortion below some requirement also requires a mirror that is thick in comparison with its width, but we must simultaneously reduce the inertia $J$ to reduce the torque $T$ required to turn the mirror:

$$T = J\ddot{\theta} \qquad [\text{N-m}] \tag{5.5}$$

where the rotational inertia $J$ for a round mirror accelerated about its center axis of rotation (as in Fig. 5.10) depends on the mirror radius $r = S/2$:

$$J = \frac{1}{4} m r^2 \qquad [\text{kg-m}^2] \tag{5.6}$$

for a mirror mass $m = \rho V$ and a volume $V = \pi r^2 h$. Reducing the mirror width $S$—as in MEMS scanners—is thus very effective at reducing the mirror distortion ($\sim S^5$), inertia ($\sim S^4$), and motor torque. However, the width is often established by the laser beam diameter, so the distortion is minimized for high-speed applications by first selecting a material with a large $E/\rho$, and then selecting the thickness to meet the distortion and torque requirements.

Mass $m$ and inertia $J$ must also be minimized, in which case beryllium has a clear advantage over silicon carbide with its higher density ρ. Unfortunately, beryllium has disadvantages with respect to toxic particulates, cost, and availability, so lightweighted SiC is often preferred instead, with vendors such as Mersen and Aperture Optical Sciences offering commercial scan mirrors.

**Table 5.2** Beryllium and silicon carbide have a large specific stiffness ($E/\rho$), and are thus preferred mirror materials for minimizing dynamic distortion for high-speed scanning.

| **Material** | **Stiffness, $E$ (GPa)** | **Density, ρ (kg/m$^3$)** | **$E/\rho$** |
|---|---|---|---|
| Aluminum | 69 | 2700 | 0.026 |
| Fused Silica | 72 | 2200 | 0.033 |
| Silicon | 131 | 2330 | 0.056 |
| Silicon Carbide | 330 | 3010 | 0.110 |
| Beryllium | 290 | 1840 | 0.158 |

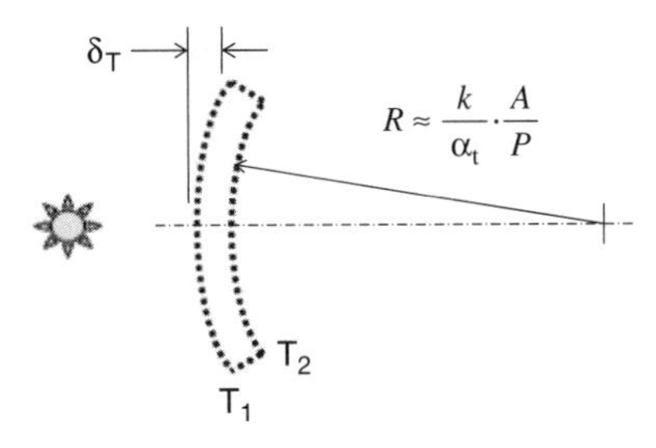


**Figure 5.11** When uniformly heated on one side with an absorbed irradiance $P/A$ (W/m$^2$)—an incident flat-top beam, for example—a flat mirror distorts with an edge deflection $\delta_T$.

In addition to dynamic distortions, thermal distortions will also occur on a much slower time scale. These occur as a result of temperature differences (gradients) across the mirror, with a larger thermal expansion of the hot side in comparison with the cool side.[15] This is shown in Fig. 5.11, where the galvo mirror has been uniformly heated with solar radiation, though a flat-top laser beam would have the same effect. The effect is to expand the hot side more than the cold, distorting the flat mirror to create a cylindrical radius $R$ about the rotation axis where the mirror is attached to a mounting shaft.

The curvature of the mirror depends on the absorbed power density $P/A$ (W/m$^2$), as well as the thermal conductivity $k$ and the thermal expansion coefficient $\alpha_t$—a larger thermal conductivity produces less curvature (increases the radius) as the temperature gradient $T_1 - T_2$ is smaller; a smaller $\alpha_t$ has the same effect, reducing the differential expansion across the mirror.

From the geometry of a cylinder, the edge distortion $\delta_T = S^2/2R$, giving

$$\delta_T = \frac{S^2}{2R} \approx \frac{S^2}{2} \frac{P}{A} \frac{\alpha_t}{k} \qquad [\mu\text{m}] \tag{5.7}$$

where the power $P$ is the average laser power absorbed by the mirror. The consequence is that the mirror is no longer flat and now has cylindrical power, diverging the reflected beam. Minimizing the thermal distortion of a flat mirror thus requires increasing the area $A$ over which the power is distributed, as well as a material with a large $k/\alpha_t$ ratio (Table 5.3). For example, a

**Table 5.3** Silicon and silicon carbide have low thermal distortion based on a large value of $k/\alpha_t$. The coefficient of thermal expansion (CTE) units are parts per million (ppm) per K, or $10^{-6}$/K.

| Material | CTE, $\alpha_t$ (ppm/K) | Conductivity, $k$ (W/m-K) | $k/\alpha_t$ |
|---|---|---|---|
| Fused Silica | 0.5 | 1.35 | 2.7 |
| Aluminum | 23.6 | 167 | 7.1 |
| Beryllium | 11.5 | 216 | 18.8 |
| Silicon | 2.6 | 137 | 52.7 |
| Silicon Carbide | 2.4 | 220 | 91.7 |

2-mm-diameter silicon carbide mirror absorbing 1% of a top-hat beam with a diameter $D = 2$ mm ($A = 3.14 \times 10^{-6}$ m$^2$) and an average power $P = 100$ W results in a thermal distortion $\delta_T = 0.5 \times (0.002 \text{ m})^2 \times [1 \text{ W}/(3.14 \times 10^{-6} \text{ m}^2)] \times (2.4 \times 10^{-6} \text{ per K}/280 \text{ W/m-K}) = 5.5 \times 10^{-9}$ m $= 5.5$ nm, or $\lambda/100$ PV at $\lambda = 550$ nm—an insignificant change from a perfectly flat mirror.

If the beam diameter does not match the mirror size, then there will be changes in both curvature and surface figure as the mirror absorbs energy. In either case, silicon carbide has significantly better thermal performance than beryllium, although SiC has a higher density $\rho$ and cannot be scanned as quickly owing to its higher inertia $J$. In addition, while absorption can be low for a mirror, a small fraction of a large incident power density is still enough to cause considerable thermal distortion. Mirror coatings must therefore be selected carefully and must also take into consideration the angular range as coating reflectivity varies with angle (Section 4.5.5).

### 5.2.2 f-θ lenses

We have mentioned a number of times in this chapter the use of a focusing lens with a scanner; in this section, we go into more detail on the characteristics and use of such lenses. While not necessary for some applications, the use of what is known as an "f-θ" lens is common. These lenses are designed with the following features useful for beam control:[16]

- Constant scan velocity: In a conventional imaging lens, distortion is corrected such that the image location $y = f \times \tan\theta$. In an f-θ lens, negative (barrel) distortion is allowed such that $y = f \times \theta$ (hence the "f-θ" name of the lens), and the scan velocity $v = \Delta y/\Delta t = f \times \Delta\theta/\Delta t$ is constant across the image plane to the degree that the scan rate $\Delta\theta/\Delta t$ is constant.
- Flat field: In all lenses, there is some degree of field curvature, i.e., the surface on which the focused spot is a minimum is not a plane but a paraboloid. As shown in Fig. 5.12, the image surface in an f-θ lens is ideally designed to be planar, minimizing the size of the focused spot on a flat image plane.
- External entrance pupil: Also shown in Fig. 5.12 is an external entrance pupil (virtual aperture) in front of the lens, so it can be located on the scan mirror. While this forces an increase in lens diameter, it also allows a flat-field design and a reduction is mirror size—a more critical consideration for scanning systems than lens diameter.
- Telecentricity: If the entrance aperture is at the front focal length of the lens, the exit pupil is at infinity, and the focused beam is perpendicular to the flat image plane (Fig. 5.12). Such a telecentric lens is useful in manufacturing systems where a round spot shape is important. Telecentricity is not required for all applications, and f-θ lenses with or without a telecentric option are commercially available.

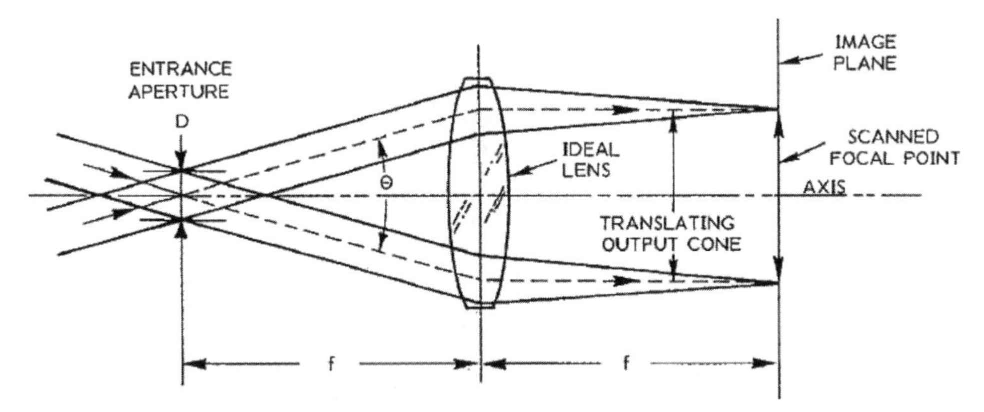


**Figure 5.12** An f-θ focusing lens has an external entrance aperture, a flat image plane, and may also be telecentric (as shown). [Reprinted from L. Beiser, *Laser Scanning Notebook*, SPIE Press, Bellingham, Washington (1992).]

As the degree of barrel distortion does not guarantee an exact f-θ relationship, the velocity linearity spec on these lenses is typically $\Delta v/v \approx 0.2$–1% over a 200 mm × 200 mm field, and is in addition to the linearity of the scanner. The lens diameter can also be fairly large, particularly for the telecentric lens whose diameter must equal the field size plus the beam diameter at the lens (see Fig. 5.12). These lenses are also relatively expensive, but this high cost is fortunately not always necessary, as mirror control software can correct for low-level scan velocity errors.

## 5.3 System Design and Trades

We have seen that beam-scanning subsystem designs entail a number of details, four of which are reviewed in more detail in this section: mirror-speed–angle–aperture trades, resolvable spots, scan velocity and PRF, and entrance pupil design.

### 5.3.1 Mirror speed, angle, and aperture trades

The directed-energy system shown in Fig. 5.1 has a number of design trades common to all beam-scanning subsystems, the primary ones being between the mirror speed (bandwidth), angle (travel), and size (aperture). Figure 5.13, for example, shows that a larger aperture cannot respond as quickly as a smaller aperture when turning a mirror with the same torque through the same angle, as the larger aperture has more rotational inertia. Alternatively, the travel angle can be reduced to keep the same speed as the aperture is increased.

An example of how these trades can also be used in subsystem design is shown in Fig. 5.14, where an afocal telescope is used as a beam expander with

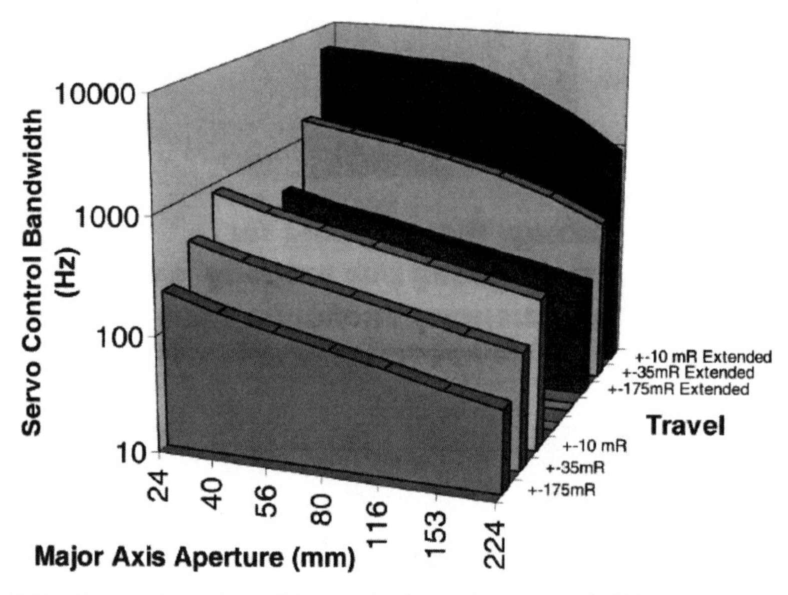


**Figure 5.13** Scan mirrors have inherent trades between bandwidth, angular travel, and aperture. (Credit: Left Hand Design Corp., Boulder, Colorado; reprinted with permission.)

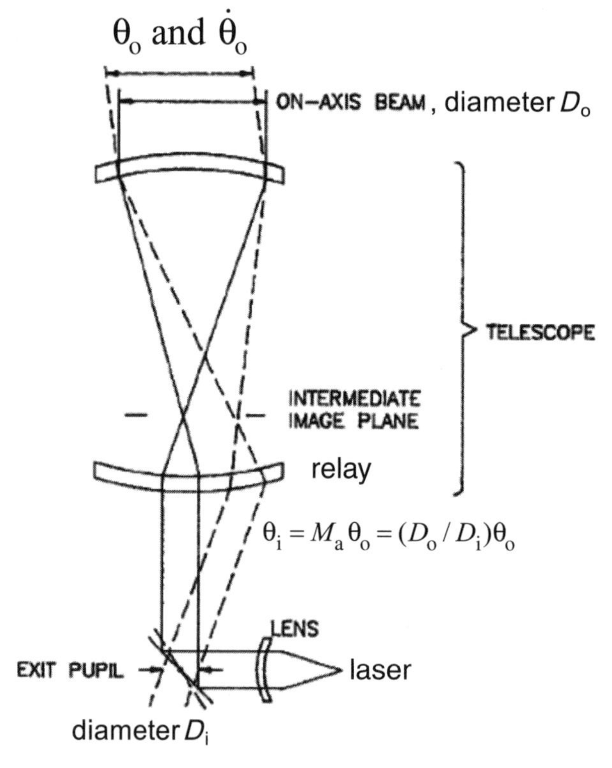


**Figure 5.14** An afocal telescope illustrates the trades between mirror aperture and scan angle. [Adapted from J. M. Lloyd, *Thermal Imaging Systems*, Plenum Press, New York (1983).]

a magnification of the beam diameter $M_a = D_o/D_i$. In addition, a scan mirror is placed before the beam expander, whose motion results in an angular scan of $\theta_o$ on the object.

With a linear ramp-up and ramp-down in scan velocity $\ddot{\theta}$, and neglecting settling time, the time $t_s$ required to turn a mirror through an angle $\theta_i$ depends on the angular acceleration ($\ddot{\theta}= T/J$) and the angle:

$$t_s \approx 2\sqrt{\frac{\theta_i J}{T}} \qquad \text{[sec]} \tag{5.8}$$

Inherent in the afocal telescope—a Keplerian design with an intermediate image plane in Fig. 5.14—is the inverse relationship between internal mirror size $D_i$ and scan angle $\theta_i = M_a\theta_o = (D_o/D_i) \times \theta_o$, so a scan angle on the object of $\theta_o$ requires a larger scan angle of the internal mirror by the afocal magnification $M_a$.[17]

The advantage of the afocal architecture is that the mirror inertia $J$ drops much faster than the scan angle $\theta_i$ increases, with the mass $m \sim D_i^3$ and $J = mD_i^2/16 \sim D_i^5$, giving a scan time $t_s \sim (D_i^5/D_i)^{1/2} \sim D_i^2$ for the same torque $T$. In practice, we also need to include the motor torque and inertia in this analysis, but these will both be reduced approximately in proportion, resulting in a clear trend to a faster scan time for smaller mirrors.

Additional advantages of using a small internal scan mirror are the reduction in dynamic and thermal distortion. The dynamic distortion varies with $S^5$, and even though the angular acceleration $\ddot{\theta}$ for the small mirror is larger—a larger angle must be covered in the same time—the net effect is a reduction in dynamic distortion for smaller mirrors [Eq. (5.4)]. In addition, the smaller mirror is easier to fabricate with an acceptable surface figure (see Chapter 4). Finally, the requirement on laser pointing stability is not as severe, as the magnification $M_a$ also reduces any change in inherent pointing angle of the laser itself.

The disadvantage of the afocal architecture is that the larger internal scan angle may not be physically possible. For example, if it's necessary to scan over a 90-deg external FOR, then $M_a = 4$ requires a 360-deg internal scan angle, an obvious impossibility requiring the use of either an external mirror or a gimbal to scan the beam over the FOR.

### 5.3.2 Resolvable spots

We saw in Section 5.1.3 that a disadvantage of analog MEMS scanners is their limited resolution. This affects the number of resolvable spots $N$ that can be seen on a laser projection screen or are available from a laser printer; with a scan distance $\Delta y$, $N$ is given by

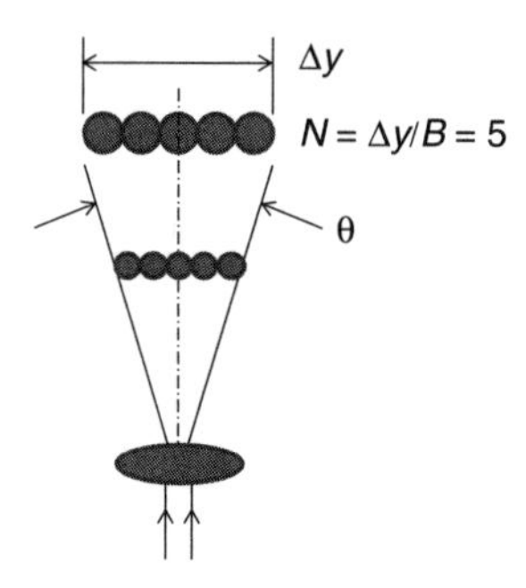


**Figure 5.15** The number of resolvable spots $N$ depends on the size of the field $\Delta y$ in comparison with the spot size $B$, but not on the distance to the screen or the focal length of the imaging lens if the scan angle $\theta$ is fixed.

$$N = \frac{\Delta y}{B} \tag{5.9}$$

for a fixed scan angle, and a large spot size $B$ limits the number of spots across the screen or field (Fig. 5.15). Typical numbers for high-resolution laser printers, for example, are $N = 3{,}000$ to 10,000, and a high-resolution graphic-arts imager may have $N = 10{,}000$ to 100,000.[4]

It sometimes happens that a designer will try to increase the number of resolvable spots by reducing the distance to the screen or the focal length of any imaging lenses. Unfortunately, this does not work as the number of spots does not depend on screen distance or focal length—a concept that is best understood by expressing the number of spots in terms of the scan angle $\theta$ and spot separation based on a FWHM spot size[18] for an untruncated beam:[19]

$$N = \frac{\Delta y}{B} \approx \frac{\theta \cdot f}{2.36\lambda f / \pi D_{1/e^2}} = \frac{\pi\theta \cdot D_{1/e^2}}{2.36\lambda} \tag{5.10}$$

where $N$ depends only on the scan angle and spot resolution based on the wavelength $\lambda$ and beam diameter $D_{1/e^2}$. Physically, the shorter distance to the screen has smaller spots, but also scans across a shorter distance $\Delta y$, as shown in Fig. 5.15; this makes $N$ dependent only on the scan angle $\theta$ and spot spacing. For example, scanning a 500-μm diameter, $\lambda = 0.5$-μm beam over an angle of 45 deg (0.786 rad) gives $N \approx \pi \times 0.786$ rad $\times$ 500 μm/(2.36 $\times$ 0.5 μm) $\approx$ 1046 spots (or a resolution of 0.75 mrad per spot)—sufficient for a 1 Mpixel display.

### 5.3.3 Scan velocity and PRF

In addition to resolvable spots, the velocity of these spots plays an important role in many beam-scanning designs. For example, the introduction of high-PRF lasers with ultrashort pulses has led to the need for ultrafast scanners to

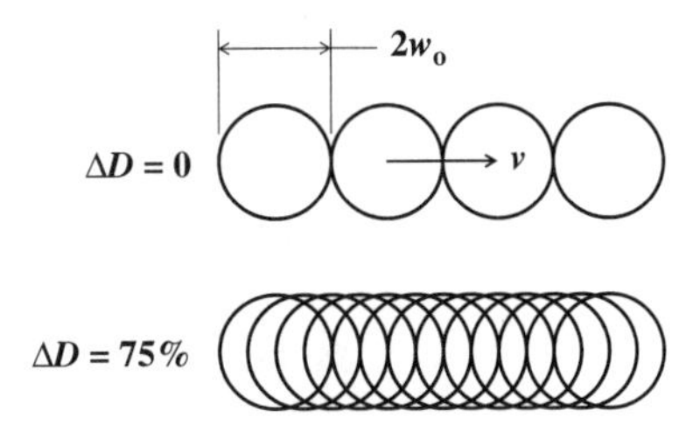


**Figure 5.16** The required scan velocity $v$ depends on the spot overlap $\Delta D$ as well as the spot size $2w_o$ and PRF.

synchronize the pulse rate with the scan velocity, enabling higher manufacturing throughput—for example, more lines scribed per second.

The required scan velocity depends on the resolvable spot size $2w_o$, their overlap $\Delta D$ in the scan direction, and how quickly the spots are generated (i.e., the laser's PRF). The dependence on overlap is illustrated in Fig. 5.16 for $\Delta D = 0$ (no overlap) and $\Delta D = 75\%$.

Quantitatively, the scan velocity $v$ required to match the laser PRF is given by

$$v = 2w_o(1 - \Delta D) \times PRF \qquad [\text{m/sec}] \tag{5.11}$$

where a small overlap, high PRF, and larger spot size require a faster scanner. This is not to say that overlap should be used to reduce the requirements on scanner velocity; instead, a large overlap such as that shown in Fig. 5.16 may be a detriment for ultrashort-pulse "cold" machining, as the long dwell time on the workpiece can result in accumulated thermal effects for materials with low thermal diffusivity, as well as reduce manufacturing throughput.

The synchronization of high-PRF lasers with the linear scan velocity can require extremely large angular scan rates. For example, a spot size $2w_o = 50$ μm for a 1-MHz PRF with a 0% overlap profile requires a scan velocity $v = 50$ μm × 1 MHz = 50 m/sec. If a focusing lens is used, then the scan rate is connected to the scan velocity by $v = f \times \dot{\theta}$, giving $\dot{\theta} = v/f =$ 50m/sec divided by 0.1 m = 500 rad/sec (28,650 deg/sec) for a lens with a commonly used focal length $f = 100$ mm. This is a very high rate that not all scan technologies can accommodate. Typical rates for COTS scanners include:

- Galvanometers: Scan rate $\dot{\theta} = 100$ rad/sec $\approx 6000$ deg/sec (optical). A usable linear scan velocity for high-resolution positioning ($\leq 5$ μm) with a 100-mm focal length lens is $\leq 10$ m/sec, insufficient for MHz-PRF lasers requiring scan speeds up to 200 m/sec.
- Resonant scanners: A 1-kHz resonant galvo with a ±60-deg optical scan angle has an average scan rate of 0.5 kHz × 60 deg (half-scan) = 30,000 deg/sec, limited to sinusoidal or triangular patterns with restricted range.

- Polygons: Scan rate $\dot{\theta} = 1{,}000$ RPM, or 12,000 deg/sec (optical) for inexpensive polygons and increasing linearly with RPM up to 100,000 RPM for very high-performance scanning. A usable linear scan velocity for high-resolution positioning ($\leq 5$ μm) with a 100-mm focal length lens is 10–200 m/sec. These are currently being used in COTS scanning heads for high-PRF, ultrashort-pulse lasers.

---

**Example 5.1**

In Section 5.3.2, we saw that the focal length has no effect on the number of resolvable spots. But given that $v = f \times \dot{\theta}$, is it perhaps the case that reducing the focal length is preferred? In this example, we show that a longer focal length is sometimes the best option.

This is the case when the scan velocity requirement is fixed, as is common in laser-based machining where a given scribe length must be covered in a minimum time to guarantee a certain manufacturing throughput. For example, if the scan velocity is fixed at $v = 5$ m/sec (let's say), then the required scan rate gets smaller as the focal length is increased, such that $v = f \times \dot{\theta}$ is a constant. So a lens with $f = 100$ mm and a scanner with $\ddot{\theta} = 50$ rad/sec could just as easily be used in this example as a lens with $f = 250$ mm and a slower scanner with $\ddot{\theta} = 20$ rad/sec.

While there is an advantage to slower scan rates, the disadvantage of the longer focal length is the larger spot size [see Eq. (3.9)]. It often happens that the focal length must also be fixed to control the spot size which, in conjunction with the fixed velocity, sets the scan rate. In such situations, the available scan technologies such as galvo, resonant, polygon, or MEMS then dictate the possible solutions.

---

### 5.3.4 Entrance pupils

Looking again at Fig. 5.14, we see that as the scan mirror swings through an angle $\theta_i$, the beam does not scan across the larger entrance lens, but instead pivots through the lens with a smaller angle $\theta_o$. This can only occur if the scan mirror and entrance lens are conjugates—i.e., images of each other.[17] When they are conjugates, a tilting of the wavefront by the internal scan mirror (exit pupil) is reproduced as a tilting of the wavefront at the conjugate image plane; the wavefronts thus pivot through the entrance lens, with the pivot angle of the mirror reduced by the magnification $M_a$ for the beam exiting the afocal telescope.

Another example is shown in Fig. 5.17, where a scanning confocal microscope scans a beam over a microscope objective that focuses the beam onto a biological specimen. To reduce the size of the objective lens, its aperture (entrance pupil) is made conjugate to the scan-mirror aperture so

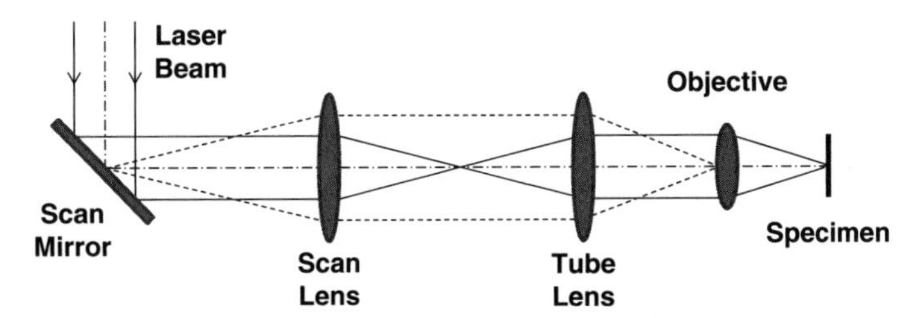


**Figure 5.17** In a scanning confocal microscope, the scan lens and tube lens combine to re-image (relay) points on the mirror aperture onto the entrance aperture of the objective lens (dashed lines).

that changes in mirror angle pivot the reflected wavefronts through the objective, rather than sweep across it.

The lens required to do the imaging—known as a relay lens because it re-images (or transfers) the aperture of the scan mirror to a lens—is shown in Fig. 5.14 as the lens between the scan mirror and the entrance lens; in Fig. 5.17, the scan lens and tube lens combine to act as a relay lens. In either case, the thin-lens equation given in Eq. (3.14) is usually sufficient for first-order estimates of the object and image conjugate distances for a relay lens with a given focal length.[17]

Relay lenses are not always necessary. Referring again to Fig. 5.3, we see that the entrance pupil for an f-θ lens is located midway between the two galvo mirrors rather than on either (or both, with additional relay optics). The first mirror thus scans the beam across the second, and the second must be large enough to accommodate the motion given the spacing between them. When a single-axis scanner can be located at an entrance pupil—such as that shown in

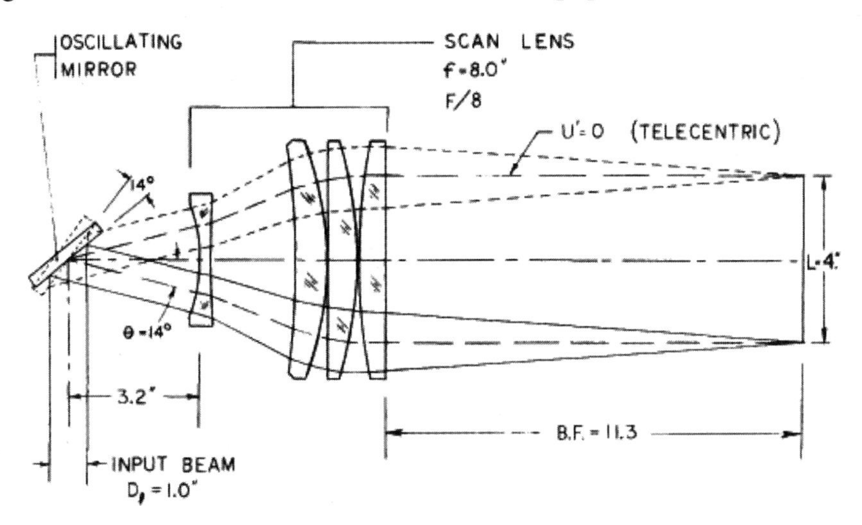


**Figure 5.18** A scan mirror placed at the entrance pupil of an f-θ lens minimizes the size of the mirror. [Reprinted from R. E. Hopkins and M. J. Buzawa, "Optics for laser scanning," *Optical Engineering* **15**(2), 150290 (1976).]

Fig. 5.18 for an f-θ lens—the mirror size is reduced, but the lens size is increased. Entrance pupils also control the amount of light entering the system, a topic we look at in more detail in Chapter 6.

## 5.4 Problems

**5.1** A vendor of closed-loop galvanometers offers a product with a positional resolution spec of 10 μm when used with a lens with a focal length $f = 100$ mm. What is the angular resolution in units of microradians (μrad) and arcseconds? What angular change (mechanical) of the galvo mirror does this correspond to?

**5.2** What is the average scan rate (units of rad/sec) for a high-end resonant scanner with a scan frequency $f_s = 18$ kHz and a ±8-deg (optical) range?

**5.3** A high-PRF laser has some uncertainty in the exact time between pulses, and therefore some uncertainty in the PRF. If a polygon scanner is used, what is the allowable percentage change in PRF if the polygon velocity stability $\Delta v / v = 0.1\%$?

**5.4** A MEMS scanner is moving a spot on a distant wall at an angular rate of 100 rad/sec. What is the scan velocity (units of m/sec) if the wall is 10 m away? What if the wall is $10^8$ m away—does the calculated velocity in this case exceed any known limitations?

**5.5** Equation (5.4) gives the dynamic mirror distortion measured as a PV value. What is the distortion measured as a RMS value? Which is more important?

**5.6** What are the advantages and disadvantages of $M_a = 10$ in the Keplerian afocal telescope shown in Fig. 5.14? Is there a different telescope architecture that gets around some of the disadvantages?

**5.7** What is the number of resolvable spots for a VGA laser projection system? For a high-definition 1080p system?

**5.8** Show that $D_{1/e^2} = 1.699 D_{FWHM}$ for a Gaussian irradiance profile such as that given by Eq. (3.1).

**5.9** What minimum spot size (units of milliradians) is required for viewing a laser-projection display with the eye? What determines that spot size?

**5.10** Referring to Fig. 5.14, if the distance from the center of the scan mirror to the relay lens is 100 mm, and from the relay lens to the exit lens of the telescope is 200 mm, what focal length is required for the relay lens? Is this reasonable?

## Notes and References


1. See, for example, Jim Hilkert's SPIE short course SC160, "Precision Stabilized Pointing and Tracking Systems."
2. P. Merritt, *Beam Control for Laser Systems*, Directed Energy Professional Society, Albuquerque, New Mexico (2011).
3. J. Montagu and H. DeWeerd, "Optomechanical Scanning Applications, Techniques, and Devices," in *The Infrared & Electro-Optical Systems Handbook*, Vol. 3, ERIM, Ann Arbor, Michigan and SPIE Press, Bellingham, Washington, Chapter 3 (1993).
4. L. Beiser and R. B. Johnson, "Scanners," in *OSA Handbook of Optics*, Second Edition, Vol. 2, McGraw-Hill, New York, Chapter 9 (1995).
5. G. A. Gibson, "Laser pointing technology," *Proc. SPIE* **4034**, 165–174 (2000) [doi: 10.1117/12.391865].
6. J. Montagu, "Galvanometric and resonant low-inertia scanners," in *Laser Beam Scanning*, G. F. Marshall, Ed., Marcel-Dekker, New York, pp. 193–288 (1985).
7. *Resolution* is the smallest step size the scanner can make and is measured in units of angle, dots per inch (dpi) for printing applications, or number of resolvable spots for video displays such as SVGA [Eq. (5.10)]. *Repeatability*—also known as precision—is the deviation from a specific angle to which the scanner has been commanded to point (10 deg, e.g.), and is usually larger than the angular resolution. *Speed* can be measured in terms of angular rate [radians per second, cycles per second (Hz), and RPM are commonly used units] or, if the distance to the image plane is known—lens focal length or screen distance, for example—as a linear speed (m/sec). *Step time* is for small angle changes, a vendor-specific definition, but typically 1% of the range (full scale); step time and speed both depend on scan angle and mirror aperture.
8. M. Freeman, M. Champion, and S. Madhaven, "Scanned laser pico-projectors: Seeing the big picture (with a small device)," *Optics and Photonics News* **20**(5), 28–34 (2009).
9. J. L. Miller, *Principles of Infrared Technology*, Van Nostrand Reinhold, New York, Section 7.2 (1994). Also see the Left Hand Design web site (www.lefthand.com) for recent data.
10. P. F. McManamon, P. J. Bos, M. J. Escuti, J. Heikenfeld, S. Serati, H. Xie, and E.A. Watson, "A review of phased array steering for narrow-band electrooptical systems," *Proc. IEEE* **97**(6), 1078–1096 (2009).

11. S. Serati and J. Stockley, "Advances in liquid crystal based devices for wavefront control and beamsteering," *Proc. SPIE* **5894**, 58940K (2005) [doi: 10.1117/12.623191]. MEMS devices known as deformable mirrors (DMs) are also available from vendors such as Boston Micromachines for controlling wavefront error across a beam, but these are not scanning devices.

12. J. Kim, C. Oh, M. J. Escuti, L. Hosting, and S. Serati, "Wide-angle non-mechanical beam steering using thin liquid crystal polarization gratings," *Proc. SPIE* **7093**, 709302 (2008) [doi: 10.1117/12.795752].

13. A. Mahjoubfar, K. Goda, C. Wang, A. Fard, J. Adam, D. R. Gossett, A. Ayazi, E. Sollier, O. Malik, E. Chen, Y. Liu, R. Brown, N. Sarkhosh, D. Di Carlo, and B. Jalali, "3D ultrafast laser scanner," *Proc. SPIE* **8611**, 86110N (2013) [doi: 10.1117/12.2003135].

14. This assumes that Poisson's ratio $\nu = 0.23$ for glass mirrors; for a different value of Poisson's ratio, the distortion scales by $(1 - \nu^2)/(1 - 0.23^2)$. See P. J. Brosens, "Dynamic mirror distortion in optical scanning," *Applied Optics* **11**(12), 2987–2989 (1972).

15. K. J. Kasunic, *Optomechanical Systems Engineering*, John Wiley & Sons, Hoboken, New Jersey, Chapter 8 (2015).

16. W. J. Smith, *Modern Lens Design*, McGraw-Hill, New York, Chapter 22 (1992).

17. K. J. Kasunic, *Optical Systems Engineering*, McGraw-Hill, New York, Chapter 2 (2011).

18. O. Solgaard, "Miniaturization of free-space optical systems," *Applied Optics* **49**(25), F18–F31 (2010).

19. The usual size of the untruncated Gaussian blur $B = 4\lambda f/\pi D_{1/e^2}$ is too large a separation for the adjacent spots for video displays. Based on the FWHM criterion, the spots can be placed closer together and still be resolved with a center-to-center spacing equal to the FWHM blur $B = 2.36\lambda f/\pi D_{1/e^2}$, where $D_{1/e^2} \approx 1.7 D_{\mathrm{FWHM}}$.

# Chapter 6
# Radiometry

Some years ago, a monochrome laser projection system was shown on the cover of one of the first "lasers and optics" magazines, illustrating the state-of-the-art in laser system R&D for future consumer products.[1] More than 30 years later, this vision has started to come to fruition in the form of large-screen IMAX theaters using high-brightness semiconductor lasers for a three-color projection system that does not use large, inefficient arc lamps. These projectors are an ongoing area of product development, with Necsel IP, Inc. winning a 2014 SPIE Prism Award for its high-power (3 W) green lasers for use in cinematic laser-projection engines. With further miniaturization and cost reduction, these large-screen systems will evolve into smaller, home-based consumer products with a much larger market potential (Fig. 6.1).

While high-brightness lasers emitting into a small divergence angle can easily be coupled to projection-system optics with small aperture and long focal length—i.e., large *f*/#—it is laser intensity (units of W/sr) that is a key requirement for the use of lasers for directed energy.[2] In this case, the laser is a source not of light but of heat, but the effectiveness of the laser depends on its power and divergence angle. Radiometric concepts are thus critical to understanding the use of lasers for laser displays, directed energy, manufacturing, laser radar, fluorescence microscopy, and so on. As we will see this chapter, it is not the laser power by itself that determines performance, but the laser's brightness (Section 6.1) and intensity (Section 6.3).

As the power available is a key component of brightness and intensity, Section 6.2 reviews how to estimate the power collected by a telescope, camera, or microscope directly from a laser, including material, truncation, and obscuration losses.

Laser brightness, intensity, and collected power are then combined in Section 6.4 to estimate radiometric performance using a systems engineering tool known as a power budget. An example power budget is illustrated with the range equation for laser radar and active imaging.

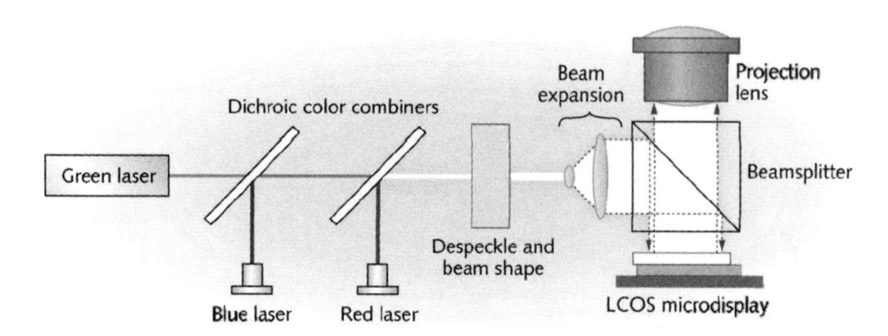


**Figure 6.1** A laser projection system for high-definition TV. [Reprinted with permission from K. M. Guttag, "Laser-LCOS microdisplays make for tiny, low-cost picoprojectors," *Laser Focus World* **46**(1) (2005); © 2005 by PennWell.]

## 6.1 Laser Brightness

Lasers are the brightest man-made sources, and in this section we first explore why this is. In the case of laser projection systems, the brightness of the screen image depends in part on that of the laser, so the use of high-brightness lasers allows the development of projection systems that are bright enough to be seen against a sunlit background.

The screen brightness depends on the area over which the image is spread, and the larger the area the lower the screen brightness. LED picoprojectors, for example, are constrained to a relatively small projection area because the brightness of the LED sources is not currently high enough for a larger area. In addition, the power will be scattered off the screen towards the viewer or audience, and the larger the scatter solid angle the lower the brightness.

Quantitatively, the screen brightness $L_s$ (or radiance, units of W/m$^2$-sr) thus depends on the incident power $P$ per unit area $A$ (or irradiance $E$, units of W/m$^2$), screen-scatter solid angle $\Omega$ (units of steradians, sr), and screen reflectivity $\rho$:[3]

$$L_s = \frac{\rho P}{A\Omega} = \frac{\rho E}{\Omega} \qquad [\text{W/m}^2\text{-sr}] \tag{6.1}$$

As we will see in this section, a brighter laser leads to a larger incident irradiance, sufficient for many single- or multimode lasers to be useful over a large screen area.

Laser brightness $L$ is defined in a similar way:

$$L = \frac{P}{A\Omega} \qquad [\text{W/m}^2\text{-sr}] \tag{6.2}$$

where the solid angle $\Omega$ is defined in Fig. 6.2, which assumes a circular emission cone with planar half-angle $\theta_o = \lambda/\pi w_o$. Radiometrically, solid angle

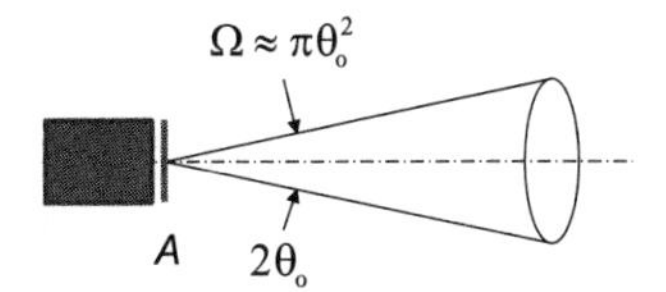


**Figure 6.2** Laser brightness depends on the laser output power $P$, emission area $A$, and solid angle $\Omega$ (units of rad$^2$, or steradians) into which the power is emitted with a half-cone angle $\theta_o$.

takes into account the fact that the power is emitted not in a plane, but typically into a circular, elliptical, or rectangular area.[4]

While lasers do not necessarily have a large output power, it is their small emission area and diffraction-limited emission angle that makes them so bright. Higher output power, however, does not guarantee higher brightness:

- Higher power may require a proportionally larger emission area, resulting in the same brightness if $M^2$ increases.
- Higher power may result in higher-order modes having sufficient energy to lase, thus increasing the solid angle $\Omega$ into which the power is emitted, and again resulting in the same (or lower) brightness.

For the same reasons, lower power does not necessarily mean lower brightness. The brightest lasers today are fiber and solid-state waveguide lasers, with $L > 1000$ GW/cm$^2$-sr.

From the perspective of laser system design, laser brightness affects far-field irradiance, and many laser applications depend on irradiance $E$ (W/cm$^2$) or fluence $F$ (J/cm$^2$). For example, a quickly diverging, low-brightness beam has a large beam area $\pi w^2(z)$ in the far field and therefore a smaller peak irradiance $E_o(z)$ incident on a target or sample.

With the exception of lasers, source brightness cannot in general be increased. That is, a laser may have a higher brightness than its pump laser, and a laser is thus sometimes described as a brightness converter. The reason is that the pump emits from a large area into a large angle; the laser output, however, is from a smaller area into a smaller angle. So brightness is a measure of geometric emission efficiency; generating laser power with few atoms (i.e., over a small area) emitting into a diffraction-limited solid angle can be much brighter than the pump laser, even with conversion inefficiencies.[5]

Once designed, however, a laser's brightness cannot be increased by the optics. For example, we saw in Chapter 4 that a beam expander can reduce the divergence of a beam, so is the expanded beam brighter? Unfortunately, the brightness has not increased; as shown in Fig. 6.3, it is the larger beam area $A$ that allows the smaller solid angle $\Omega$ *for a given laser mode*. So it is the product of the two—the $A\Omega$ product (or *étendue*) in the denominator of Eq. (6.2)—that may be conserved, and this is the physical basis for conservation of brightness.

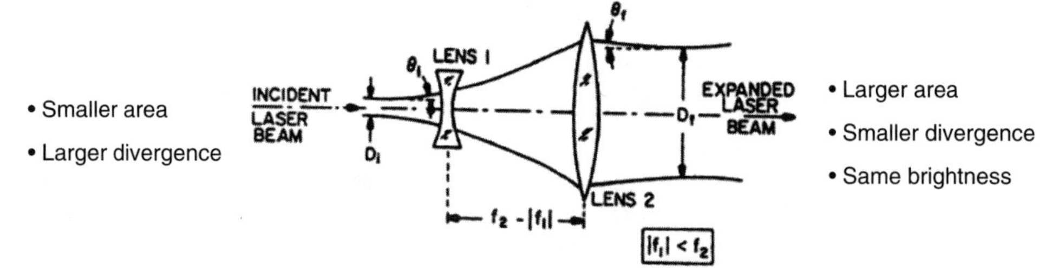


**Figure 6.3** Neglecting transmission losses, an expanded laser beam has the same brightness as the incident beam due to conservation of étendue. (Adapted with permission from the 8th edition of *Electro-Optical Systems Design*; © 1976 by PennWell.)

Similarly, for a diffraction-limited beam with the smallest-possible BPP, brightness is conserved at focus, but the irradiance (or fluence) is not. For example, we saw in Chapter 4 that a small beam divergence $\theta_1$ can be focused to a smaller spot $w_{02} \approx \theta_1 f$, giving a larger peak irradiance $E_o = 2P/\pi w_{02}^2$ or peak fluence $F_o = E_o \Delta t$. So the irradiance and fluence of the focused and far-field beam can be controlled with the use of a beam expander, but brightness cannot.

Beam quality and BPP, however, affect laser brightness and thus far-field and focused irradiance. For example, the two lasers shown in Fig. 6.4 emit Gaussian beams from the same emission area, but one has an $M^2 > 1$ and a larger divergence angle, and therefore a lower irradiance at focus. From the definition of brightness given in Eq. (6.2), we see that lasers with $M^2 > 1$ are not as bright as those with diffraction-limited $M^2 = 1$. The beam quality thus directly affects the irradiance at focus and after propagation.

Quantitatively, brightness for aberrated Gaussian beams with $M^2 > 1$ depends on $w_o \times \theta_o$:

$$L = \frac{P}{A\Omega} = \frac{P}{\pi w_o^2 \cdot \pi \theta_o^2} = \frac{P}{(\lambda M^2)^2} \qquad [\mathrm{W/m^2\text{-}sr}] \qquad (6.3)$$

where the BPP $= w_o \times \theta_o = \lambda M^2/\pi$ was used to obtain the expression on the RHS. As expected, $M^2 > 1$ reduces the brightness; also shown in Eq. (6.3) is

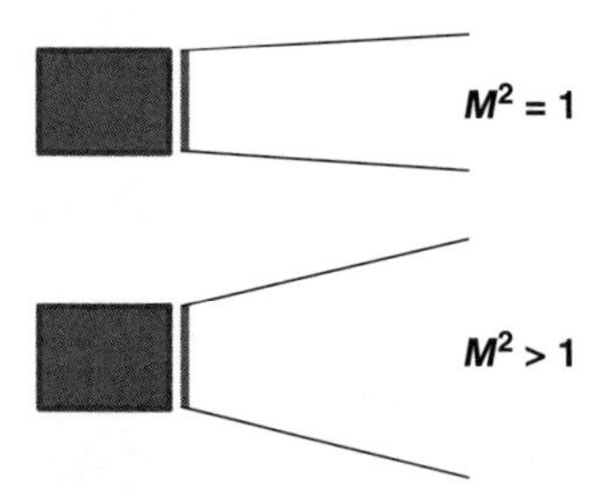


**Figure 6.4** A beam quality $M^2 > 1$ increases the laser's beam divergence $\theta_o$ and solid angle $\Omega$ to greater than diffraction limited and therefore reduces its brightness [see Eq. (6.3)].

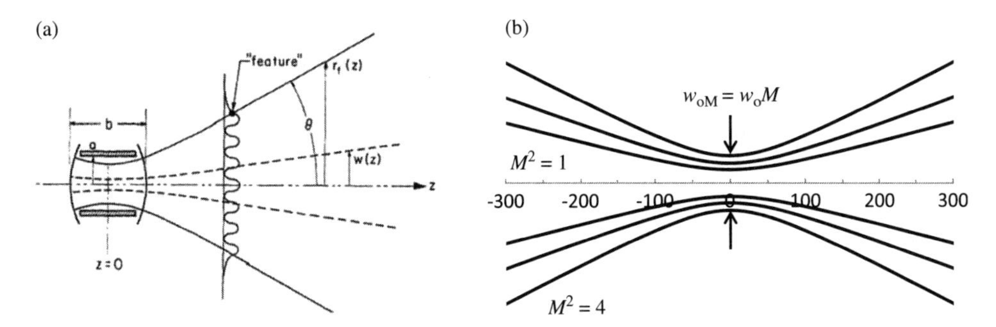


**Figure 6.5** (a) Wavefront errors across a laser beam cause it to diverge at an angle $\theta > \theta_o$, (b) increasing the BPP and thus diminishing laser brightness. [Part (a) reprinted with permission from W. B. Bridges, "Divergence of high-order Gaussian modes," *Applied Optics* **14**(10), 2346–2347 (1975).]

that the far-field brightness is $\sim 1/\lambda^2$, so UV lasers—with their smaller beam divergence—are inherently brighter than IR lasers for the same power and beam quality. Also note that *brightness is not conserved when comparing modes*. That is, the larger area of the non-diffraction-limited beam also has a larger $\Omega$ when compared with the mathematical idealization of an "embedded Gaussian"—i.e., both $w_o$ and $\theta_o$ increase by $M$ in Fig. 6.5(b)—increasing $A\Omega$. This is also illustrated in Fig. 3.7, where it is seen that either the waist $w_o$ or far-field angle $\theta_o$ increases by $M^2$, and thus the brightness decreases by $w_o^2$ or $\theta_o^2$, i.e., a factor of $(M^2)^2$.

Finally, the concepts of spectral brightness $L_\lambda$ or $L_\nu$ are used to describe the brightness in a narrow wavelength band $\Delta\lambda$ or spectral width $\Delta\nu = c|\Delta\lambda|/\lambda_o^2$:

$$L_\lambda = \frac{P}{A\Omega \cdot |\Delta\lambda|} \qquad [\text{W/m}^2\text{-sr-nm}] \tag{6.4}$$

That is, the power in a laser is confined to a narrow $\Delta\lambda$, and this determines the laser's effectiveness for certain applications (spectroscopy, for example). When lasers are described as being "brighter" than the Sun, it is spectral brightness that is being referred to, as the Sun's power is distributed over a large wavelength band and thus has lower spectral brightness.

---

## Example 6.1

In this example, we illustrate how it is laser brightness that determines the far-field heating of a target, not the power itself. Because the surface area that power is distributed over determines in part how hot it will get,[6] an important directed-energy metric for heating a target is the power density (or *irradiance*, units of W/m$^2$) incident on the object. Looking at Fig. 6.6, which of the two lasers shown has a higher far-field irradiance: a 1-W laser with $M^2 = 1$ or a

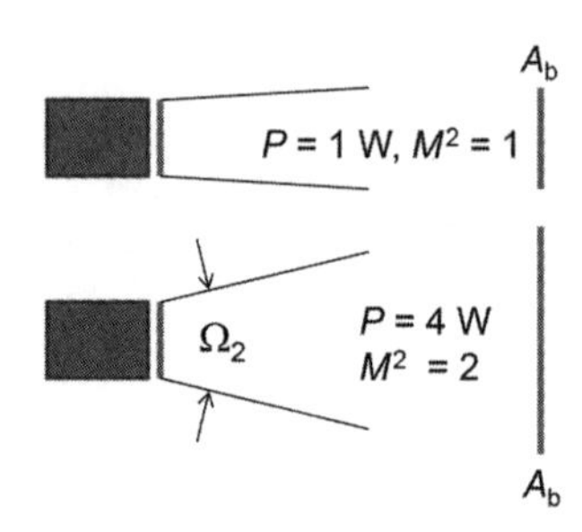


**Figure 6.6** A high-power, aberrated-Gaussian laser is compared with a fundamental-mode, low-power laser for their effectiveness at placing power on a target area.

4-W laser with $M^2 = 2$? Both lasers are emitting from the same aperture area and at the same wavelength.

From Eq. (6.3), laser brightness $L = P/(\lambda M^2)^2$. For the same wavelength $\lambda$, the brightness then varies with $P/(M^2)^2 = 1$ for both lasers. The brightness and apertures are the same, and thus the far-field irradiance is also the same.

To understand why, we see from Chapter 3 that the beam propagation equation for far-field illumination shows the far-field angle $\theta_o \sim M^2$; the solid angle $\Omega$ and illuminated beam area $A_b$ are thus $\sim (M^2)^2$. The average far-field irradiance $E = P/A_b \sim P/(M^2)^2 = 1$ for both lasers.

So even though one laser has 4× the power of the other, the power is distributed over 4× the area; the far-field irradiance is thus the same because the brightness and apertures of the lasers are the same. While this does not indicate anything about the optimum irradiance profile or the laser damage threshold of the target (Section 4.5.4), we can conclude that *higher laser power does not guarantee higher power where it matters (such as over an area).*

## 6.2 Power-in-Bucket

The concept of irradiance has a number of applications other than that illustrated in Example 6.1. A focused beam, for example, also has less surface area to dissipate heat—and the material exposed to the beam thus becomes hotter as the beam size and area are reduced.[6] As well, the excitation of material fluorescence and nonlinearities may also depend on the irradiance. It is thus important to know the size of the "bucket"—a lens or target, for example—collecting the power, and in this section we look at this concept as it applies to both far-field and focused irradiance.

With the irradiance $E(r, z)$ of an ideal Gaussian beam given by[7]

$$E(r, z) = \frac{2P}{\pi w^2(z)} e^{-2r^2/w^2(z)} \qquad [\mathrm{W/m^2}] \tag{6.5}$$

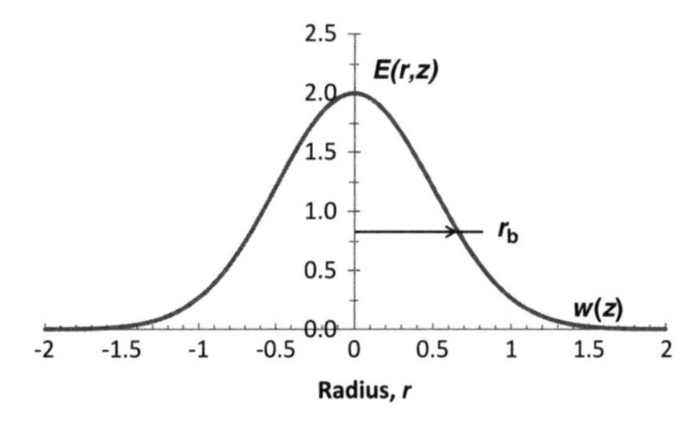


**Figure 6.7** The PIB depends on the size $r_b$ of the circular bucket and the beam size $w(z)$.

we see that the peak irradiance drops as the beam propagates [due to the increase in the beam area $\pi w^2(z)$]. In addition, the peak irradiance at the center of the beam ($r = 0$) is 2× higher than expected from the total power $P$. As shown in Fig. 6.7, the power-in-bucket (PIB) $P_b$ for a given collection area varies with bucket radius $r_b$ and is the integrated irradiance:

$$PIB(r) = \int_0^{r_b} E(r,z)dA = P[1 - e^{-2r_b^2/w^2(z)}] \qquad [W] \tag{6.6}$$

Equation (6.6) is plotted in Fig. 6.8, where the curve shows an increase in power collected as the bucket radius $r_b$ increases in comparison with the beam size $w(z)$. Also known as the *encircled power* or *encircled energy* when measured with circular detectors—and also sometimes recommended as a measure of beam quality[8]—the PIB plot (also seen in inverted form as power loss in Fig. 3.13) has a number of useful design features. For example, we see that if the bucket size $r_b = w$ (i.e., one beam radius based on the $1/e^2$ size), then the collected power is 86.5% of the incident. In addition, the plot also shows that if we use a lens or telescope aperture $r = 1.5w$ (or $D = 1.5D_{1/e^2}$) to avoid

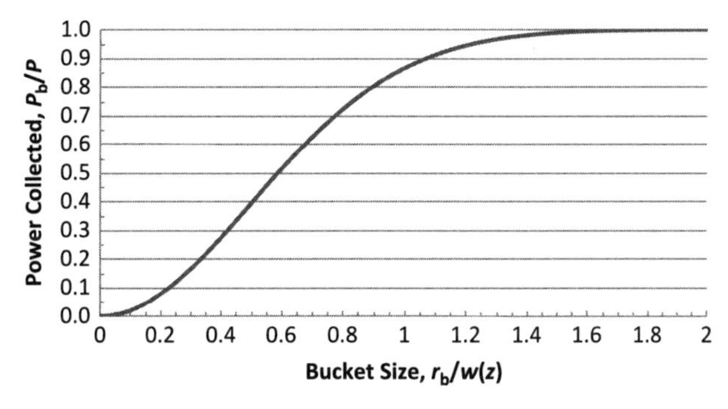


**Figure 6.8** The fraction of power collected (or transmitted) by a bucket centered on an ideal Gaussian beam depends on the radius $r_b$ in comparison with the beam size $w(z)$.

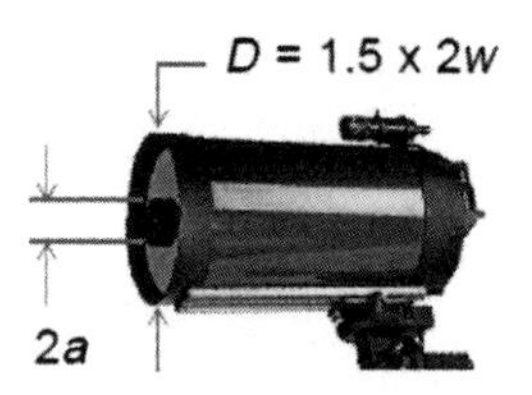


**Figure 6.9** A central obscuration can block a large fraction of the incident power of an ideal Gaussian beam. (Photo credit: CGE 1400 telescope, courtesy of Celestron, LLC.)

truncation effects on spot size (Section 4.2.2), the power transmission is very close to 99%, and only 1% is lost to truncation clipping.

The PIB plot is thus useful for estimating truncation losses for both obscured and unobscured apertures. For example, we can estimate the central-obscuration losses for a telescope such as that shown in Fig. 6.9, where the aperture $D = 1.5D_{1/e^2}$; the PIB curve gives a truncation of only 1% of the incident power based on the entrance aperture. Including a central obscuration ratio $\varepsilon = 2a/D = a/1.5w = 0.2$, on the other hand, gives $a/w = 0.3$ with 16.5% of the incident power blocked by the central obscuration "anti-bucket." The net transmission into the telescope for an ideal Gaussian beam is thus $\approx 1.0 - 0.01 - 0.165 = 82.5\%$. This contrasts with the blockage of only $\varepsilon^2 = 4\%$ of the light for an incident plane wave—the difference being that the Gaussian beam carries much of its power in the center where it is stopped by the obscuration. Table 6.1 summarizes how the obscuration ratio affects the fractional PIB of a centered Gaussian beam.

We also need to estimate not just the fraction of power $P_b/P$, but the absolute power (watts) collected by the bucket. Equation (6.6) allows us to do this for both truncation and obscuration losses if we look at the term in brackets on the RHS as a power transmission $T$. That is, $\mathrm{PIB}(r) = P \times T_{\mathrm{trunc}}$ for the transmitted power after truncation, where $T_{\mathrm{trunc}} = 1 - \exp[-2r^2/w^2]$, and $P$ is the power incident on the aperture of radius $r = D_{\mathrm{EP}}/2$ of an optical system collecting light directly from a laser.

For the obscuration losses, the power in the bucket is now blocked, so $1 - \exp[-2a^2/w^2]$ is a loss $\gamma_{\mathrm{obs}}$ (or power-*not*-in-the-bucket) for an

**Table 6.1** With an entrance-aperture truncation loss of 1% and an obscuration loss from Eq. (6.6) for $D = 1.5D_{1/e^2} = 3w$, the power collected by a centrally obscured telescope drops quickly.

| Obscuration Radius, $a/w$ | Obscuration Ratio $\varepsilon = 2a/D$ ($D = 3w$) | Power Obscuration, $P_{\mathrm{obs}}/P$ | Collected Power |
|---|---|---|---|
| 0.1 | 0.067 | 2.0% | 96.9% |
| 0.2 | 0.133 | 7.7% | 91.2% |
| 0.3 | 0.200 | 16.5% | 82.5% |
| 0.4 | 0.267 | 27.4% | 71.5% |
| 0.5 | 0.333 | 39.4% | 59.5% |

obscuration of radius $a$. From energy conservation, $\gamma_{obs} = 1 - T_{obs}$, giving $T_{obs} = \exp[-2a^2/w^2]$. Putting everything together, the PIB transmission due to truncation and obscuration is

$$T_{PIB} = T_{trunc} - \gamma_{obs} = e^{-2a^2/w^2(z)} - e^{-2r^2/w^2(z)} \tag{6.7}$$

Including atmospheric and optical attenuation losses, the net transmission of laser power through the optical system is then

$$T = T_{atm} T_{opt} T_{PIB} \tag{6.8}$$

where the transmission terms may be wavelength dependent. The use of these equations for estimating power collected is illustrated in Example 6.2.

---

**Example 6.2**

Free-space laser communication (lasercom) terminals are becoming more common when the high modulation rate is required to reduce the transmission time of large data sets. In this example, we look at the radiometry of designing such systems.

As shown in Fig. 6.10, the problem starts with a fundamental-mode ($M^2 = 1$) transmit (Tx) laser emitting a power $P = 1$ W into a half-angle $\theta_o = 1$ mrad towards a distant receiver (Rx) telescope at a range $R = 500$ m. The aperture diameter collecting laser photons is $D_{EP} = 2r = 1$ m, and the obscuration radius $a = 0.2$ m (not shown). The problem is to determine the power collected by the Rx telescope, including truncation and obscuration losses.

The truncated power depends on the size of the beam diameter $D_{1/e^2}$ in comparison with the telescope aperture $D_{EP}$, with $D_{1/e^2} = 2w(R) \approx 2\theta_o R = 2 \times 0.001 \text{ rad} \times 500 \text{ m} = 1$ m. The beam diameter and telescope aperture are thus equal, for which Eq. (6.6) gives $T_{trunc} = 86.5\%$.

For the obscuration loss, the normalized obscuration radius $a/D_{EP} = 0.2/1$, and Eq. (6.6) gives $\gamma_{obs} = 7.7\%$, a relatively low loss for obscurations.

From Eq. (6.7), the net transmission is thus $T_{PIB} = T_{trunc} - \gamma_{obs} = 78.8\%$. After ignoring the atmospheric transmission and including an optical

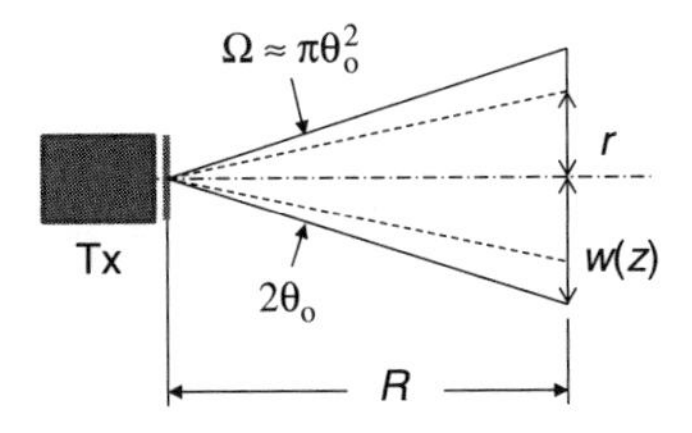


**Figure 6.10** A free-space lasercom terminal consists of a laser transmitter (Tx) and a receiver (Rx) telescope aperture with radius $r$ on which is incident a $1/e^2$ beam radius $w(z)$.

transmission $T_{opt} = 0.8$, Eq. (6.8) shows that the net transmission of optical power through the telescope is $T = 0.8 \times 0.788 = 0.63$—a large loss of 37%.

To reduce the losses, we can increase the collection aperture $D_{EP}$ (it's already pretty big, so not likely an option) or reduce the optical losses. We might also consider reducing the range $R$ (likely fixed by customer requirements) or decreasing the laser emission angle with a beam expander, both of which reduce the beam size incident on the telescope. Unfortunately, while a halving of $\theta_o$ to 0.5 mrad (for example) reduces the truncation losses from 13.5% to 0.03%, the obscuration losses increase—the beam radius $w(R)$ is smaller so a larger fraction of power is obscured with the same telescope dimensions—from 7.7% to 27.4%. The net transmission is then $T = 0.58$ for the smaller divergence angle, a *reduction* in collected power.

An unobscured telescope will perform better as the divergence angle decreases, as the truncation losses will get smaller, and there are no obscuration losses to increase. This feeds back into the telescope design, but, in general, obscurations should be avoided in laser system optics. This is not always possible, and there will be an optimum telescope design for a given obscuration ratio (see Problem 6.6)—an unexpected result that emphasizes the need for an integrated approach to laser systems engineering, and not just designing components in isolation.

---

A disadvantage of the PIB is that the bucket averages the irradiance variations—variations that may be useful for heating or utilizing material nonlinearities, but that are lost in the averaging. For example, the homogenized top-hat profile shown in Fig. 6.11 has approximately the same total power as a nearly untruncated Gaussian with a peak irradiance that is 4.5× higher than the top-hat, but has almost the same PIB for a bucket size $r \geq 1.5w_o$. We look at how to maximize the peak irradiance of a laser system in Section 6.3. In addition, there are many laser systems where we are not collecting power directly from the laser, but rather reflected from a target, projection screen, or biomedical sample. We look in detail at the radiometry of such situations in Section 6.4.

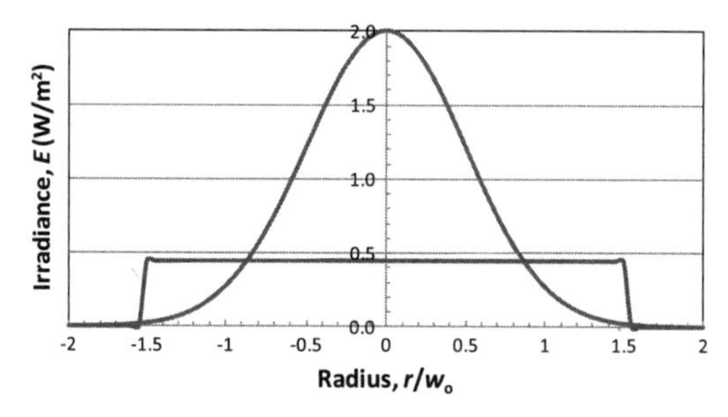


**Figure 6.11** The PIB is nearly the same for both the Gaussian and the flat-top irradiance profiles for $r = 1.5w_o$, yet the Gaussian peak irradiance is more effective for microscopy, laser radar, nonlinear harmonic generation, etc.

## 6.3 Laser Intensity

In Example 6.1, we compared two lasers with the same aperture but different beam quality and found that the brightness and far-field irradiance can be the same for both lasers. In this section, we look at two lasers with the same beam quality but different apertures to determine which of these design options has the larger irradiance in the far field (Fig. 6.12).

Looking at Eq. (6.5), we see that the irradiance of a Gaussian beam varies inversely with the beam size $w(z)$—a larger beam size distributes the power over a larger area and thus has a smaller irradiance. From Eq. (3.8), however, the far-field beam size $w(z) \approx \theta_o z = \lambda z / \pi w_o$, so a smaller waist $w_o$ diverges the beam at a larger angle and thus results in a larger beam area and smaller irradiance.

Putting these two results together, the irradiance in the far field of a Gaussian beam increases with the average power $P$ and waist area $\pi w_o^2$ (and also varies as $1/\lambda^2 z^2$). As a result, *the laser with the larger aperture in Fig. 6.12 has the larger irradiance (peak or average) in the far field*, whether incident on an object or collected by a lens or some other bucket. This is an important result, illustrating the advantage of using beam expanders for increasing far-field irradiance (even though the brightness is not increased).

We can look at this result from another perspective, namely, by using a radiometric property known as laser *intensity*. Unlike laser brightness, intensity does not depend inversely on the area of the aperture; similar to brightness, intensity does depend on the solid angle into which power is emitted. That is, average laser intensity $I = P/\Omega$ and is measured in units of W/sr.

Intensity is not a conserved quantity and can be modified with beam expanders that change the far-field divergence angle $\theta_o$. It can also be degraded for multimode beams such that the divergence angle increases by $M^2$ and the solid angle $\Omega$ by $(M^2)^2$, giving $I = P/[\Omega \times (M^2)^2]$.

The solid angle for an $M^2 = 1$ beam depends on the divergence angle of the beam, giving $\Omega = \pi\theta_o^2 = \lambda^2/\pi w_o^2$ (Fig. 6.12). Laser intensity is therefore $I = P/\Omega = P \times \pi w_o^2/\lambda^2$. Note that this expression is identical to the irradiance in the far field except for the $1/z^2$ propagation factor.

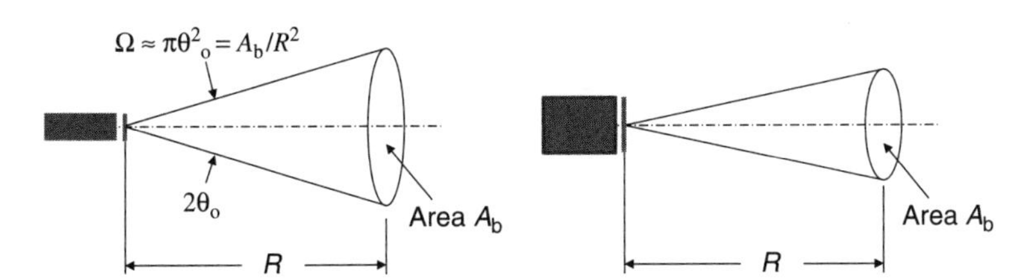


**Figure 6.12** Does the laser with the smaller or the larger aperture have the higher irradiance in the far field? Both lasers have $M^2 = 1$ and the same average power $P$ and average radiance $L$.

The average irradiance in the far field depends on the power and the $1/e^2$ beam area $A_b$, giving $E = P/A_b$. The laser intensity required to create this irradiance can be estimated by using an alternative equation for $\Omega \approx A_b/z^2$, giving $E = P \times \pi w_o^2/\lambda^2 z^2 = I/z^2$. This is an extremely useful result indicating that a high-intensity laser or a beam expander should be used to maximize laser-plus-optics intensity and far-field irradiance—and therefore power collected if the (unobscured) collecting aperture is fixed in size [see Eq. (6.6) and Problem 6.8]. Example 6.2 illustrated the consequences of using obscured apertures, and how the smallest divergence (and highest intensity) is not always optimum. In either case, laser intensity plays a role only through the solid angle but not the aperture area; as we will see in Section 6.4, however, screen or target brightness is important for applications such as laser projection, laser radar, and active illumination—all requiring reflected illumination.

## 6.4 Power Budgets

The problem of how much laser power is reflected or emitted by a screen, target, or sample has a number of applications, including laser-based projection systems, biomedical microscopy, laser radar, active imaging, etc. In addition, we must also determine how much reflected power is collected by an optical system, as this determines the strength—and thus the usefulness—of the signal measured with the detector. The collected power depends on:

- The power reflected off of the target and into a solid angle
- The optical transmission of the receiving optics
- The radiometric capacity (étendue, or $A\Omega$) of the receiving optics

In addition, there will almost always be sources of light that are not signal but background noise, and the optical system must also reject these extraneous photons. The purpose of this section is to walk through step-by-step the methodology needed to estimate photons collected by a telescope, lens, microscope, etc., from a laser beam reflected off an object (Fig. 6.13).

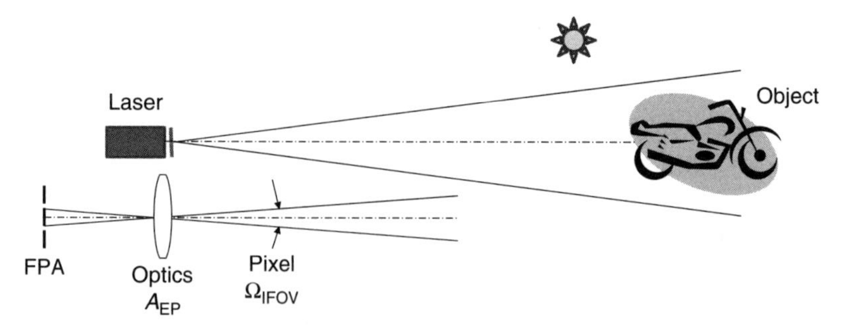


**Figure 6.13** Both signal photons from the laser beam reflected off of the object and background photons from the Sun contribute to the optical power collected by the focal-plane array (FPA) with a pixel solid angle $\Omega_{IFOV}$ and optics with an aperture area $A_{EP}$.

Unless the object is a conventional mirror, the power collected by the bucket (telescope) is now from an extended source, and the radiometry is different from direct illumination with a point source (the laser itself). What's different from direct illumination is that:

- Scattered, diffuse reflection of laser light off a specimen, screen, or target is not a coherent beam, even if the incident irradiance pattern is a $TEM_{00}$ Gaussian.
- The diffuse reflection also creates a source of radiance, rather than laser power directly illuminating the bucket.
- Unwanted background light from the Sun (direct or reflected) or the target's own infrared emission can obscure the signal trying to be measured.

Other design parameters remain the same—optical transmission, truncation, obscuration, etc.—and we will also use these to develop a power budget to be used in Chapter 7 for estimating the signal-to-noise ratio (SNR) of the detector.

### 6.4.1 Reflected power and radiance

The first step in developing a power budget is to estimate the radiance reflected from a screen or target. This will then be used in Section 6.4.2 to estimate the power collected by the optics.

We have seen in Section 6.1 that even though laser power may be relatively low, lasers are very bright because they emit from a small area into a small solid angle. Even though lasers are bright, however, their reflected light may not be. For example, beams spread out into a larger area—a big projection screen, for example—are not as bright. In addition, beams scattering into a large solid angle are also not as bright.

We can quantify the reflected signal by assuming that the reflecting surface diffusely scatters into a lobe (Fig. 6.14). Using a projection screen to illustrate, the power reflected from a screen with reflectivity $\rho$ is $P_r = \rho P_{inc}$ (units of watts). This is a simple enough result, but is not the final answer we need because the power has been *diffusely scattered* by the screen—not specularly reflected as with a conventional mirror. As a result, brightness (radiance) and étendue are *not* conserved, and the power collected cannot be estimated using the PIB methods of Section 6.2.

If the "screen" were a mirror, the specular reflection would be almost as bright as the incident beam (the difference being the reflection loss), and in that case the equations of Section 6.2 would be valid. What's needed, then, is a measure of how big a solid angle the light is scattered into, as well as from how large of an area. Along with the reflected power, these determine the brightness of the screen and, ultimately, the power collected by the optical subsystem.

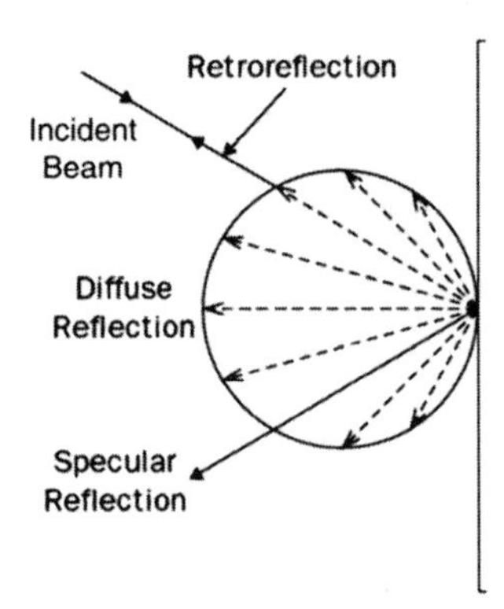


**Figure 6.14** Light is reflected from a diffuse surface such as a projection screen, biomedical sample, scene, or target into a lobe of scattered light, including specular and retroreflected components.

The image area $A_\mathrm{i}$ is easy enough to determine, and, when combined with the reflected power, the image irradiance (also known as *exitance*) can be estimated as $E_\mathrm{i} = \rho P_\mathrm{inc}/A_\mathrm{i}$ (units of W/m$^2$).

The final step in determining the brightness is some estimate of the solid angle into which the screen scatters. A commonly used assumption is that the screen is Lambertian—i.e., looks equally bright from all angles.[9] Mathematically, it can be shown that this is equivalent to saying that the screen scatters into a projected solid angle $\Omega = \pi$ sr, giving a Lambertian-screen image radiance $L_\mathrm{i}$ from Eq. (6.1) as

$$L_i = \frac{\rho P_\mathrm{inc}}{\pi A_\mathrm{i}} \qquad [\mathrm{W/m^2\text{-}sr}] \tag{6.9}$$

As we will see in Section 6.4.2, this is an extremely important result for estimating the power collected. Figure 6.15 illustrates the difference between collecting power directly from a radiant source and collecting power from a scattering surface; this difference includes the use of optical components with a transmission $T$ that affect the incident power and image radiance $L_\mathrm{i}$.

While the assumption of Lambertian reflection from a flat screen is common, the concept of *optical cross-section* (OCS) can be used for other geometries and scattering profiles.[10] For example, an optical component known as a corner cube reflects light directly back towards the source with a diffraction-limited angle that depends on the size of the cube. In this case, light is not scattered into $\pi$ sr, but is specularly reflected into a much smaller solid angle, and the watts per steradian (intensity) is correspondingly higher.

The optical cross-section is thus a measure of the reflected intensity $I$ (W/sr) in comparison with the incident irradiance $E$ (W/m$^2$), where a large OCS $\equiv I/E$ (m$^2$/sr) reflects or scatters into a small solid angle for a given cross-sectional area (m$^2$) *of the incident beam* (which may or may not be the same as

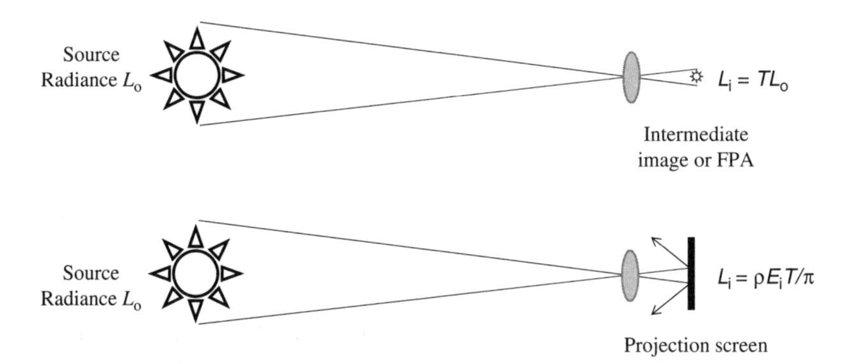


**Figure 6.15** Aside from the transmission loss $T$, source brightness (radiance) and étendue are conserved when there is no scattering (top figure), while Eq. (6.9) determines the brightness of a diffuse surface such as a projection screen, biomedical sample, scene, or target (bottom figure).

the target area—see Fig. 6.21). For example, the OCS of a flat Lambertian screen is found using the fact that the reflected screen intensity $I = L \times A_b = \rho E A_b/\pi$, giving $\text{OCS} = I/E = \rho A_b/\pi$ (or $\text{OCS} = \rho A_b/\Omega$ for the more general case of scattering into $\Omega$ sr).

Another example is the OCS of a flat mirror or corner cube. In this case, the reflected power is not scattered but instead diffracted into a solid angle that depends on the diameter of the mirror. If the beam fills the mirror, the diffraction-limited divergence angle $\theta = \lambda/\pi w$ [Eq. (3.8)], and the reflected solid angle $\Omega = \pi\theta^2 = \lambda^2/\pi w^2$. For a beam area $A_b = \pi w^2$, the general OCS equation in the previous paragraph gives $\text{OCS} = \rho(\pi w^2)^2/\lambda^2$ for a flat circular mirror.

Independent of whether the target is an ideal reflector, ideal scatterer, or something between the two, a known OCS is used to obtain the intensity $I = \text{OCS} \times E_{inc}$—a useful result when estimating the far-field irradiance from a reflecting screen or target (as in Section 6.3). Alternatively, $L = I/A_b = \text{OCS} \times E_{inc}/A_b$, which can be used as a replacement for Eq. (6.9) when the OCS can be measured for those "in-between" cases.

### 6.4.2 Power collection

To understand the use of Eq. (6.9) in determining the power collected by an optical subsystem, Fig. 6.16 compares two different cameras: one with a small FOV, and another with a larger FOV. The radiance $L$ (or spectral radiance $L_\lambda$) of the source is the same in both cases, as is the aperture diameter and *f*/# of the cameras; the problem to be solved is: Which camera collects more power from the source?

Given that the aperture diameter and *f*/# of the cameras are the same, we might at first think that the optical power collected by both cameras is the same. This is not correct; the camera with the larger detector and FOV collects more power from the source. To see why, we can think of the source

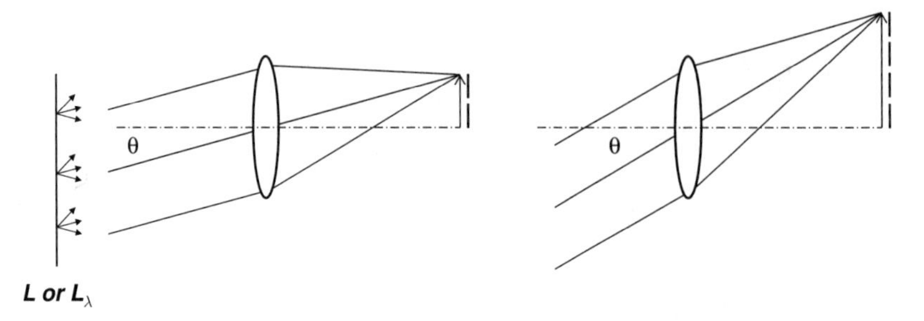


**Figure 6.16** Even though the aperture and *f*/# of the cameras are the same, the larger FOV (right figure) collects more power from a source with radiance $L$ that covers the full FOV = 2θ.

as an array of smaller sources—LEDs, for example—and the camera with the larger FOV will image more of these LEDs. More LEDs emit more power, and more power emitted equates to more power collected.

A larger aperture will of course also collect more power, as it intercepts more of the wavefront carrying energy from the source. The power $\Phi$ collected thus depends on both the aperture *and* the FOV:[4]

$$\Phi = T \cdot L A_{\mathrm{EP}} \Omega_{\mathrm{FOV}} \qquad [\mathrm{W}] \tag{6.10}$$

where $L$ is the source radiance estimated from Eq. (6.9), $T = T_{\mathrm{atm}} T_{\mathrm{opt}} T_{\mathrm{PIB}}$, $A_{\mathrm{EP}}$ is the area of the entrance pupil of the optics, and $\Omega_{\mathrm{FOV}}$ is the solid angle of the FOV [as seen in Fig. (6.17) and whose product $A_{\mathrm{EP}}\Omega_{\mathrm{FOV}}$ is the étendue of the camera].

A key assumption in the use of Eq. (6.10) is that the source uniformly illuminates the entire aperture and covers the entire FOV; a small, highly directional source such as a laser may not meet these criteria, while a laser scattered from a screen can easily do so. An additional complication that shows up in practice is that the radiance may vary over the FOV; we will see in Section 6.4.5 how to address this detail.

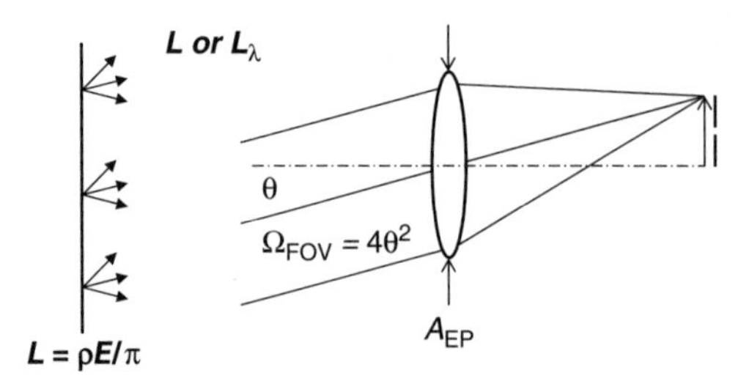


**Figure 6.17** Power collected from a radiant source with brightness $L$ depends on both the area $A_{\mathrm{EP}}$ of the entrance pupil and the solid angle $\Omega_{\mathrm{FOV}} = 4\theta^2$ for a square FOV = 2θ.[4]

### 6.4.3 Atmospheric transmission

In propagating from a laser to a target—and back to the optical subsystem—light may travel over a significant range $R$ and thus suffer atmospheric losses. The losses depend on wavelength (Fig. 6.18), and have a Beer's law attenuation similar to that found for optical materials:

$$T_{\text{atm}}(\lambda) = e^{-\alpha(\lambda)R} \tag{6.11}$$

for an atmospheric attenuation coefficient $\alpha(\lambda)$. The transmission $T_{\text{atm}}$ is thus highly dependent on range, and the numbers shown in Fig. 6.18 illustrate trends, not absolute values. Once an absolute value for $\alpha(\lambda)$ is established at the laser wavelength(s)—see Ref. 11, for example—the two-way atmospheric transmission is found using $2R$ in the exponent in Eq. (6.11).

In addition to loss, atmospheric propagation has a number of intricacies—scintillation, coherence diameter, atmospheric turbulence that affects beam pointing, etc.—that can affect performance for systems such as long-range laser-radar and free-space laser communications. This is an ongoing area of research, an overview of which can be found in Ref. 12.

### 6.4.4 Background and stray light

While the laser power reflected from the target, screen, or sample is considered to be "signal," there are also sources of photons that can overwhelm the detector with "background" noise. For example, if we are trying to measure light from an 800-nm laser reflected off of an object in the presence of sunlight (Fig. 6.13), the solar background can easily be much stronger than the laser itself. Similarly, if the system is using midwave infrared (MWIR) or long-wave

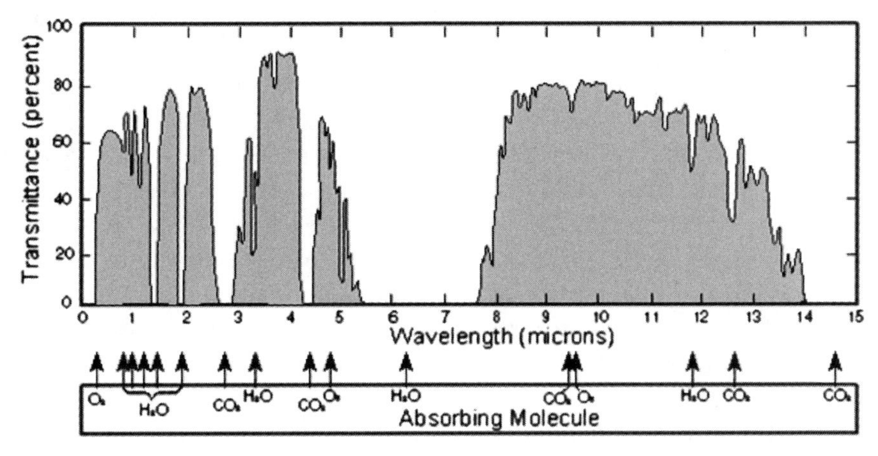


**Figure 6.18** Atmospheric transmission depends on wavelength; the numbers in this plot assume a range $R = 1.8$ km. (Credit: Wikipedia, Public Domain: https://en.wikipedia.org/wiki/Transmittance.)

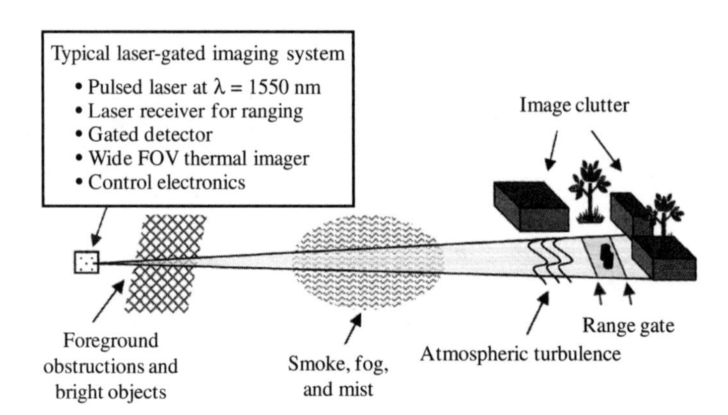


**Figure 6.19** Range gating in time allows exclusion of backscattered laser light, while a small pinhole (confocal aperture in Fig. 1.6) excludes photons in space. [Reprinted from I. Baker, S. S. Duncan, and J. W. Copley, "A low-noise laser-gated imaging system for long-range target identification," *Proc. SPIE* **5406**, 133–144 (2004).]

infrared (LWIR) wavelengths, then the infrared emission from the target[4] may be sufficient to dominate the measurement.

The laser itself can also be a source of background photons that obscure the signal, examples of which are shown in Fig. 6.19, where smoke, fog, and mist in the laser's path scatter light backwards towards the detector, possibly overwhelming the weak signal from the target. In this case, the detector can be temporally *range gated* to allow measurement only after the time interval $t_R$ when the target's reflections have traversed the range $R = c \times t_R$, thus excluding backscattered stray light from nearby fog, smoke, or other objects from being detected.

In Fig. 1.6, on the other hand, a microscope is difficult to time gate for nearby objects, but a confocal geometry allows a similar exclusion of unwanted laser photons. Specifically, the confocal microscope uses a small pinhole (confocal aperture) to "gate" photons in space, only allowing in-focus light near the specimen plane to be imaged by the detector.

In another example of how the laser can be a source of unwanted photons, Fig. 6.20 shows that backscatter from the optics themselves can be retroreflected back towards the detector. We have seen in Section 4.2.6, for example, that surface roughness of a lens or mirror creates a total integrated scatter (TIS) into a diffractive lobe of diffuse light. If the same optics are used for transmitting the laser as are used for receiving the reflected power from the target—a *monostatic* system—some of this total will be retroreflected and may be incorrectly measured as signal if it is within the detector's FOV.[4]

Estimating the background power $\Phi_b$ for these situations starts with a modification of Eq. (6.10):

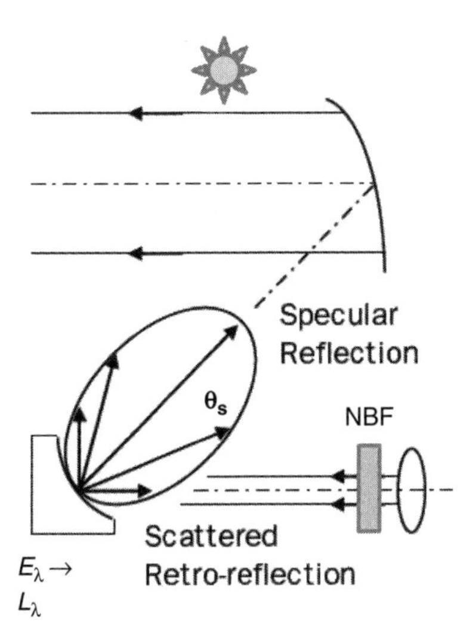


**Figure 6.20** Laser light reflected off of a mirror may scatter as a retroreflection back into the FOV of the detector where it is incorrectly measured as signal.

$$\Phi_b = T \cdot L_\lambda A_{EP} \Omega_{FOV} \cdot \Delta\lambda \qquad \text{[W]} \tag{6.12}$$

where the spectral radiance $L_\lambda$ (units of W/m$^2$-sr-nm) is commonly used for many background sources (such as the Sun or IR radiation), and the bandwidth $\Delta\lambda$ (units of nm) of the spectral filter is available from vendors in a range of values on the order of 10 nm down to $<0.1$ nm for a narrow-band filter (NBF).

In addition to the use of a NBF, Eq. (6.12) shows that another method for reducing background and stray light is to reduce the FOV of the receiver. This is commonly employed in long-distance, free-space lasercom systems where the detector sensitivity is on the order of a single photon, and even small amounts of noise will result in false alarms and data-transmission errors.[13] Chapter 7 has more detail on quantifying detector noise and sensitivity.

Not obvious from Eq. (6.12) are methods for reducing $L_\lambda$. In particular, the backscattered radiance in Fig. 6.20 depends on the spectral irradiance $E_\lambda$ from the laser and the surface roughness and cleanliness of the mirror. How much the mirror scatters in a particular direction—no surface is perfectly diffuse or perfectly specular—is summarized by a mirror property known as the bidirectional scatter distribution function (BSDF), giving $L_\lambda = \text{BDSF} \times E_\lambda$. As a result, reducing the BSDF by increasing the off-axis scatter angle $\theta_s$ or polishing the mirror to a low surface roughness reduces the scattered radiance and thus the background and stray light. Additional details can be found in Ref. 4.

### 6.4.5 The range equation

While not used for all laser system designs, the range equation is a common example of a power budget for laser radar, active imaging, and other applications for estimating the number of photons returned to the detector after propagating a given distance (or range). In this section, we develop the range equation as an example to illustrate how much power reflected by a target is collected by a laser radar system. The result will be used in Chapter 7 to determine the SNR, a key performance metric for many laser systems.

The particular application used in this example is for self-driving vehicles such as those being developed by Apple, Google, and others. These vehicles rely on knowing the distance to other vehicles, pedestrians, buildings, etc., in a scene, where pulsed lasers are used to determine the time of flight $t_f$ and thus range $R$ based on $2R = c \times t_f$ for the speed of light $c$. The system architecture is the same as that given in Fig. 6.13, showing laser, object, and optics for collecting reflected light onto an FPA with pixels with an instantaneous FOV (IFOV).

System parameters for a notional system are given in Table 6.2, including the laser, Rx optics, and detector subsystems. Items of interest include the use of a "flash" laser radar, where all of the power in a pulse is distributed over the entire FOV—as distinct from a scanned laser radar, where the power in each pulse is contained in each spot, a distinction that has important implications for the range at which objects can be measured. The desired range $R$ is $\leq$ 100 m.

**Table 6.2** Power budget parameters summarized for an autonomous (self-driving) vehicle ranging system using flash laser radar.

| Subsystem | Parameter | Value |
|---|---|---|
| Laser | Wavelength, $\lambda$ | 1064 nm |
| | Peak power, $P_{peak}$ | 1 kW |
| | Beam divergence, $\theta_o$ | 3.67 deg |
| | Beam waist, $w_o$ | 0.1 mm |
| Atmosphere | Range, $R$ | 100 m |
| | Transmission, $T_{atm}$ | 1.0 |
| Target | Reflectivity, $\rho$ | 0.2 |
| | Scatter solid angle, $\Omega$ | $\pi$ steradians |
| | Solar background, $E_\lambda$ | 593 W/m$^2$-$\mu$m |
| Rx optics | Aperture, $D_{EP}$ | 25 mm |
| | Focal length, $f$ | 50 mm |
| | Half-FOV, $\theta$ | 3.67 deg |
| | Transmission, $T_{opt}$ | 0.8 |
| | Spectral filter, $\Delta\lambda$ | 10 nm |
| Detector | Pixel size, $d_p$ | 50 $\mu$m |
| | FPA format | 128 $\times$ 128 |
| | Pixel sensitivity, NEP | 1 nW |

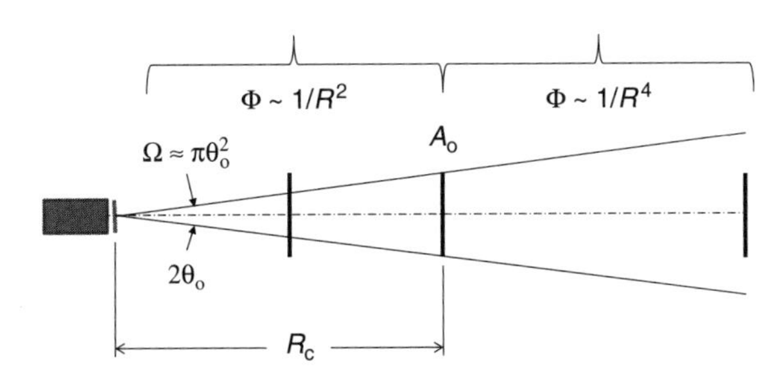


**Figure 6.21** At a critical range $R = R_c$, the object area $A_o$ equals the laser's 1/e$^2$ beam area $A_b = \pi w^2(R)$. For a range $R < R_c$ the object is underfilled ($A_b < A_o$), while for $R > R_c$ the object is overfilled ($A_b > A_o$)—a distinction that has significant effects on the power $\Phi$ collected by the receiver.

Looking first at a scanned single-pixel detector whose FOV matches the laser's 1/e$^2$ beam diameter on the object at a critical range $R = R_c$ (Fig. 6.21), the detector collects all of the scattered power except for the 1/e$^2$ truncation losses of 13.5% ($T_{\text{trunc}} = 0.865$).

From Eq. (6.10), the power collected $\Phi = T \times L \times A_{\text{EP}} \times \Omega_{\text{FOV}}$. Breaking down the terms in this equation, we find from Eq. (6.9) that the spatially averaged $L = \rho E_{\text{avg}}/\pi = \rho P/\pi A_b$, where $A_b = \pi w^2(R)$. Next, we know from the definition of solid angle that $\Omega_{\text{FOV}} = A_b/R^2$ *for the illuminated area* $A_b$ *from which light is reflected* (not the area of the object). Putting these terms together, the range equation for critically filled illumination in the far field is

$$\Phi = T \cdot \frac{\rho P}{\pi A_b} \cdot A_{\text{EP}} \cdot \frac{A_b}{R^2} = T \cdot \frac{\rho P}{\pi R^2} \cdot A_{\text{EP}} \qquad [\text{W}] \qquad (6.13)$$

illustrating that the power we can expect to collect with the Rx subsystem for a target at a given range $R$ varies with $1/R^2$. Physically, this is a result of the inverse-square dependence of the irradiance incident on the object, as given in the denominator of Eq. (6.13), where the 1/e$^2$ far-field beam area $A_b = \pi w^2(R) = \pi \cdot (\theta_o R)^2$. Surprisingly, scanning a smaller spot—obtained with a smaller beam divergence $\theta_o$—has no *radiometric* advantage over a larger spot as the larger irradiance is cancelled by the smaller beam area and solid angle over which light is collected.

The transmission $T$ in Eq. (6.13) includes material, truncation, obscuration, and atmospheric losses. As shown in Fig. 6.22 and Table 6.3, we can estimate the truncation losses on reflection using Eq. (6.6), where $T_{\text{trunc}} = 1 - \exp[-2r^2/w^2] = 1 - \exp[-2A_o/A_b]$.

As the object is moved in towards the laser ($R < R_c$), truncation losses decrease and the incident irradiance increases, while the solid angle from which scattered light is collected does not change—and is the same as the

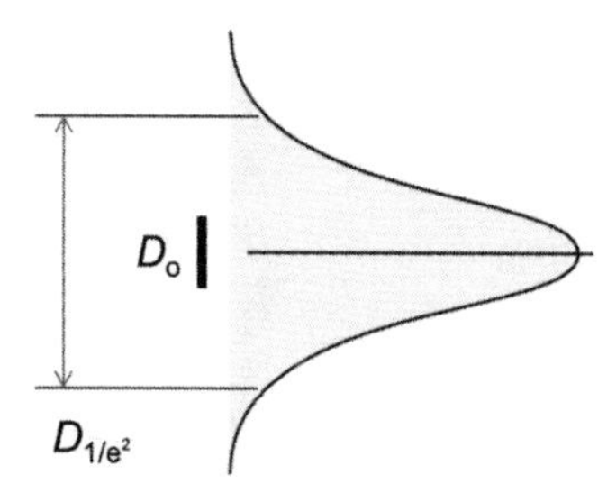


**Figure 6.22** The comparison of the object diameter $D_o$ with the $1/e^2$ beam diameter determines the truncation losses on reflection.

**Table 6.3** The power reflected from a Gaussian-illuminated object is reduced by the truncated transmission $T_{trunc}$.

| $D_o/D_{1/e^2}$ | $T_{trunc}$ |
|---|---|
| 0.25 | 0.118 |
| 0.50 | 0.394 |
| 0.75 | 0.675 |
| 1.00 | 0.865 |
| 1.50 | 0.989 |
| 2.00 | 0.999 |

laser's illumination solid angle, since $\Omega_{FOV} \approx A_b/R^2 = \pi(\theta_o R)^2/R^2 = \pi\theta_o^2$. The net result is that the range equation for $R < R_c$ is the same as Eq. (6.13), with the power collected $\Phi \sim 1/R^2$ for the entire span due solely to the change in incident irradiance (neglecting the reduction in truncation losses as the object moves closer).

For the situation where the laser's $1/e^2$ beam diameter overfills the object, however—i.e., for $R > R_c$ in Fig. 6.21—the laser-illuminated beam area from which light is scattered no longer matches the object area, and by using Eq. (6.10), this mismatch changes the range equation to

$$\Phi = T \cdot \frac{\rho P}{\pi A_b} \cdot A_{EP} \cdot \frac{A_o}{R^2} \qquad [\mathrm{W}] \tag{6.14}$$

showing a $1/R^4$ dependence due to the $1/R^2$ dependence of both the beam area and collection solid angle. That is, the far-field beam area $A_b = \pi(\theta_o R)^2$ is growing in size as the range increases, reducing the incident irradiance on the object. This is in addition to the smaller solid angle $\Omega_{FOV}$ for the illuminated area $A_o$ from which the detector collects reflected light—also proportional to $1/R^2$, as shown in the last term on the RHS of Eq. (6.14)—with the net effect neglecting truncation losses being the $1/R^4$ dependence for targets smaller than the beam size.

Note that the laser power $P$ in Eqs. (6.13) and (6.14) refers to the spatial average (as in the top-hat profile in Fig. 6.11), as a single-pixel detector cannot resolve the irradiance profile. In addition, if the detector cannot resolve the pulse width, then it is the time-averaged power that is used; for a laser radar system, however, the detector would be selected to be fast enough to measure each pulse, in which case it is the peak power $P_{\text{peak}}$ that determines the detector's output current—the reason that short-pulse lasers with high peak powers are commonly used.

For self-driving vehicles (and many other applications), scanning a small field-of-illumination (FOI) beam over the larger field of regard (FOR) leads to the underfilled situation for the power collected with a $1/R^2$ dependence [Eq. (6.13)]. Unfortunately, scanning requires more time and additional hardware, so a flash system is an option for quickly acquiring range data over the FOR. That is, the FOR is simultaneously illuminated over its entire area, and the power is collected with a FPA for pixel-by-pixel measurement of power and time-of-flight $t_f$ to remove the need for a scanning subsystem.

For such a flash-based laser radar, diffuse reflection of the laser off of the object makes the object a source of radiance $L_o(r)$ that varies radially over the object due to the incident Gaussian irradiance profile $E(r)$. This is shown in Fig. 6.23, where each point that is illuminated by the laser scatters light into a lobe, and the power collected by each individual detector (pixel) on the FPA depends on the incident irradiance. As a result, pixels that are centered on the peak of the Gaussian illumination collect more power, while those at the edges receive very little.

Since the beam area is spread over the entire FPA and the detector area collecting light is the much-smaller size of an individual pixel, Fig. 6.21 shows that Eq. (6.14) for overfilled pixels applies to flash laser radar. It's also useful to express the power in terms of optical subsystem parameters. Neglecting the Gaussian irradiance profile and using a top hat instead, the radiometric object area $A_o$ is the pixel area $A_p$ projected out onto the object, with similar triangles (and solid angles) giving $A_o/R^2 = A_p/f^2$ for a lens or mirror with a focal length $f$.

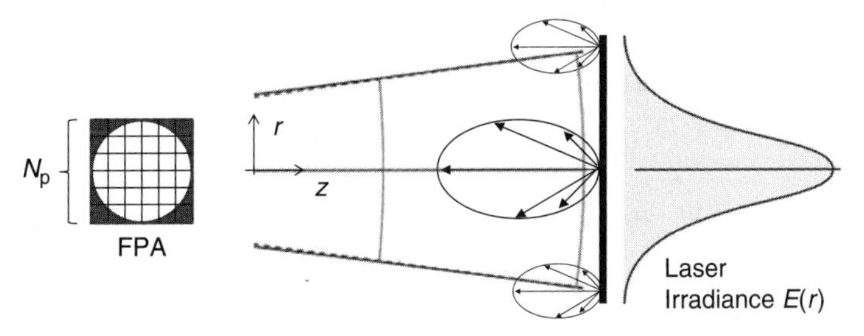


**Figure 6.23** The radiance reflected from an object back towards the FPA depends on the irradiance profile; in this case, the laser's 1/e$^2$ beam diameter on the object (white circle on FPA) matches the size of the FPA's horizontal (and vertical) FOV.

In addition, the beam area on the object can be expressed in terms of the beam area on the FPA, with similar triangles again giving $A_b/R^2 = A_{FPA}/f^2$ for a beam area $A_{FPA} = \pi(N_p d_p)^2/4$ on the FPA when using a square FPA with a pixel size of $d_p$ and $N_p$ pixels in each dimension (for a total pixel count of $N_p^2$).

Putting everything together, Eq. (6.14) for a flash system with flat-top illumination that covers the entire FOV of the FPA becomes

$$\Phi = T \cdot \frac{\rho P}{\pi N_p^2 R^2} \cdot D_{EP}^2 \qquad [\mathrm{W}] \tag{6.15}$$

showing that the power collected *per pixel* varies inversely with the total pixel count $N_p^2$, as more pixels equate to less power per pixel for a given beam area. As a result, FPA formats for flash laser radar, range-gated imaging, microscopy, etc., are generally restricted to relatively small pixel counts—for example, a 128 × 128 FPA giving $N_p^2 = (128)^2 = 16{,}384$ pixels, a small number compared with currently available megapixel FPAs for consumer cameras.[4]

Summarizing, comparing a scanned system with the same FOV as a flash-FPA pixel IFOV, the time to collect data is reduced by a factor of at least $N_p^2$—and likely an additional 2× smaller given the time required for stepping and settling. On the other hand, comparing Eq. (6.15) with Eq. (6.13) shows that $N_p^2$ times more power is required for the flash system under the best-case scenario of a flat-top profile. We will see the significance of this result in Chapter 7.

---

**Example 6.3**

A scanned system clearly has radiometric benefits; in this example, we illustrate these benefits by estimating the power collected by a raster-scanned laser radar system and compare it with that of a flash system.

To maintain the same spatial resolution for both the scanned and flash systems, we scan using a single-pixel detector whose FOV equals that of a pixel in the flash system, giving $\theta = 50\ \mu\mathrm{m}/0.05\ \mathrm{m} = 1$ mrad and $\Omega_{FOV} = \theta^2 = 10^{-6}$ sr. Using the properties given in Table 6.2, Eq. (6.13) shows that the power collected by the detector subsystem is $\Phi = 0.8 \times [0.2 \times 10^3\ \mathrm{W}/(\pi \times (100\ \mathrm{m})^2)] \times \pi(0.025\ \mathrm{m})^2/4 = 2.5\ \mu\mathrm{W}$. This power far exceeds the value given in Table 6.2 for the detector's sensitivity (noise-equivalent power, or NEP—see Chapter 7), indicating that the scanned laser power is more than sufficient for the given range and lens aperture.

For the flash system, Eq. (6.15) shows that the power collected per pixel for an unobscured telescope is $\Phi = 0.8 \times [0.2 \times 10^3\ \mathrm{W}/(\pi \times (128)^2 \times (100\ \mathrm{m})^2)] \times (0.025\ \mathrm{m})^2 \approx 0.2$ nW. This is significantly smaller than the detector's sensitivity which, as we will see in Chapter 7, excludes the use of a flash system with the parameters given in Table 6.2. Possible design changes to make the flash system feasible include a detector with a better (smaller) sensitivity, an FPA with fewer pixels (and therefore smaller FOV), a laser with a higher peak power, or a lens with a larger collection aperture.

In addition to laser power reflected from the object, we must also estimate the background power, as it may overwhelm the return signal. The solar background at sea level is given in *The Infrared & Electro-Optical Systems Handbook* as $E_\lambda \approx 593$ W/m$^2$-μm at $\lambda = 1064$ nm,[14] giving a worst-case ($\rho = 1$) $L_\lambda = E_\lambda/\pi \approx 189$ W/m$^2$-sr-μm; Eq. (6.12) shows that $\Phi_b = T \times L_\lambda A_{EP} \Omega_{FOV} \times \Delta\lambda = 0.8 \times 189$ W/m$^2$-sr-μm $\times\, \pi(0.025\text{ m})^2/4 \times 10^{-6}$ sr $\times\, 10^{-2}$ μm $\approx 0.75$ nW for either the single-pixel scan or FPA flash system. This exceeds the signal power for the flash system by a factor of almost four—increasing the false-alarm rate or obscuring the important signal that a pedestrian is in the way of the car—indicating yet again that the $128 \times 128$ FPA format will need to be scaled down to increase the signal power per pixel, at the expense of reducing the FOV.

In addition to solar background, either type of laser radar system will need to control the backscatter from fog and rain as well as speckle noise, a complication looked at in more detail in Chapter 7.

---

Summarizing, this chapter has introduced a number of concepts useful for estimating the radiometric performance of a laser system, including brightness, PIB, intensity, and power budgets. The fundamental properties used in these estimates for a fundamental-mode ($M^2 = 1$) Gaussian beam in the far field at the $1/e^2$ irradiance level are given in Table 6.4. We next look in Chapter 7 at using these radiometric properties to calculate the signal and noise associated with the different types of detectors useful in laser systems.

**Table 6.4** Summary of radiometric properties for analyzing fundamental-mode Gaussian beams in the far field.[7,15]

| Radiometric Property | Value ($1/e^2$ Gaussian) |
|---|---|
| Laser power, $P$ (W) | $10^{-9} \rightarrow 10^{+4}$ |
| Far-field half-angle divergence, $\theta_o$ | $\lambda/\pi w_o$ |
| Far-field beam radius, $w(z)$ | $\lambda z/\pi w_o$ |
| Average irradiance, $E$ (W/m$^2$) | $P/\pi w^2(z) \sim 1/z^2$ |
| Peak irradiance, $E_o$ (W/m$^2$) | $2P/\pi w^2(z) \sim 1/z^2$ |
| Average fluence, $F$ (J/m$^2$) | $Q/\pi w^2(z) \sim 1/z^2$ |
| Laser solid angle, $\Omega$ (sr) | $\lambda^2/\pi w_o^2$ |
| Laser intensity, $I$ (W/sr) | $P/\Omega$ |
| Laser étendue (m$^2$-sr) | $A\Omega = \lambda^2$ |
| Laser radiance, $L$ (W/m$^2$-sr) | $P/A\Omega = P/\lambda^2$ |
| Laser spectral radiance, $L_\lambda$ (W/m$^2$-sr-nm) | $L/\Delta\lambda = P/(\lambda^2 \cdot \Delta\lambda)$ |

## 6.5 Problems

**6.1** Is the brightness of a bar of semiconductor diode lasers (Fig. 2.18) the same, lower, or higher than the brightness of each individual laser?

**6.2** If the output power and beam quality stay the same, does the brightness of a diffraction-limited laser increase, decrease, or stay the same as the aperture area $A$ increases?

**6.3** Can a high-order Hermite–Gaussian beam with poor $M^2$ be homogenized to have better beam quality? Hint: If so, what does this imply about the homogenized beam brightness?

**6.4** A low-power semiconductor laser ($\lambda = 1.5$ μm) has an emission area of 1 μm × 3 μm. What is the solid angle Ω into which such lasers are emitting?

**6.5** In Section 6.2, we estimated the PIB of a Gaussian beam collected by a circular bucket. What is the PIB for a Gaussian beam collected by a rectangular bucket?

**6.6** Numerically or algebraically find the optimum beam divergence for the conditions given in Example 6.2. If we change the obscuration ratio to $\varepsilon = 0.3$, how does the optimum angle change?

**6.7** In Section 6.2 it was stated that "…the homogenized top-hat profile shown in Fig. 6.11 has the same total power as a nearly untruncated Gaussian with a peak irradiance that is 4.5× higher than the top-hat." Can you prove this statement?

**6.8** Plot the PIB versus far-field beam radius for a laser with a beam waist $w_o = 1$ mm and $w_o = 2$ mm. Which laser reaches a fractional PIB of 99% at a smaller radius? How is the 99% radius mathematically related to the waist size? What does this imply about the dependence of the far-field irradiance on initial beam size?

**6.9** In Fig. 6.20, a NBF is used to exclude solar irradiance from the detector. Does the surface roughness of this filter need to be specified? What might happen if it is not?

**6.10** In Table 6.2, what is the $M^2$ of the laser used for the flash laser radar system?

**6.11** In Section 6.4.5, the range equation is derived to estimate the laser power collected by an optical system from a scattering target [Eq. (6.13)]. Show that the power collected is less than the power incident on the target.

**6.12** In Section 6.4.5, how does the power Φ collected depend on range $R$ if the object is overfilled in one dimension but underfilled in the other (telephone wires, for example)?

## Notes and References


1. *Lasers and Applications*, March 1984.

2. See, for example, "U.S. Navy Laser Weapon Shoots Down Drones in Test," *Scientific American*, http://www.scientificamerican.com/article.cfm?id=laser-downs-uavs (19 July 2010).

3. If the "screen" were a mirror, then the brightness of the reflected image would be slightly less than the brightness of the laser (depending on the reflection loss). Since the screen scatters, however, brightness is not conserved, and Eq. (6.1) must be used to estimate $L_s$.

4. K. J. Kasunic, *Optical Systems Engineering*, McGraw-Hill, New York (2011).

5. Brightness can also be increased by combining laser power. For example, if the wavefronts from $N$ different lasers are combined incoherently such that the combined beams emit *from the same aperture with the same solid angle*—using fiber wavelength multiplexing, for example—the power (and therefore brightness) increases by no better than a factor of $N$. Alternatively, if the lasers are coherently combined in phase for constructive interference of the electric field amplitudes, then the brightness increases by no better than a factor of $N^2$. For more details, see T. Y. Fan, "Laser beam combining for high-power, high radiance sources," *IEEE J. Sel. Top. Quantum Electronics* **11**(3), 567–575 (2005).

6. Compare, for example, the temperature of your hand just in front of a lens imaging the Sun versus the temperature of your hand placed at the focus of the lens. For more details, see K. J. Kasunic, *Optomechanical Systems Engineering*, John Wiley & Sons, Hoboken, New Jersey, Chapter 8. (2015).

7. Many laser design and optics books incorrectly call the irradiance $E$ (units of W/m$^2$) the intensity $I$. This is based on historical usage and is not consistent with current ISO standards, where intensity $I$ is measured in units of W/sr.

8. A. E. Siegman, "How to (maybe) measure beam quality," *Diode-Pumped Solid-State Lasers: Applications and Issues*, OSA Annual Meeting (Oct. 1997).

9. In Fig. 6.14, we see that power is scattered in all directions with the scatter lobe producing no power along the screen surface. If the power drops off with angle at exactly the same rate as the projected area ($\sim \cos\phi$ for an off-axis angle $\phi$), then $P/A$ is constant, and this constant-brightness surface is said to be Lambertian. See Ref. 4 for more details.

10. The optical cross-section is not the same concept as the laser radar cross-section used by some authors.

11. M. E. Thomas and D. D. Duncan, "Atmospheric Transmission" in *The Infrared & Electro-Optical Systems Handbook*, Vol. 2, F. G. Smith, Ed., ERIM, Ann Arbor, Michigan and SPIE Press, Bellingham, Washington, Chapter 1 (1993).

12. R. K. Tyson and B. W. Frazier, *Field Guide to Adaptive Optics*, Second Edition, SPIE Press, Bellingham, Washington (2012) [doi: 10.1117/3.923078].

13. For example, an FOV of only 17 μrad (3.5 arcsec) is used in an analysis of an extremely demanding Mars-to-Earth lasercom system requiring minimum stray-light collection. For more details, see W. J. Hurd, B. E. MacNeal, R. V. Moe, J. Z. Walker, M. L. Dennis, E. S. Cheng, D. A. Fairbrother, B. Eegholm, and K. J. Kasunic, "Exo-atmospheric telescopes for deep space optical communications," *IEEE Aerospace Conference*, Paper #1557 (2006).

14. D. Kryskowski and G. H. Suits, "Natural Sources," in *The Infrared & Electro-Optical Systems Handbook*, Vol. 1, G. J. Zissis, Ed., ERIM, Ann Arbor, Michigan and SPIE Press, Bellingham, Washington, Chapter 3, Table 3-3 (1993).

15. Many laser design and optics books incorrectly call the intensity $I$ (units of W/sr) the brightness $B$. This is based on historical usage and is not consistent with current ISO standards, where brightness (or radiance $L$) is measured in units of W/m$^2$-sr or W/cm$^2$-sr.

# Color Plates

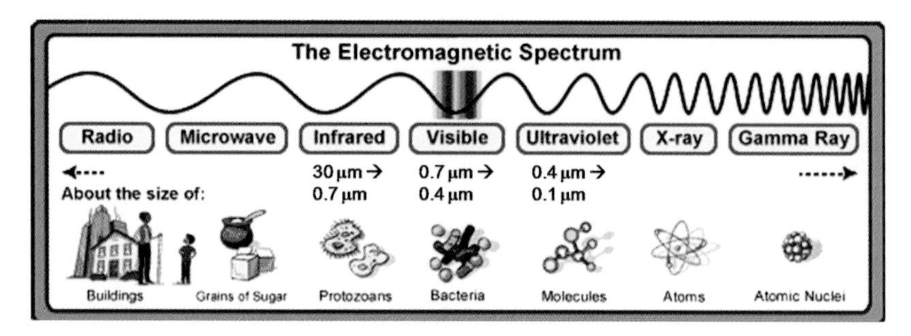


**Plate 1.1** Optical electromagnetic wavelengths ("light") can be divided into infrared, visible, and ultraviolet bands. [Credit: NASA (www.nasa.gov)].

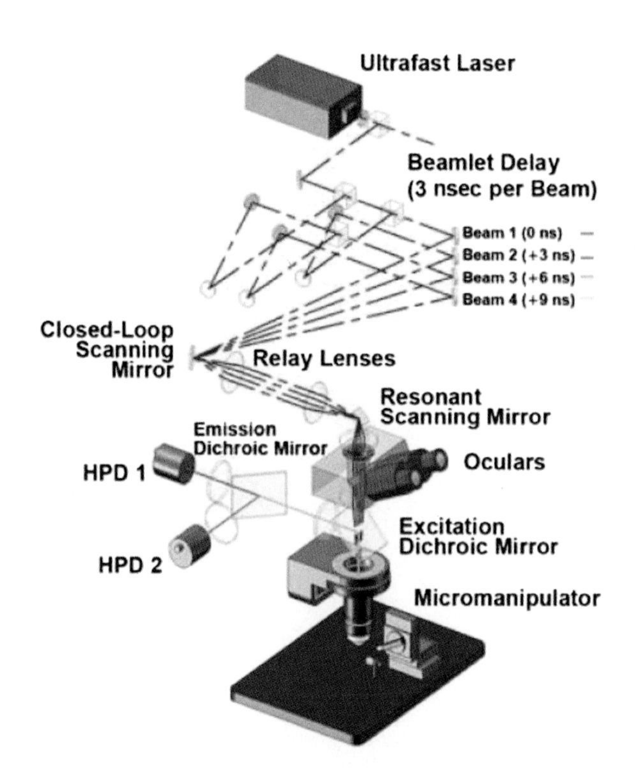


**Plate 1.2** Typical laser system components include lasers, optics, scanners, and detectors. [Reprinted with permission from: A. Cheng et al., "Simultaneous two-photon calcium imaging at different depths with spatiotemporal multiplexing," *Nature Methods* **8**, 139–142 (2011).]

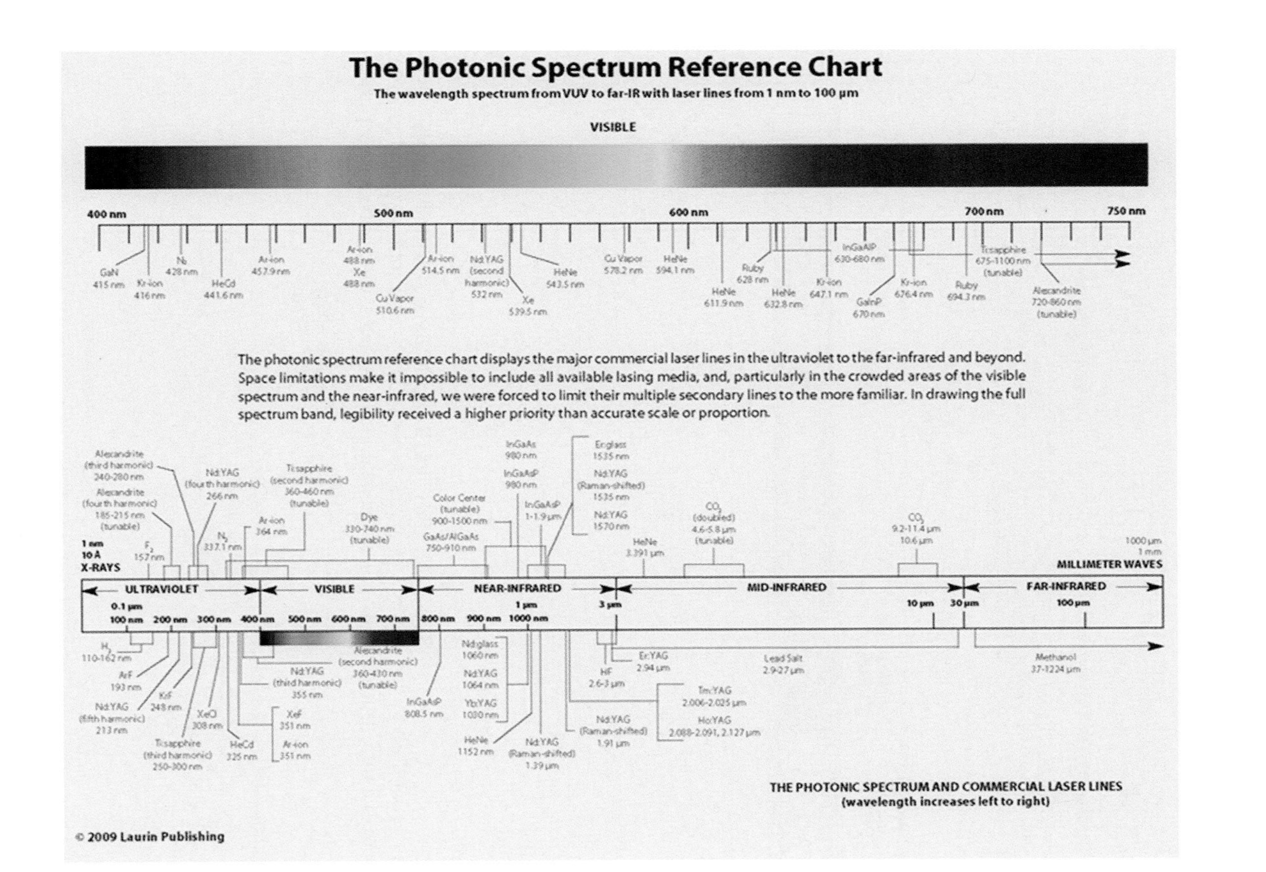


**Plate 1.3** The large number of laser types and wavelengths makes laser selection for system development a complex task. (© 2009 Laurin Publishing; reprinted with permission.)

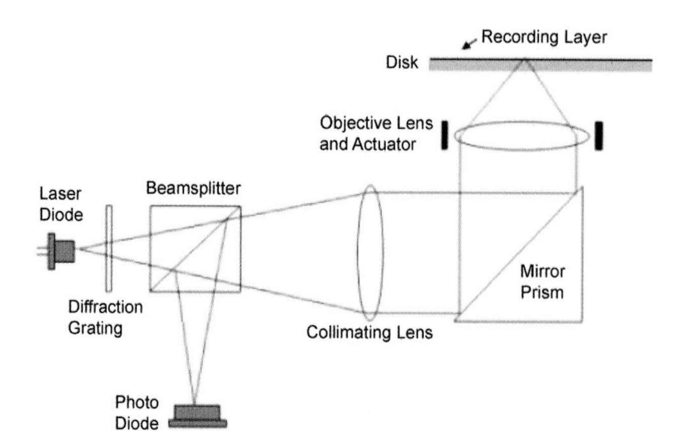


**Plate 1.4** Optical data storage requires lasers with beams that can be focused to the smallest possible spot size. [Reprinted from W.-S. Sun et al., "Compact HD-DVD pickup head with a lens-prism," *Proc. SPIE* **5174**, 128–135 (2003).]

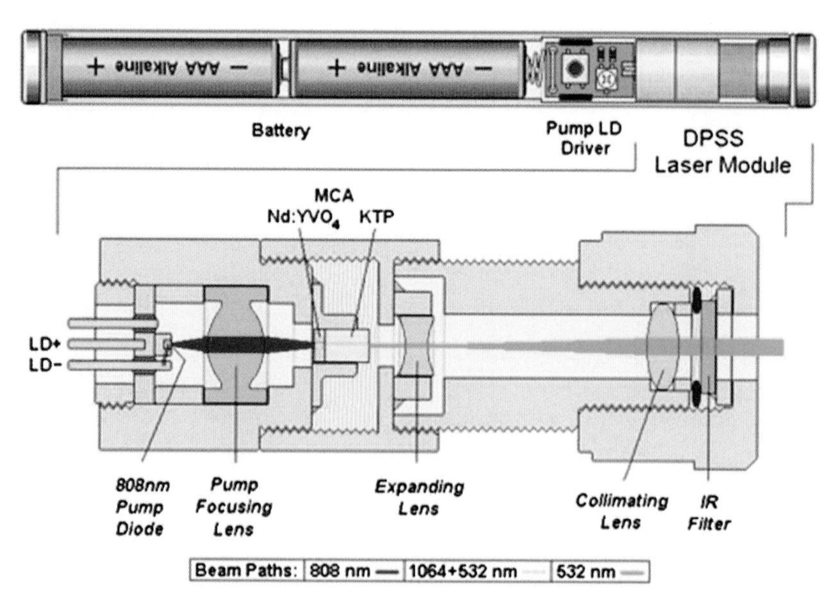


**Plate 1.19** Second-harmonic generation (SHG) of 1064-nm photons from a Nd:$YVO_4$ laser into 532-nm photons uses a nonlinear crystal such as KTP. (Credit: Chris Chen, Wikimedia Commons.)

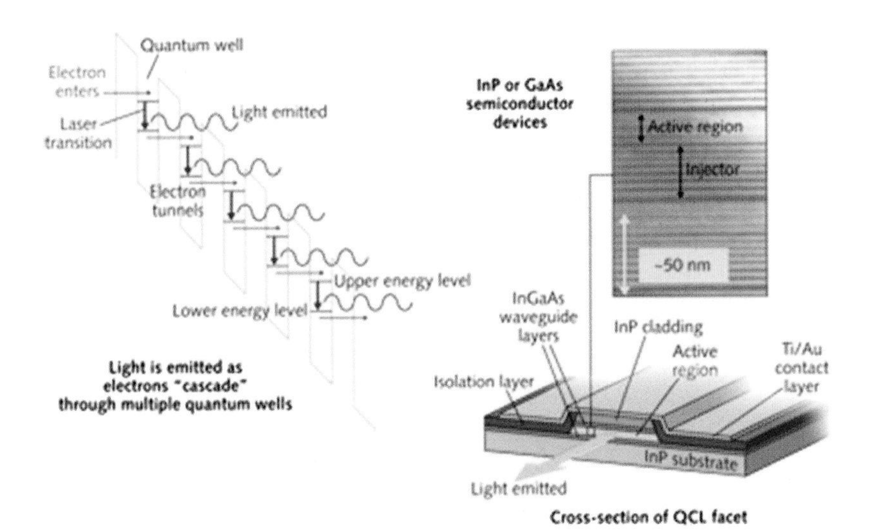


**Plate 2.22** Closely stacked quantum wells allow an electron that has changed its energy state by emitting a photon to cascade through the wells. (Credit: Prof. Jerome Faist, ETH Zurich.)

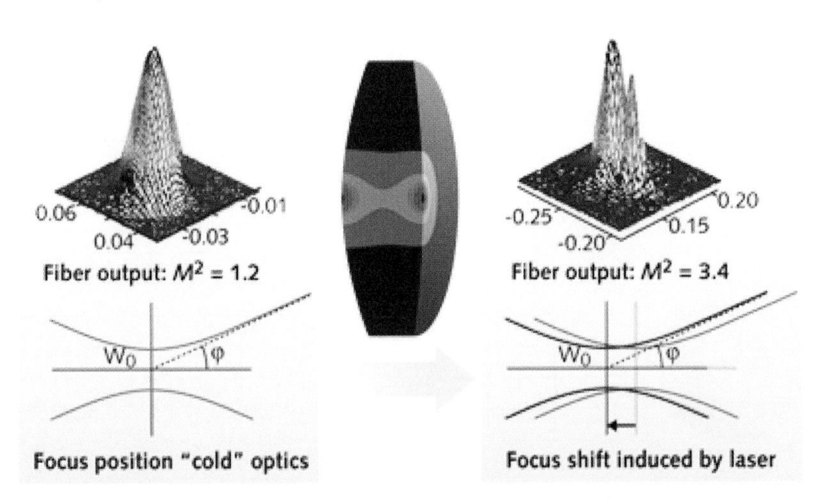


**Plate 2.24** Thermal lensing from a non-uniform temperature distribution changes both the focus position and transmitted beam quality. (Reprinted with permission from the 49th edition of *Laser Focus World*. © 2013 PennWell.)

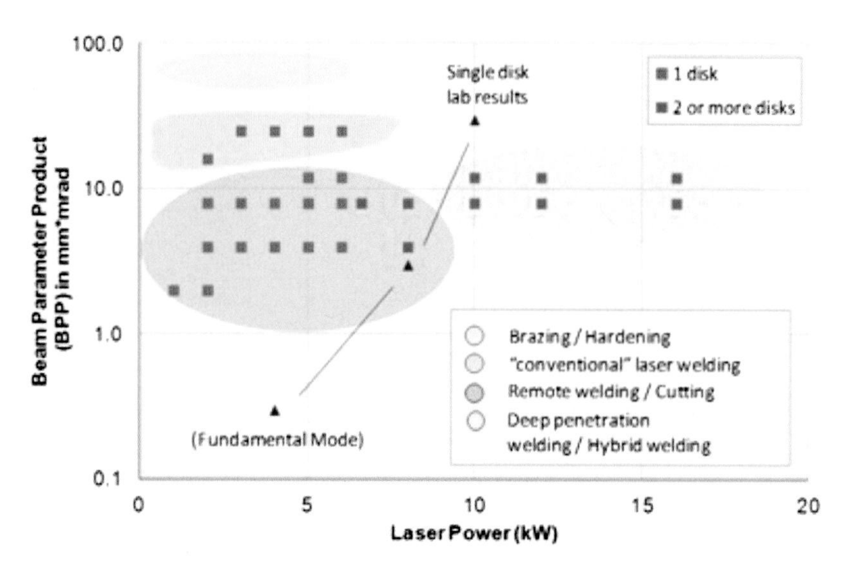


**Plate 2.27** Kilowatt-class CW disk lasers are currently restricted to applications such as welding that do not require good beam quality. (Reprinted from Ref. 33.)

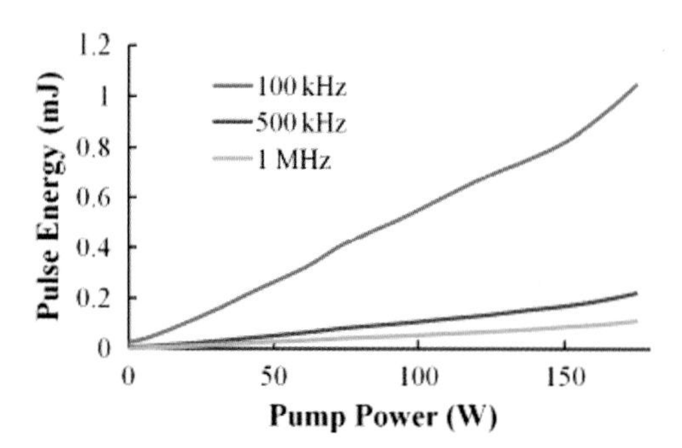


**Plate 2.31** With the same average pump power, pulse energy decreases as PRF increases per Eq. (2.6). [Reprinted with permission from P. Wang et al., "All fiber-based Yb-doped high energy, high power femtosecond fiber lasers," *Optics Express* **21**(24), 29854–29859 (2013).]

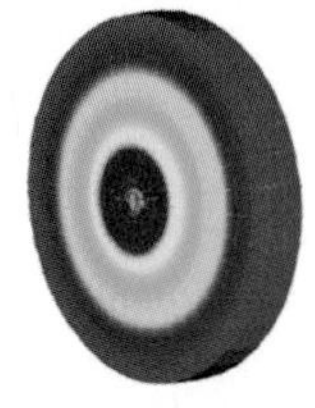

| Material | Index | CTE (ppm/K) | $dn/dT$ (ppm/K) | Wavelength | $G$ (ppm/K) |
|---|---|---|---|---|---|
| N-BK7 | 1.52 | 7.1 | 3.0 | 541.6 nm | 6.7 |
| Fused Silica | 1.46 | 0.5 | 10.2 | 541.6 nm | 10.4 |
| Sapphire | 1.77 | 5.3 | 13.1 | 541.6 nm | 17.2 |
| Silicon | 3.40 | 2.6 | 162 | 3–5 μm | 168 |
| Germanium | 4.00 | 6.1 | 385 | 8–12 μm | 403 |

**Plate 4.4** The thermo-optic constant $G$ shows that N-BK7 is less sensitive to radial thermal gradients compared to fused silica.[4] [Image reprinted from K. B. Doyle, V. L. Genberg, and G. J. Michels, *Integrated Optomechanical Analysis*, Second Edition, SPIE Press, Bellingham, Washington (2012).]

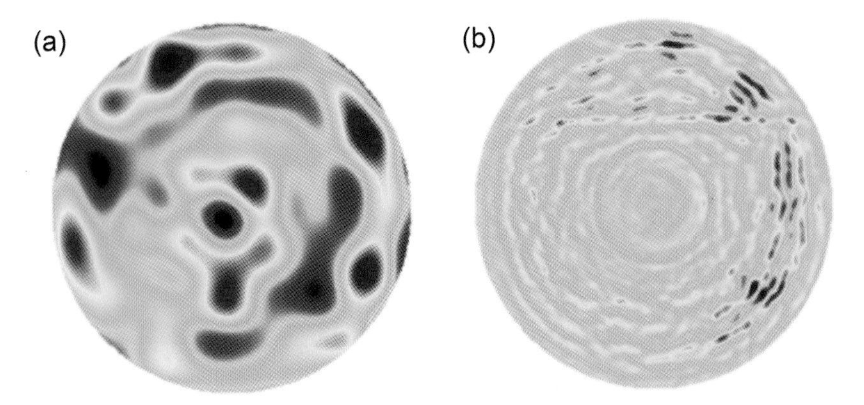


**Plate 4.27** (a) Low-spatial-frequency errors and (b) mid-spatial-frequency ripple errors from the fabrication process. (Reprinted from Ref. 19.)

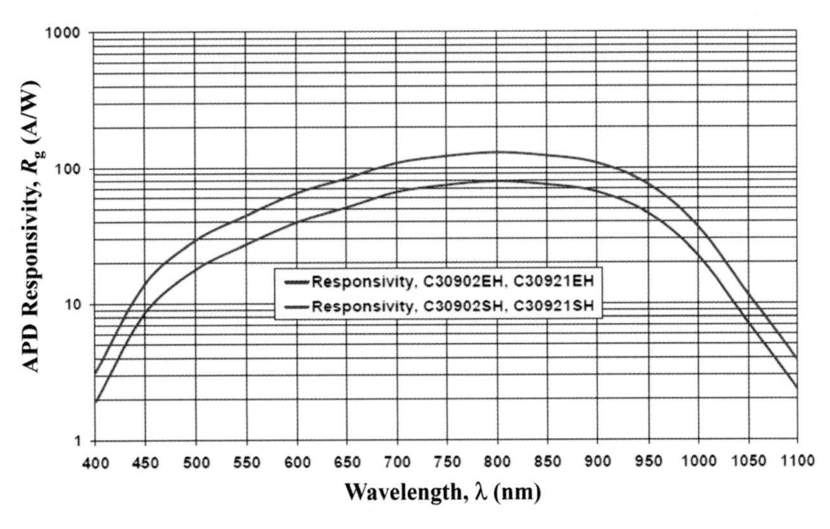


**Plate 7.7** APD responsivity $R_g \equiv R_o G$ is significantly higher than that of the PIN photodiode. (Courtesy of Excelitas Canada Inc., C30902 Series silicon APD data sheet; reprinted with permission.)

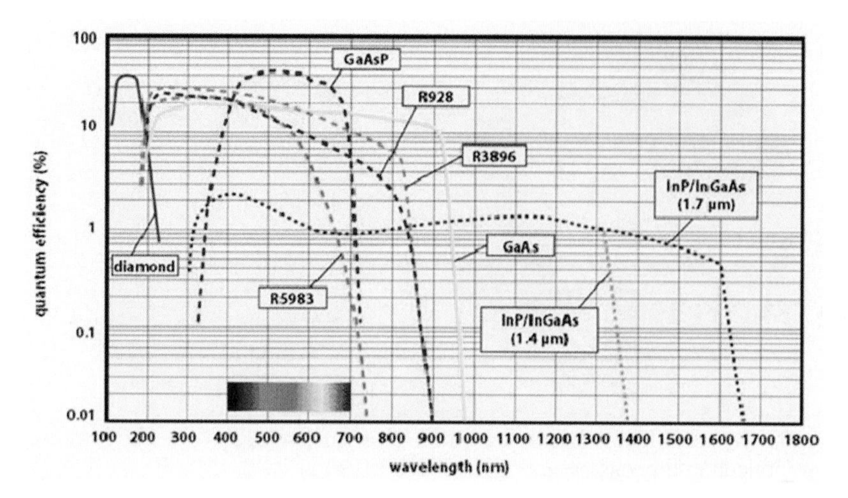


**Plate 7.16** The average QE spectrum of various PMT photocathode materials. (Reprinted with permission from Hamamatsu Photonics.[21])

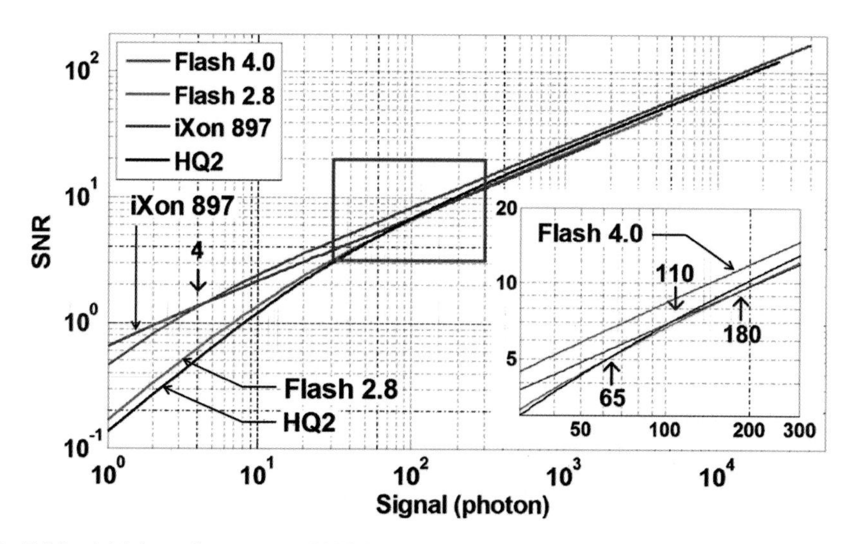


**Plate 7.26** A high-performance sCMOS array (Flash 4.0) has a better SNR than other FPA technologies for a signal photon number greater than 4. [Adapted with permission from F. Long, S. Zeng, and Z.-L. Huang, "Localization-based super-resolution microscopy with an sCMOS camera Part II: Experimental methodology for comparing sCMOS with EMCCD cameras," *Optics Express* **20**(16), 17741 (2012).]

# Chapter 7
# Detectors

When asked to describe the most important detector used in laser systems, most people will not mention the human eye (Fig. 7.1). With a dynamic range still unmatched by technology, the human eye is also the most common detector in or near the system. Laser safety officers spend many hours training employees on how to protect their eyes from laser damage, as the optical gain of the eye can increase the irradiance on the retina by a factor of 100,000 in comparison with that incident on the cornea, easily resulting in localized damage or even complete blindness using surprisingly low-power or low-energy lasers.

While the detector technologies developed to date are also susceptible to damage from low-power lasers, the purpose of this chapter is to review the options available for photon detection, not damage protection (aka *laser hardening*). These options include a choice of detector materials, detector types, detector geometry, and FPA technologies. For example, a laser-scanning microscope used to obtain images of biomedical samples typically scans a single-pixel, high-sensitivity detector to collect power over the FOV of the specimen. A flash laser radar system, on the other hand, relies on an FPA

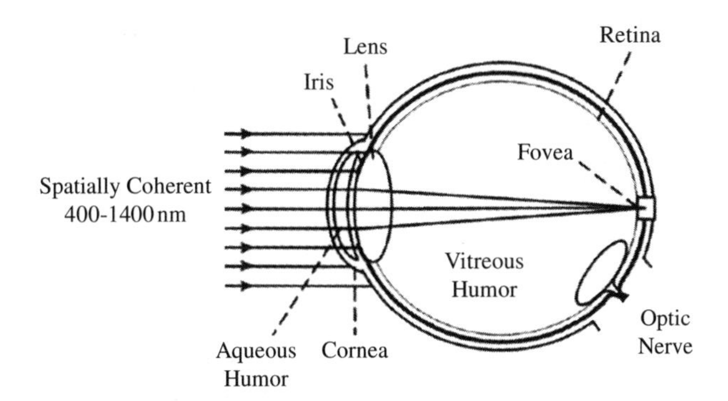


**Figure 7.1** The human eye can focus spatially coherent laser light (400–1400 nm) onto a small spot on the retina. [Adapted from D. Sliney and M. Wolbarsht, *Safety with Lasers and Other Optical Sources*, Plenum Press, New York (1980).]

to collect both power and time-of-flight information for each pixel in the array.

One of the most basic choices for detector selection, then, is single-pixel versus FPA geometry—a choice that is influenced as much by the detector options as it is by the other subsystems (laser, optics, and beam scanning) that must be included in the overall system design. In this chapter, we first review the available single-pixel types for photon detection: PIN photodiodes (Section 7.1), avalanche photodiodes (Section 7.2), and photomultiplier tubes (Section 7.3). In Section 7.4, we then look at the unique aspects of incorporating PIN and avalanche photodiodes into laser-system FPAs. Section 7.5 closes the chapter with a review of single-pixel and FPA noise limitations, photon sensitivity, and detector selection.

## 7.1 PIN Photodiodes

The most common detector technology used in laser systems is a photon detector; i.e., it is sensitive to photon energy, not thermal energy. There are also detectors that are sensitive to thermal energy; known as thermopiles and pyroelectrics, these detectors are almost always used for test-and-measurement tasks such as laser power characterization, but the goal of this chapter is a review of the detectors commonly used in the design of the laser system itself, not its measurement. In this section, we first review the basic concepts behind photon detectors, and then describe the principles and laser-system specs for *p-n* junction and PIN photodiodes.

### 7.1.1 Photon detectors

A photon detector measures the number of incident photons or photons per second. This can range anywhere from single-photon sensitivity to more than $10^{21}$ photons per second, corresponding to a kilowatt of optical power at visible wavelengths. What allows the measurement of photons is the use of a semiconductor such as silicon. For these materials, absorbed photons can transfer their energy to electrons that are normally bound to an atom, giving those electrons enough energy to move around the material and ultimately be measured as either accumulated or moving charge (i.e., current).

Each incident photon ideally produces one electron, converting photons per second into current (electron charge per second). In practice, the number of electrons created from an incident photon is less than one, with losses occurring because of Fresnel reflection at the detector surface (the reflected photons never make it into the absorption layer), incomplete absorption (due to a thin absorption layer), and poor material quality (which causes electrons to be lost before they can be measured as current).

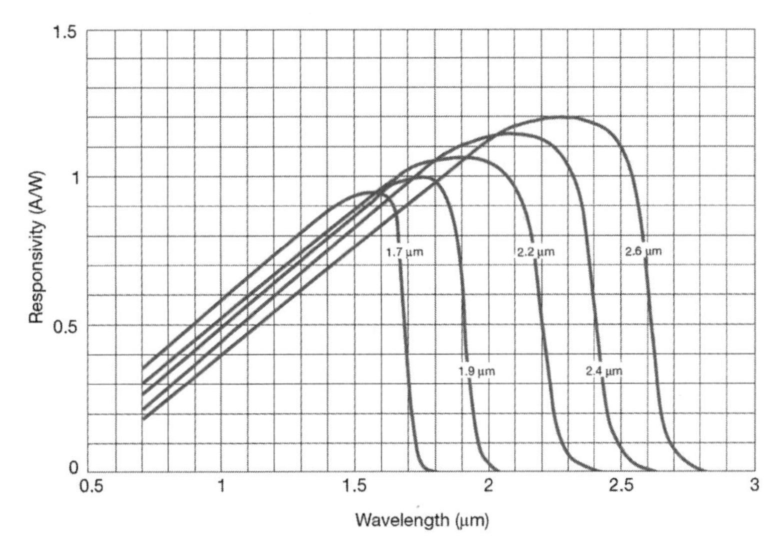


**Figure 7.2** For photon detectors, the current produced per watt of incident photons varies with wavelength; the numbers shown for each curve are the cutoff wavelengths for different varieties of InGaAs. (Credit: Teledyne Judson Technologies; reprinted with permission.)

A detector specification that takes all of these effects into account is known as the responsivity $R_o$. Responsivity is a direct measure of how efficiently a watt of peak optical power at a specific wavelength produces detector current, and it is often measured in units of amps per watt (A/W) of incident optical power. Figure 7.2 shows how responsivity varies with wavelength for indium gallium arsenide (InGaAs, pronounced "in gas") devices, a typical semiconductor material for detecting SWIR wavelengths. If the responsivity and laser power $\Phi$ incident on the detector at a particular wavelength are known, then the detector photocurrent $i_d = R_o\Phi$.

There are a couple of features in Fig. 7.2 that must be understood when designing photon detectors into laser systems. The first is the initial increase in responsivity with wavelength. Chapter 4 showed that material absorption depends on wavelength; since the absorption of semiconductors is typically smaller at longer wavelengths, one might expect their responsivity to be smaller as well. Instead, responsivity increases with wavelength (up to a certain cutoff point), as determined by the photon energy $E_p$:

$$E_p = \frac{hc}{\lambda} \qquad [\text{J}] \tag{7.1}$$

showing that photon energy is smaller at longer wavelengths, and more photons per second are therefore needed to create one watt of optical power $\Phi$. Quantitatively, the number of photons per second $N_p$ at a given wavelength is given by

$$N_{\mathrm{p}} = \frac{\Phi}{E_{\mathrm{p}}} \qquad [\text{photons/sec}] \qquad (7.2)$$

where the optical power is measured at a specific wavelength and the photon energy associated with this wavelength is given by Eq. (7.1). For example, 1 W of optical power at $\lambda = 0.5$ μm ($E_{\mathrm{p}} = 3.98 \times 10^{-19}$ joules/photon) in the visible corresponds to approximately $2.5 \times 10^{18}$ photons per second, whereas 1 W of power in the MWIR ($\lambda \approx 5$ μm) requires 10× as many photons per second, with each photon having only one-tenth the energy of those in the visible.

Since the number of electrons created in a photon detector is directly proportional to the number of incident photons, it follows that 1 W of longer-wavelength photons creates more photocurrent than 1 W of shorter-wavelength photons—initially resulting in an increase in responsivity with wavelength.

The second feature of interest in Fig. 7.2 is that the increase in responsivity with wavelength for photon detectors doesn't increase forever. The peak occurs when the photon energy, as it becomes less and less at longer wavelengths, is no longer sufficient to give electrons enough energy to conduct. At that point, the low material absorption dominates the responsivity, and $R_{\mathrm{o}}$ quickly decreases to zero.

The point at which responsivity is essentially zero is controlled by a semiconductor material property known as the bandgap energy. That is, the energy of an absorbed photon must be greater than the bandgap energy $E_{\mathrm{g}}$ in order for the semiconductor's electrons to have enough energy to conduct (i.e., $E_{\mathrm{p}} > E_{\mathrm{g}}$). The photon wavelength associated with this bandgap energy is the cutoff wavelength, beyond which detector responsivity is reduced to essentially zero.

An equally important point on the curves plotted in the figure is the peak responsivity, which occurs at about 90% of the cutoff wavelength.[1] For example, the cutoff wavelength for InGaAs with a bandgap energy of 0.75 eV (= $1.2 \times 10^{-19}$ J) is 1.24 eV-μm/(0.75 eV) = 1.65 μm. The peak responsivity then occurs at a wavelength of approximately $0.9 \times 1.65$ μm $\approx 1.5$ μm, as seen in the curve labeled "1.7 μm" in Fig. 7.2.

An efficient laser system matches, as best it can, the wavelength of the peak responsivity with the laser's output spectrum (Table 7.1). Silicon and InSb are photon-detector materials with a fixed bandgap and peak wavelength, but the bandgap for other material systems—e.g., InGaAs and mercury cadmium telluride (or HgCdTe, pronounced as "mer cad tel" or simply "mer cad")—can be controlled. Using HgCdTe as an example, there is no such thing as a unique "HgCdTe" detector. The complete description is actually $Hg_{1-x}Cd_xTe$, where $x$ denotes the fraction of cadmium atoms in the semiconductor that determines the bandgap of the material. For example, 200 atoms of the semiconductor $Hg_{0.7}Cd_{0.3}Te$ would consist of 70 atoms of

**Table 7.1** Photon detector materials most commonly used for a given laser wavelength band, listed alphabetically within the band.[3]

| Wavelength (μm) | Band | Detector Materials |
|---|---|---|
| 0.1–0.4 | UV | InGaN, Si, SiC |
| 0.4–0.7 | VIS | CdS, Ge, HgCdTe, Si |
| 0.7–1 | NIR | CdSe, Ge, HgCdTe, InGaAs, Si |
| 1–3 | SWIR | Ge, HgCdTe, InGaAs, InAs, PbS, Si |
| 3–5 | MWIR | HgCdTe, InSb, PbSe |
| 8–12 | LWIR | HgCdTe, QWIP, Si:As |

mercury, 30 atoms of cadmium, and 100 atoms of tellurium; its net bandgap energy is approximately 0.25 eV at 77 K.[2] Similarly, "InGaAs" is most often $In_{0.53}Ga_{0.46}As$—although, as seen in Fig. 7.2, other compositions are also used to shift the peak responsivity to different wavelengths.

### 7.1.2 Reverse-bias PINs

The PIN photodiode is the first type of detector to be considered in designing a laser system. It is fast and relatively sensitive to low-power levels, and is readily available in FPA formats for imaging. Applications include high-speed, single-pixel detectors for measuring data communications (datacom) pulses and active imaging using laser illuminators and silicon and InGaAs PIN photodiode FPAs.

The PIN photodiode is based on the semiconductor *p-n* junction. That is, a photodiode is created when a *p*-doped and *n*-doped layer of semiconductor are grown on top of each other (Fig. 7.3). These layers are often made of the same semiconductor (e.g., silicon), but each layer is doped with additional materials that have either extra electrons (the "n" layer in Fig. 6.6) or extra holes (the "p" layer). Without going into the details, this produces a large electric field across the interface where the *p*-layer and *n*-layer meet

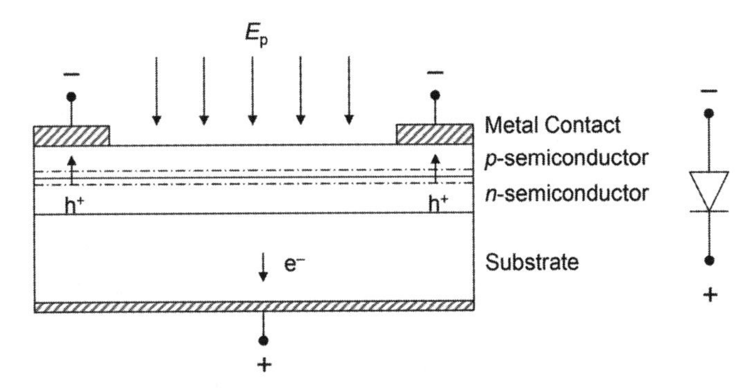


**Figure 7.3** A semiconductor *p-n* junction allows the mobile electrons ($e^-$) and holes ($h^+$) created by absorbed photons to be collected at metal contacts and measured as photocurrent.

(the *p-n* junction); this field is in response to a charge redistribution and resulting voltage drop across a thin layer surrounding the junction from which charge is depleted (the depletion region), shown as the area between the dashed lines in Fig. 7.3.[4]

The large electric field pulls electrons (and holes) away from the junction, where they are collected as current at electrical contacts. This phenomenon is referred to as the photovoltaic (PV) effect and is useful for converting photons into electrical power. Unfortunately, the efficiency with which photons are converted to conduction electrons is limited in part by the low absorption of the thin depletion region. Photons are also absorbed outside the junction, but those photoelectrons can be lost (recombine with holes) in the time it takes for them to move (diffuse) toward the contacts.

For better performance, the electric field is made larger by applying a negative voltage (a reverse bias) across the junction. This results in a slightly thicker depletion region, which yields a modest improvement in conversion efficiency; the larger field near where photons are absorbed also increases the speed at which the electrons are moved away from the junction and measured at the contacts as current. In this case, we could say that the photodiode is being used in *photoconductive* mode. However, there is obviously some potential for verbal confusion with photoconductive detectors,[5] so a better term to use is *reverse-bias* mode.

Better absorption efficiency and higher speed can be obtained by adding a third layer between the *p* and *n* layers (Fig. 7.4). This extra layer is not doped and thus creates an undoped (intrinsic) layer where absorption occurs; the result is a three-layer *p-i-n* photodiode (often written as PIN). This additional layer is quite a bit thicker ($\approx$ 1–10 $\mu$m) than the *p-n* junction depletion region; it thus provides more absorption in the vicinity of the electric field and also results in a lower capacitance and much higher speed—exceeding 10 GHz for optimized designs.[6]

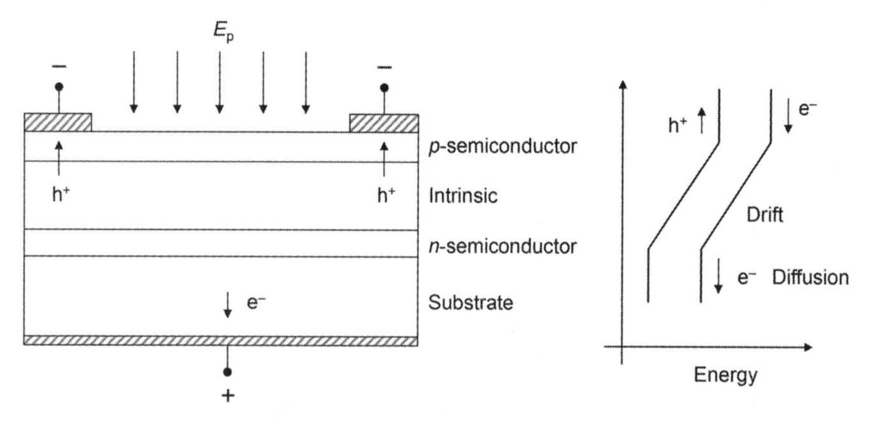


**Figure 7.4** The thick intrinsic layer in a PIN photodiode results in higher speed and greater responsivity than is possible with simple *p-n* junction detectors.

An applied voltage—a reverse bias $V_b < 0$—also helps separate the charge carriers and increase the speed, while also preventing the voltage from drifting as photons are absorbed and create free carriers. Unfortunately, the reverse bias also allows more dark current to flow in the absence of photons—a source of noise that can affect sensitivity (see Section 7.5).

### 7.1.3 PIN detector specifications

Just as there were for lasers, there are a number of important specs that a detector must meet. In this section, we review those that are relevant to reverse-bias PINs; other specs specific to avalanche photodiodes, photo-multiplier tubes, and FPAs will be looked at in more detail in Sections 7.2, 7.3, and 7.4, respectively.

**Responsivity and Quantum Efficiency.** As we have seen, responsivity is one of the most important specs for detectors. An equally common measure of detector output for photon detectors is the quantum efficiency (QE). Rather than measuring current per watt of optical power, QE measures the related quantity of how many electrical quanta (electrons) are produced for each optical quantum (photon) absorbed. Even if the electrons are later amplified, as in an avalanche photodiode (APD) or electron-multiplying CCD detector, the number of electrons produced by photon absorption can be no more than 1.0 and is typically less than 0.95. As shown in Fig. 7.5, the QE is fairly constant with wavelength across the absorption range of the detector material (1–1.5 μm); this is because, unlike the

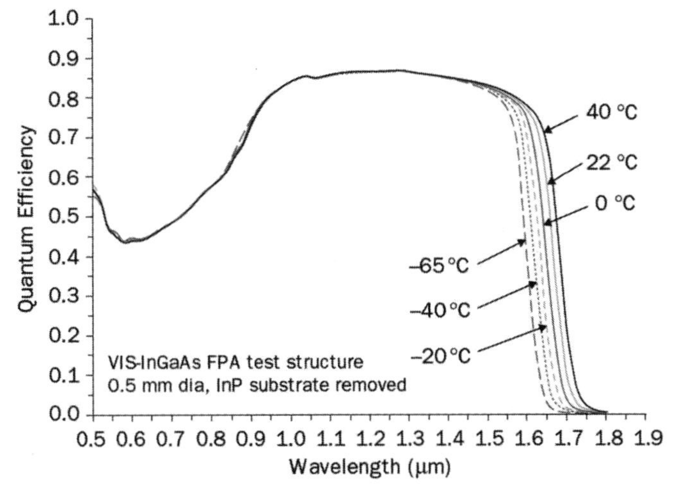


**Figure 7.5** In contrast to the responsivity shown in Fig. 7.2, the quantum efficiency is more or less constant over a range of wavelengths. [Reprinted from H. Yuan, G. Apgar, J. Kim, J. Laquindanum, V. Nalavade, P. Beer, J. Kimchi, and T. Wong, "FPA development: from InGaAs, InSb, to HgCdTe," *Proc. SPIE* **6940**, 69403C (2008).]

responsivity plotted in Fig. 7.2, QE does not depend on the absolute number of absorbed photons.

Responsivity is an engineering spec that's easily measured, whereas QE is derived from that measurement. Given that QE is defined as the number of electrons generated ($n_e$) per number of photons absorbed ($n_p$), it can be converted to responsivity once we realize that detector current equals coulombs per second ($i_d = n_e q/\Delta t$) and optical power equals photon energy per second ($\Phi = n_p h\nu/\Delta t$). Thus, the relation between responsivity $R_o$ and quantum efficiency $\eta_{QE} \equiv n_e/n_p$ for photodiodes can be expressed as

$$R_o = \frac{i_d}{\Phi} = \frac{n_e q/\Delta t}{n_p h\nu/\Delta t} = \frac{\eta_{QE} q}{h\nu} = \frac{\eta_{QE} q\lambda}{hc} = \frac{\eta_{QE}\lambda}{1.24} \quad [\text{A/W}] \tag{7.3}$$

where the wavelength $\lambda$ must be measured in units of microns for the constant $hc/q = 1.24$ eV-μm = 1240 eV-nm. As expected, the responsivity for photodiodes increases linearly with wavelength for a constant QE, since proportionally more photons are required to produce a watt of optical power at longer wavelengths.

Because of this wavelength dependence, comparing responsivity and QE can lead to incorrect conclusions regarding detection efficiency. For example, InGaAs has a QE of 80% at a wavelength of 1.55 μm, which Eq. (7.3) shows corresponds to a responsivity $R_o = 1.0$ A/W. A comparable VIS detector with the same QE at $\lambda = 0.5$ μm, on the other hand, has a responsivity of only 0.32 A/W. Quantum efficiency is thus the more fundamental measure for detector comparisons; additional details on the use and limitations of QE can be found in Ref. 5.

**Bandwidth.** How quickly a detector needs to respond depends on the application, with speeds ranging from 60-Hz video rates for FPA active imaging up to 10 GHz for measuring datacom pulses. Video rates do not need to discriminate between the pulses used for active-imaging illumination, and the detector in that case only needs to respond to slow changes in average power.

Laser systems that measure peak power and pulse energy, however (datacom, lasercom, and laser radar signals, e.g.) require a detector response time that is fast enough—and an associated electrical bandwidth that is wide enough—to pass the pulse spectrum and not attenuate it. Fourier analysis indicates that creating a rapidly changing signal requires a spectrum extending out to higher-frequency sinusoids;[7] shorter pulses thus require more bandwidth. Depending on the pulse shape, the electrical bandwidth $\Delta f$ is often approximated by[8]

$$\Delta f \approx \frac{1}{2\Delta t} \qquad [\mathrm{Hz}] \qquad (7.4)$$

where $\Delta t$ is the laser pulse width ($\Delta t = \Delta t_p$). For example, Nd:YAG pulses of 10-nsec duration require an electrical-system measurement bandwidth $\Delta f \approx 1/(2 \times 10 \times 10^{-9}$ sec) = 50 MHz. Measuring the pulse shape (and not just its energy), however, requires a faster response time $\Delta t$ so that the temporal details of the pulse form—rise time, fall time, etc.—can be extracted.

PIN photodiodes have the fastest available response time; they can measure peak power or changes in pulse energy at rates of 10 GHz and higher, depending on material type. The InGaAs PINs in particular have been optimized for very high speeds, given their high responsivity at a wavelength of 1.5 μm and resulting applicability for use in high-speed fiber-optic networks.

**Sensitivity.** While the highest-possible detector bandwidth may be an important spec, the smallest possible power that can be measured may also govern the system design. As we have seen in Section 1.3, for example, a common systems engineering design trade is to use a less-powerful laser when a more-sensitive detector is available.

One metric for determining the sensitivity of a detector is the signal needed to equal the detection noise. The sources of noise that can overwhelm the signal are many—the signal itself, background fluctuations, detector dark current, post-detector amplifier noise, speckle, and so on—and when the signal current $i_s = R_o \Phi_s$ equals the total noise current $\sigma_n$, the sensitivity is given by $\Phi_s$ and is known as the noise-equivalent power (NEP). As we will see in more detail in Section 7.5, a simple example is when the amplifier noise $\sigma_{amp}$ is much larger than the others; the NEP in that case is given by

$$NEP_{amp} = \frac{NSD\sqrt{\Delta f}}{R_o} \qquad [\mathrm{W}] \qquad (7.5)$$

where a noisier amplifier [i.e., an increase in the amplifier's noise spectral density (NSD)] and a wider measurement bandwidth $\Delta f$ make the detector less sensitive (higher NEP), and a higher responsivity makes it more sensitive (smaller NEP). Note that NEP values listed on vendor spec sheets will sometimes be listed in units of $W/Hz^{1/2}$ over a given frequency range ($pW/Hz^{1/2}$, for example), which is obtained by dividing both sides of Eq. (7.5) by $\Delta f^{1/2}$.

It would seem from Eq. (7.5) that the only way to improve the sensitivity of an amplifier-limited laser system is to use a quieter amplifier, smaller bandwidth, or higher-responsivity detector. Once this is done for a PIN photodiode, the need for even better sensitivity pushes the system design to a different type of detector, namely, an avalanche photodiode (APD).

## 7.2 Avalanche Photodiodes

The APD has internal gain that increases the responsivity in Eq. (7.5) to something on the order of 10–100× larger, thus decreasing the NEP by the same factor. Applications for APDs include the detection of very weak, single-photon return signals by space-based laser radar instruments collecting Earth-science environmental data, as well as receivers for long-distance fiber-optic communications that measure Internet data at bandwidths greater than 10 GHz.

APDs can be classified into two types based on applied voltage: linear mode (Section 7.2.1) and Geiger mode (Section 7.2.2). In addition, only two detector materials dominate the COTS products at this point: silicon for VIS–NIR APDs and InGaAs for SWIR APDs.

### 7.2.1 Linear-mode APDs

Avalanche photodiodes add to the basic PIN structure yet another layer that provides electron gain, with one photon producing more than one electron (Fig. 7.6). After a high voltage is applied, the additional layer has a large electric field strength across it; this forces conduction electrons to move quickly through the layer, where they may impact nonconduction electrons with enough energy to make them conductive. Each impact doubles the number of conduction electrons, a process that can "avalanche" to produce an extremely large number of electrons—a function of the applied voltage.

The resulting ratio of electrons to absorbed photons is known as the APD gain (symbol $G$), with optimum values of $G \approx 100$–$200$ for a "quiet" material such as silicon, and $G \approx 10$–$20$ for a noisier material such as InGaAs. Hence the gain-multiplied responsivity can be large, with a peak value $R_g \equiv R_o G \approx 1.0$ A/W $\times$ $100 = 100$ A/W for AR-coated silicon APDs (Fig. 7.7). If an APD

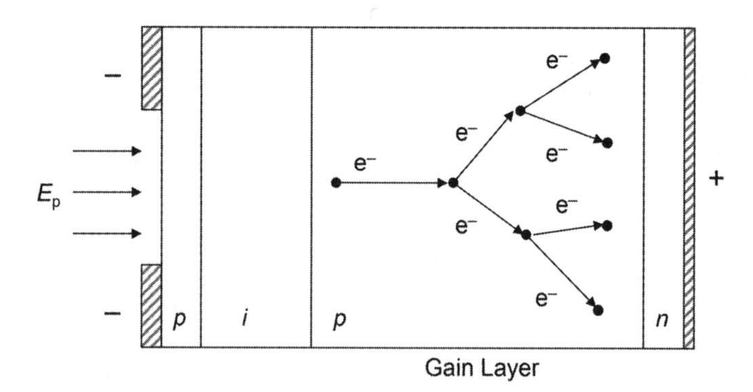


**Figure 7.6** Avalanche photodiodes (APDs) rely on momentum transfer via mechanical impact to give electrons enough energy to conduct. Each impact doubles the number of electrons, thereby creating an "avalanche." The gain $G$ illustrated in this figure is $G = 4$.

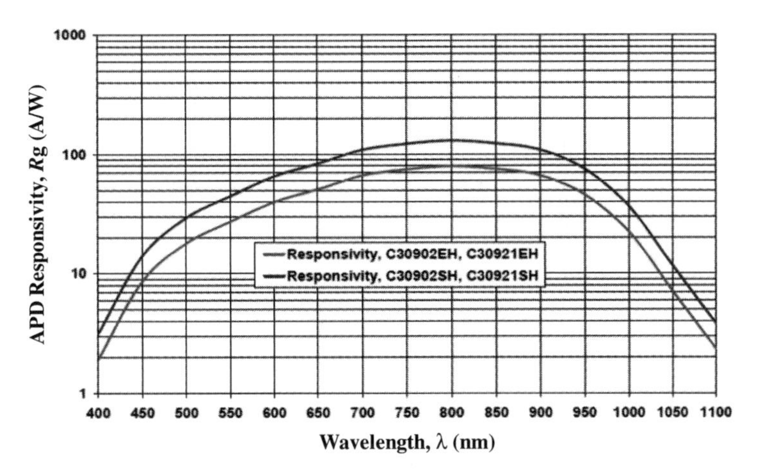


**Figure 7.7** APD responsivity $R_g \equiv R_o G$ is significantly higher than that of the PIN photodiode. (Courtesy of Excelitas Canada Inc., C30902 Series silicon APD data sheet; reprinted with permission.) (See color plate.)

is used in a laser system where the amplifier noise dominates even at high gain, Eq. (7.5) still applies, with $R_g$ substituted for $R_o$, and the NEP is improved (reduced) by the gain.

There are three costs to be paid for this gain. The first is that obtaining gain with a large electric field requires a higher voltage than is needed for a PIN, with 300–350 V for $G = 100$ being common for silicon APDs (in comparison with the 1–10 V needed for silicon PINs).

The second cost is the effect of gain on bandwidth. That is, we have seen in Section 7.1.3 how the bandwidth of a PIN photodiode can exceed 10 GHz. The same is true for APDs, with an important exception: the bandwidth varies inversely with gain at high gain, as it takes more time for avalanching to occur. This is described in terms of a gain–bandwidth product $G{\cdot}\Delta f$ that is constant at high gain; for example, an InGaAs APD may have $G{\cdot}\Delta f = 100$ GHz for $G = 10$–50. As a result, the bandwidth of such an APD is $\Delta f = G{\cdot}\Delta f / G = 100$ GHz/10 = 10 GHz at best, and lower by as much as a factor of 5 at higher gain. At moderate gain, however, the bandwidth is more-or-less independent of gain, as it depends on the carrier transit time or RC time constant, not avalanche time.

The third cost is that APDs add current-fluctuation noise to the system, which may be much larger at higher gains. This means that the gain can't be increased indefinitely; instead, there's an optimum gain whose value is determined by the material, amplifier noise, and electrical bandwidth. Below that optimum, the APD noise is still lower than the bandwidth-dependent amplifier noise (see Section 7.5); above the optimum, the APD noise is higher. Both noises are equal at the optimum, resulting in a detector with higher responsivity than a PIN photodiode. For high-bandwidth systems such as long-distance fiber-optic networks with large amplifier noise, the sensitivity of an optimum-gain APD can thus be better than that of a PIN.

For most semiconductors, the APD noise is associated with electrons and holes avalanching independently of each other. Known as excess noise, most APD materials exhibit a gain-dependent excess-noise factor $F(G)$ given by the McIntyre equation:[9]

$$F(G) = kG + (1 - k)\left(2 - \frac{1}{G}\right) \tag{7.6}$$

where the impact ionization ratio $k$ depends on how easily holes are ionized in comparison with electrons.[10] This equation is plotted in Fig. 7.8; typical values of $k$—with larger values resulting in a noisier APD—are $\approx 0.002$–$0.02$ for silicon, $\approx 0.2$–$0.5$ for InGaAs, and *undefined* for HgCdTe, which shows an ideal $F(G) = 1$ for *all* values of gain $G$, and is thus not explained by the McIntyre equation.

From the perspective of the laser systems engineer, the important features of Fig. 7.8 are the values of $F(G) \approx 2$ for small $k$ and large $G$, as well as the value of $F(G) \approx 1$ for HgCdTe (aka MCT). This indicates that MCT has near-noiseless gain—an almost unheard of concept in the world of amplifiers, but one that is confirmed by experiment (Fig. 7.9). While single-pixel APDs based on such MCT single-carrier (electron) ballistic gain are rarely available for the commercial market, high-cost products have been developed for military and aerospace applications in FPA format (see Section 7.4). The use of the excess-noise factor $F(G)$—noiseless or otherwise—will be illustrated with a system-design example in Section 7.5.1.

The dynamic range of APDs can vary from nanowatts to single-photon detection. The development of single-photon APDs—also known as single-photon avalanche diodes, or SPADs—has been particularly impressive over the last decade, with SPADs available as off-the-shelf products from

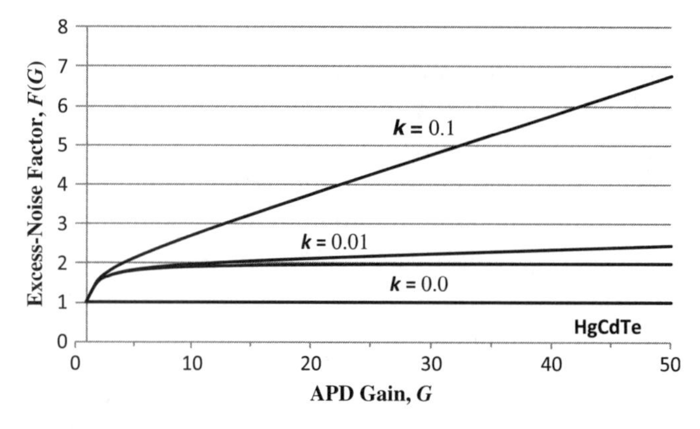


**Figure 7.8** Plot of Eq. (7.6) for various values of the impact ionization ratio $k$.

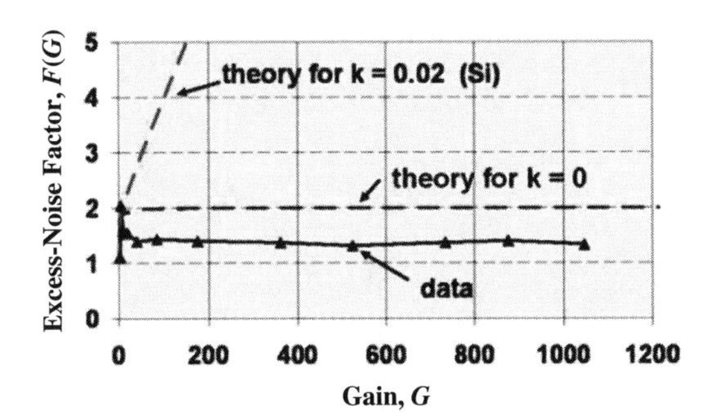


**Figure 7.9** HgCdTe APDs have near-noiseless gain with $F(G) < 2$. [Reprinted from J. Beck, J. McCurdy, M. Skokan, C. Kamilar, R. Scritchfield, T. Welch, P. Mitra, X. Sun, J. Abshire, and K. Reiff, "A highly sensitive multi-element HgCdTe e-APD detector for IPDA lidar applications, *Proc. SPIE* **8739,** 87390V (2013).]

companies such as Excelitas Technologies Corp. (Si SPADs) and ID Quantique (InGaAs SPADs).

One application requiring an NEP near the single-photon level is the fluorescence detection of biomedical samples. That is, after the inefficiencies of excitation laser absorption and fluorophore emission, there may be only a few photons remaining for detection.[11] Another application for SPADs is laser radar for self-driving vehicles, where laser pulses must be of a low enough energy to be eye safe at $\lambda = 905$ nm, possibly requiring a high-sensitivity detector.

Two types of SPADs have been developed: linear mode and Geiger mode. As shown in Fig. 7.10, the linear mode is obtained when the bias voltage $V_b$ is less than the APD breakdown voltage $V_{br}$, resulting in a proportional increase in detector current and responsivity $R_g = R_o G$ with

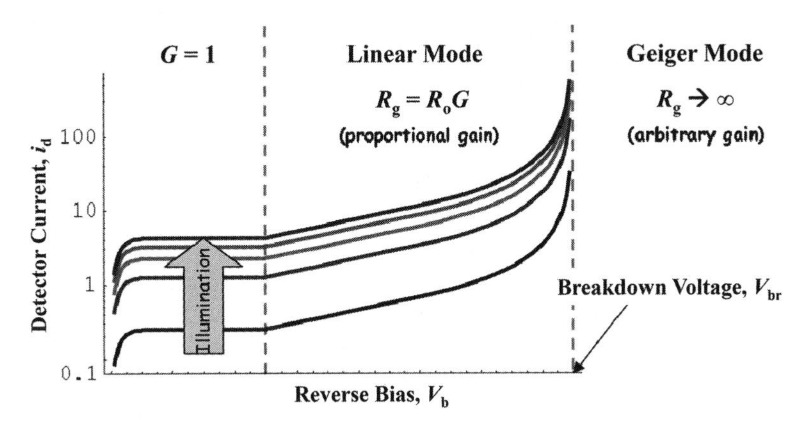


**Figure 7.10** APDs can be used in either linear mode or Geiger mode to obtain single-photon gain. [Adapted from G. Williams and A. Huntington, "Probabilistic analysis of linear mode vs. Geiger mode APD FPAs for advanced LADAR enabled interceptors," *Proc. SPIE* **6220**, 622008 (2006).]

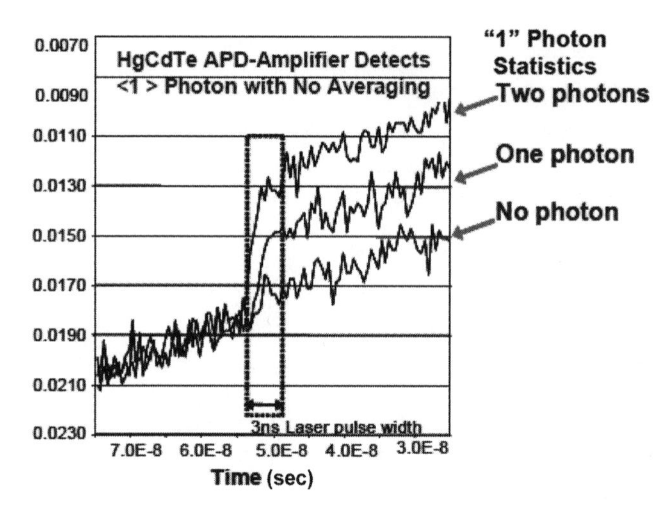


**Figure 7.11** A photon-counting linear-mode APD can discriminate between zero, one, two, etc., photons. [Reprinted from M. Jack, G. Chapman, J. Edwards, *et al.*, "Advances in ladar components and subsystems at Raytheon," *Proc. SPIE* **8353**, 83532F (2012).]

gain $G$ (but not $V_b$). Geiger-mode operation with $V_b \geq V_{br}$ will be reviewed in Section 7.2.2.

To date, linear-mode SPADs have been obtained with silicon APDs using a high-gain (near-breakdown) bias voltage[12] or low-voltage MCT APDs.[13,14] The concept of photon-number discrimination using linear-mode SPADs is illustrated in Fig. 7.11, where zero-, one-, and two-photon inputs are used to measure a proportional change in detector current for 3-nsec pulses at $\lambda = 1064$ nm. Despite the benefits of linear-mode SPADs over the Geiger-mode SPADs reviewed in the next section—e.g., photon-number discrimination and dynamic range, no quenching circuitry, relatively insensitive to dark counts (false positives), faster recovery times given the absence of afterpulsing, and so on—products have not yet made their way to the commercial market, given the limitations of cost and cryogenic cooling (180 K). Nonetheless, extremely expensive, moderate-format MCT FPAs have been developed for military and aerospace applications.[13–15]

### 7.2.2 Geiger-mode APDs

Another option for single-photon detection is the Geiger-mode APD, and here there are a number of commercial products available, both as single-pixel APDs and as FPAs, in both silicon and InGaAs—but only used as SPADs, not conventional APDs. As shown in Fig. 7.10, the reason is that the Geiger mode is obtained for a reverse bias $V_b \geq V_{br}$, which results in a nearly infinite responsivity when a photon is absorbed. The distinction between a conventional and a Geiger-mode APD is also determined by the detector design, where the vendors must use proprietary semiconductor structures to

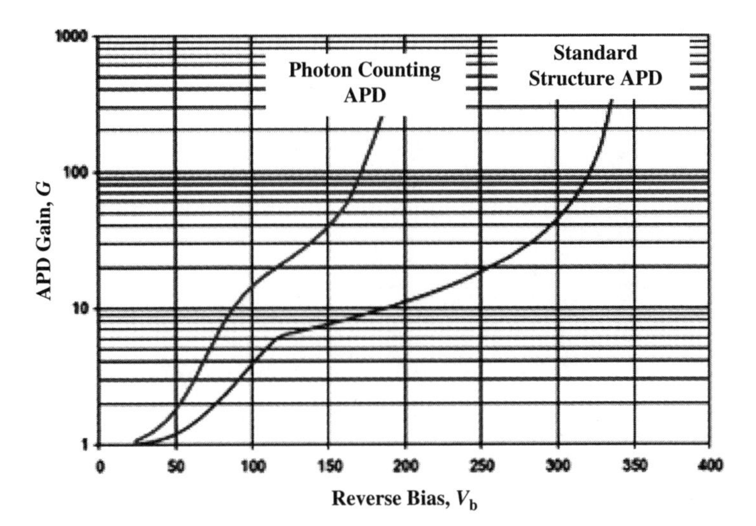


**Figure 7.12** APD gain $G$ reaches breakdown at a lower voltage for photon-counting APDs in comparison with standard-structure APDs. [Courtesy of Excelitas Canada Inc., "Avalanche Photodiodes: A User Guide" (2011); reprinted with permission.]

ensure single-photon sensitivity at relatively low breakdown voltage, resulting in performance differences between the different types of APDs (Fig. 7.12).

The benefit of using a Geiger-mode APD (GM-APD) is that a large pulse of current is created that is easily detected even in the presence of large amplifier noise. The disadvantages, however, are many, including:

- Unlike the linear-mode photon-counting APD illustrated in Fig. 7.11, the GM-APD cannot discriminate between one, two, or more photons. The detector avalanches as soon as one or more photons are absorbed, outputting an extremely large current pulse in response. The GM-APD, then, is a photon detector but not a single- or multiple-photon *counter*.
- The GM-APD is also extremely susceptible to any other "event" (or upset) that initiates avalanching, most notably dark counts, where electrons become mobile not by photon absorption but by thermal excitation. Such "false positives" indicate the presence of photons when, in fact, there are none.
- Whether initiated by photons or dark counts, the GM-APD is a "hairy beast" and continues to pulse output current well after the event has occurred (Fig. 7.13). Such afterpulsing requires an active quenching circuit to minimize and places a limitation on the smallest time allowed—the required holdoff time (or "dead time")—between pulses, determining the allowable laser PRF.

As we will see in Section 7.4, there are additional limitations on the use of GM-APDs in FPAs.

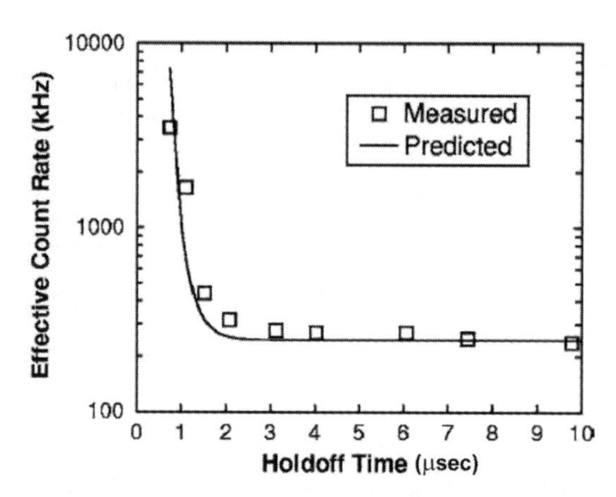


**Figure 7.13** The holdoff time (aka dead time or reset time) after a photon or dark-count event has initiated avalanching determines how quickly an APD can be "re-armed" (i.e., re-set to $V_b > V_{br}$) for the next measurement. [Reproduced with permission from K. E. Jensen, P. I. Hopman, E. K. Duerr, et al., "Afterpulsing in Geiger-mode avalanche photodiodes for 1.06 μm wavelength," *Applied Physics Letters* **88**, 133503 (2006). © 2006, AIP Publishing LLC.]

In practice, Geiger-mode avalanching requires attention to a number of operational details to obtain the performance specs promised by the vendors. The first of these is the timing and level of a gating voltage. That is, to reduce dark-count avalanching, the GM-APD voltage is held below breakdown and then momentarily increased ("armed") to some level above $V_{br}$ during a timing window synchronized with the laser PRF. The degree of bias above breakdown is called the excess bias (or overbias) voltage (Fig. 7.14); this voltage determines the photon detection efficiency (PDE), defined as the product of the QE and the efficiency $\eta_{GM}$ with which an absorbed photon results in a sustained avalanche, i.e., PDE $= \eta_{QE} \times \eta_{GM}$.[16] Unfortunately, the excess bias also allows more electrons and holes to conduct, thus increasing the dark-count rate.

The second operational detail is detector cooling to reduce the dark-count rate (DCR) for a given excess bias. Since dark counts compete with "light" counts (i.e., photons), the NEP for a Geiger-mode APD increases with the DCR:[17]

$$NEP_{GM} \approx \frac{2hv}{PDE}\sqrt{DCR \cdot \Delta f} \qquad [\mathrm{W}] \tag{7.7}$$

where the energy of a single photon is now expressed as an energy per unit time, i.e., the NEP.

Dark counts are measured in units of electron counts per second (cps or Hz) and increase exponentially with temperature. Thermoelectric coolers (TECs) operating at 220–250 K or so are thus sufficient for significantly

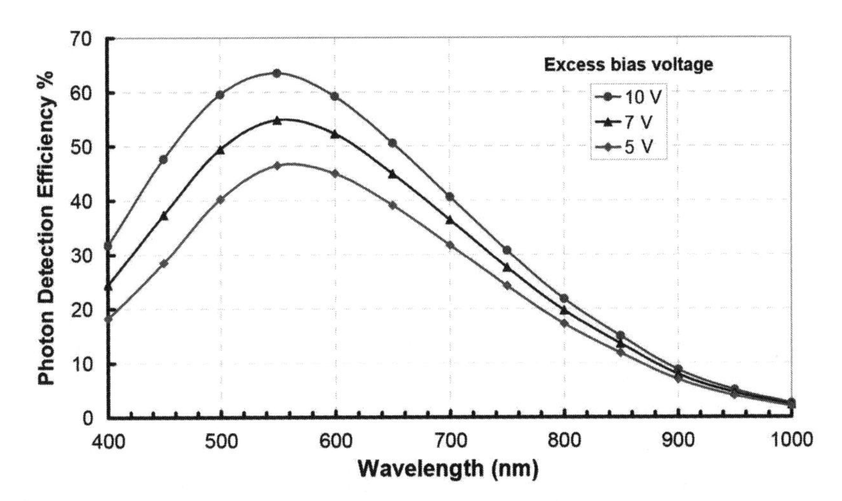


**Figure 7.14** The excess bias voltage above the APD breakdown voltage affects the photon detection efficiency and dark-count rate. [Reprinted from S. Cova, M. Ghioni, F. Aappa, I. Rech, and A. Gulinatti, "A view on progress of silicon single photon avalanche diodes and quenching circuits," *Proc. SPIE* **6372**, 63720I (2006).]

reducing the DCR and NEP. Typical dark-count rates for cooled silicon are 50–500 Hz (larger detectors have more atoms to generate dark current) at $T = 250$ K, while InGaAs—with its smaller bandgap energy—is inherently more susceptible to dark counts than silicon, with an InGaAs DCR $\approx$ 5–500 kHz at $T = 250$ K and a 4-V over-bias.

A third GM-APD spec—closely connected to the laser PRF—is the maximum count rate allowed by the dead time. That is, if the dead time required to settle down to a minimum count rate is 1 μsec for InGaAs (e.g.), then the pulse rate cannot be any faster than $1/10^{-6}$ sec = 1 MHz, thus placing a restriction on the laser PRF (or a reduced multiple). With silicon having a much shorter dead time of approximately 30–50 nsec, the laser PRF can be higher by at least a factor of 20, potentially influencing the process of laser and detector selection (Section 7.5).

A fourth design detail when using GM-APDs is the overload that can occur when a detector that is designed for single-photon sensitivity collects many orders of magnitude more. SPADs can easily be damaged by an excess of incident optical power, and a narrow-bandpass optical filter centered at the laser wavelength is required in such cases. For example, laser radar systems operating in the field have the potential for ambient sunlight—direct, glint, or scattered—to be collected by the receiver optics, and an optical filter with a wavelength bandpass $\Delta\lambda \approx 1$ nm has been found to be useful in preventing detector damage for InGaAs GM-APDs.[18]

In addition to the specs and details reviewed in this section, there are others that may or may not be of importance—timing jitter, breakdown-voltage tolerance and temperature dependence, etc.—depending on the particular application. In general, GM-APDs are a mature technology with commercial products available from more than one vendor for both silicon (400–1000 nm) and InGaAs (1000–1600 nm) single-photon detection.

---

**Example 7.1**

We can use Eq. (7.7) to determine the allowable DCR for single-photon detection in a pulse. Using a Nd:YAG solid-state laser at $\lambda = 1064$ nm, the energy of a single photon is $E_p = h\nu = hc/\lambda = 6.626 \times 10^{-34}$ J-sec $\times 3 \times 10^8$ m/sec/$(1064 \times 10^{-9}$ m$) = 1.87 \times 10^{-19}$ J. For a rectangular pulse width $\Delta t_p =$ 10 nsec, the peak power $P_{peak} \approx E_p/\Delta t_p = (1.87 \times 10^{-19}$ J)/$(10 \times 10^{-9}$ sec$) =$ $1.87 \times 10^{-11}$ W, which is the Geiger-mode NEP. Substituting in Eq. (7.7) and using Eq. (7.4) for the bandwidth $\Delta f$, we find that the $DCR = [PDE \times NEP_{GM}/2h\nu]^2/\Delta f = 4.5$ MHz for InGaAs with a PDE = 30% at $T = 250$ K. This compares favorably with the 5- to 50-kHz DCR found in commercially available gated SPADs, indicating the possible suitability of cooled InGaAs for single-photon detection.

---

Another disadvantage of the SPAD is the relatively small area of the detector. As we have seen in Chapter 6, this affects the power and energy collected for a given *f*/# (see Example 6.3). A recent innovation to address this problem for silicon SPADs is the multipixel photon counter (MPPC). Also known as the silicon photomultiplier (SiPM), these devices increase the effective area by placing a number of individual SPADs in a 2D array.[19]

MPPCs are not FPAs, as the individual SPADs cannot independently measure single photons to create an image. Instead, each SPAD collects light over a small IFOV, and its Geiger-mode electrical pulse is added to that from the other SPADs during the measurement time to give a composite signal for the entire array, rather than a pixilated image.

Since each SPAD is operating as a GM-APD, it cannot discriminate between the number of photons collected over its IFOV; however, the number of single- or multiple-photon *detector events*—but not the total number of photons—across the entire FOV can be determined if the photons fall on different SPADs, thus allowing pulse-height (but not photon) discrimination when the SPAD outputs are added together.

Typical MPPC array sizes range from 10 SPADs $\times$ 10 SPADs to $40 \times 40$, each with a passive-quenching resistor to limit afterpulsing; the resistor unfortunately results in a relatively long settling time for an avalanche event. By using a complementary metal-oxide-semiconductor (CMOS) manufacturing process, breakdown voltages are low (30–40 V) but will be sensitive to changes in detector temperature if not TEC stabilized. Specifications such as crosstalk and uniformity that are specific to pixel arrays will be reviewed in Section 7.4.

## 7.3 Photomultiplier Tubes

Another common option for single-photon detection with a large-area detector is the photomultiplier tube (PMT). While PMTs are often used in biomedical instruments found in laboratories where ruggedness and low-voltage operation are not critical requirements,[11] they have also been qualified for use in space-based laser radar instruments.[20]

As shown in Fig. 7.15, the PMT is based on the photoelectric effect, where photons incident on a photocathode material give the cathode's electrons enough energy to escape the material. These so-called primary electrons are then amplified by a sequence of internal PMT components known as dynodes, sheets of metal covered with a thin layer of material that is different from the photocathode; the impact of a high-energy electron with each dynode ejects 5–50× secondary (gain) electrons, thus providing an overall PMT gain as high as $10^8\times$. The entire process of photocathode emission and dynode amplification occurs in an evacuated tube, where the electron loss is minimal.

PMTs are classified by their photocathode material and resulting wavelength response. For example, a PMT with a gallium arsenide (GaAs) photocathode has the QE shown in Fig. 7.16; GaAs and other materials have a relatively large QE for UV and VIS wavelengths—a common reason for selecting PMTs. For comparison, the InGaAs PMT has a peak QE at $\lambda = 400$ nm ($\approx 2.5\%$) that is 18× smaller than the silicon-based single-photon counting module (SPCM) SPAD offered commercially by Excelitas.

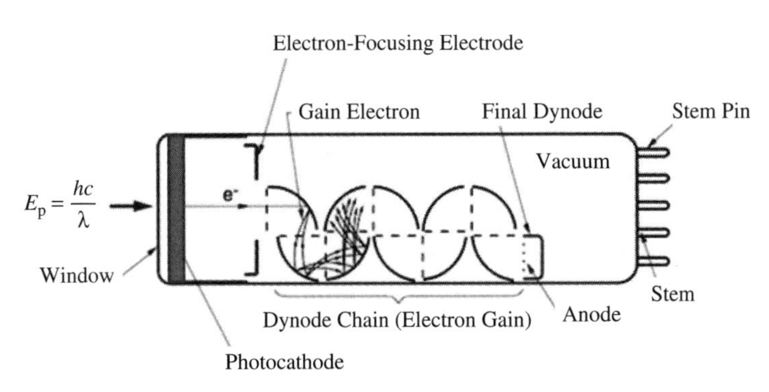


**Figure 7.15** The photocathode in a PMT ejects an electron towards a sequence of dynodes where the number of electrons is amplified, providing low-noise gain. (Adapted with permission from Hamamatsu Photonics.[21])

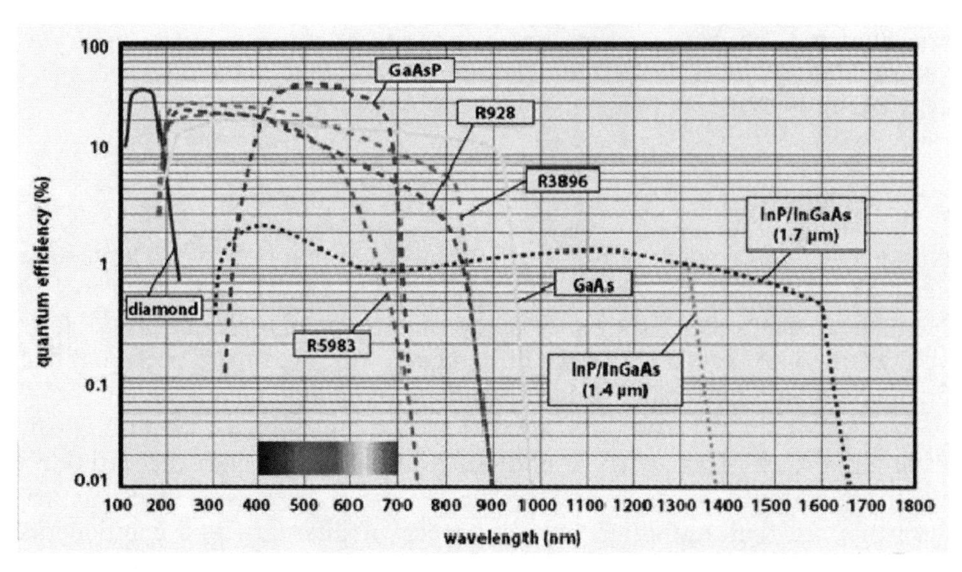


**Figure 7.16** The average QE spectrum of various PMT photocathode materials. (Reprinted with permission from Hamamatsu Photonics.[21]) (See color plate.)

It is sometimes the case that the relatively low QE shown for PMTs in Fig. 7.16 is a dominant factor in selecting SPADs over PMTs. The low QE of PMTs, however, is not always as big a disadvantage as is commonly thought. Specifically, with the large active area in comparison with APDs—around 1–10 mm for PMTs compared with only 50–100 μm for SPADs—the optical power collected can be much larger, resulting in the same total detector current given that $i_d = R_g\Phi$ and $\Phi = TLA_d\Omega$ [Eq. (6.10)]. As a result, the large PMT detection area $A_d$ may be able to compensate for the smaller QE and responsivity $R_g$, giving the same detector current if the optical system can collect power from—and the laser power is distributed over—the larger FOV associated with the larger detector area (for a fixed *f*/# of the optics).

For example, the PDE at $\lambda = 1550$ nm for an InGaAs PMT is $\approx 0.005$, while that for a linear-mode APD (LM-APD) is 0.2, which is 40× better than the PMT. But the size of the active area is 1.6 mm for the PMT and only 40 μm for the APD—1600× less collection area than the PMT. In addition, PMT gains on the order of $10^6\times$ can also increase the PMT current well beyond that of the APD. What is necessary for system design, then, is not a simplistic comparison of PDE but a complete photon or power budget of the type reviewed in Section 6.4. We will come back to this topic again in Section 7.5.1.

Like the LM-APD, PMTs can also be used for photon counting, not just photon detection. That is, the PMT does not have a breakdown voltage and thus does not avalanche in the same manner as a GM-APD into an uncontrollable cascade. Instead, while the gain may be extremely large, it is known and can be measured, thus allowing single- and multiple-photon discrimination via pulse-height analysis of the type seen in Fig. 7.11.[21] As with HgCdTe LM-APDs, the excess-noise factor for PMTs varies slightly with gain, but $F(G) \approx 1.2$ is a good number to use for initial system-design calculations.

The dark current—or dark counts for photon counting—due to thermal (thermionic) emission of electrons from the photocathode is generally very low and depends on photocathode material, area, and temperature; typical numbers are 5–500 cps at $T = 25$ °C. Dark counts can also be increased by orders of magnitude after exposure to an excessively bright source such as sunlight or a high-peak-power laser. The maximum allowable output current based on CW or peak power is $\approx 0.1$–100 μA, possibly requiring a narrow-bandpass optical filter to avoid, or a recovery time on the order of hours before the PMT is again usable after over-exposure. In extreme cases, the photocathode can be damaged to the point where even a long recovery time cannot reduce the dark counts, and the PMT must be replaced.

The time response of PMTs is very fast—on the order of 1–20 nsec, giving measurement bandwidths of 25–500 MHz. Gated versions are also available to reduce background noise or when multiple lasers wavelengths are used in the same system,[22] with gate widths of 30–100 nsec and gate repetition frequencies of 10–100 kHz.

While the benefits of PMTs include single-photon sensitivity, relatively high QE for UV and VIS wavelengths, and a large collection area, there are disadvantages to their use as well. These include:

- A common technique for photon counting is pulse-height discrimination, where pulse amplitudes that exceed a certain threshold value are counted as a photon. Unfortunately, photocathode QE (and dynode gain) in a PMT can have a large statistical variance, resulting in significant pulse-height variations. For example, PMTs using bi-alkali photocathode materials are preferred for low pulse-amplitude noise, while S25 cathodes are to be avoided.[23]
- Like the almost-obsolete cathode-ray tube (CRT) display, the motions of PMT electrons moving through a vacuum tube are susceptible to magnetic fields.
- As many PMTs are evacuated glass tubes, they may break in difficult vibration and shock environments as may be found in aerospace applications. Metal-package PMTs are available, however, with low-performance versions in housings as small as a TO-8 can used for compact, field-portable instruments—see Section 13.4 of Ref. 21—and having the additional benefit of good immunity to magnetic fields.

- A high voltage (1–3 kV) is required to obtain the high-speed electrons required for dynode gain. Packaged PMTs may use a power supply with only 15–20 V, but the voltage applied to the PMT inside the box is ≈ 1–3 kV.

---

**Example 7.2**

A typical photon collection (or "dwell") time in laser fluorescence microscopy is 1 μsec. If a PMT is used as the detector, how many dark counts are created during the gating time, and will these counts be a problem?

With a PMT DCR of 100 cps, there are 100 cps × 1 μsec = $10^{-4}$ counts per sample measurement. The sample is then scanned with a galvo to obtain a 1-Mpixel image; there are thus $10^{-4}$ counts/pixel × $10^6$ pixels = 100 dark-count errors in the image.

Is this significant? While the NEP is sufficiently low based on these dark counts, the consequences of a dark-count "false alarm" may be important, depending on the application. If used to count photons, for example, a PMT dark count looks the same as a photon, indicating fluorescence in a part of the image where there may be none. With 100 of these errors randomly distributed over the 1-Mpixel image, there is a probability of false alarms of 1 part in $10^4$.

Whether or not this is significant depends on the system requirements for overall image fidelity; if such a rate is a problem, reductions in the dark counts can be obtained by cooling the PMT, typically with a TEC. In addition, a reduction in the number of false alarms is possible by obtaining an additional 1-Mpixel image for comparison with the first; most of the randomly distributed dark counts can then be identified and subtracted from the composite image.

---

Variations on the PMT theme are numerous. One of these is the hybrid photodetector (HPD), which combines a PMT photocathode with "electron-bombardment" amplification. That is, electrons ejected by the photocathode are accelerated to a very high velocity onto a semiconductor, rather than a dynode chain; the semiconductor then provides electron gain of 50,000× in the same manner as an APD—see Ref. 21, Chapter 11. This is essentially a single-dynode device with a correspondingly low variance in the pulse-height distribution, enabling a more-precise count of photon number than a conventional PMT.

Another variation is the micro-channel plate (MCP) for ultrafast, single-photon imaging on each pixel of an array. The channels are micro-capillary glass tubes approximately 5–20 μm in diameter and 300 μm in length, arranged in a 2D array; the walls of each tube provide PMT-type dynode gain of $10^5$–$10^7$×. This is extremely good performance in a small package, with the short channel length allowing a fast response time with bandwidths exceeding 1 GHz—see Ref. 21, Chapter 10. While the spatial resolution of the array is high, so is the impact on the budget; in the next section, we look at other imaging options that are much less expensive.

## 7.4 Focal Plane Arrays

The *p-n* junction, PIN, and avalanche photodiodes reviewed in the previous sections are also available as 2D arrays of individual detectors (or pixels), typically used at the image (or focal) plane of an optical or laser system (Fig. 7.17). The primary advantage of such FPAs is that a scanning subsystem—as in Fig. 5.3, for example—is not necessary for obtaining images, resulting in a significant reduction in system size, weight, and complexity (though not necessarily cost). Alternatively, scan mirrors can be used in conjunction with an FPA to acquire an image over a field of regard (FOR) that is larger than the FOV of the FPA.

Typical applications for FPAs in laser systems include biomedical microscopes using moderate-sensitivity *p-n* junction photodetectors, as well as high-sensitivity imaging microscopes using intensified or electron-multiplying FPAs.[11] Laser-illumination ("active") imaging for night-time viewing under low-light-level (LLL) conditions has also been developed using

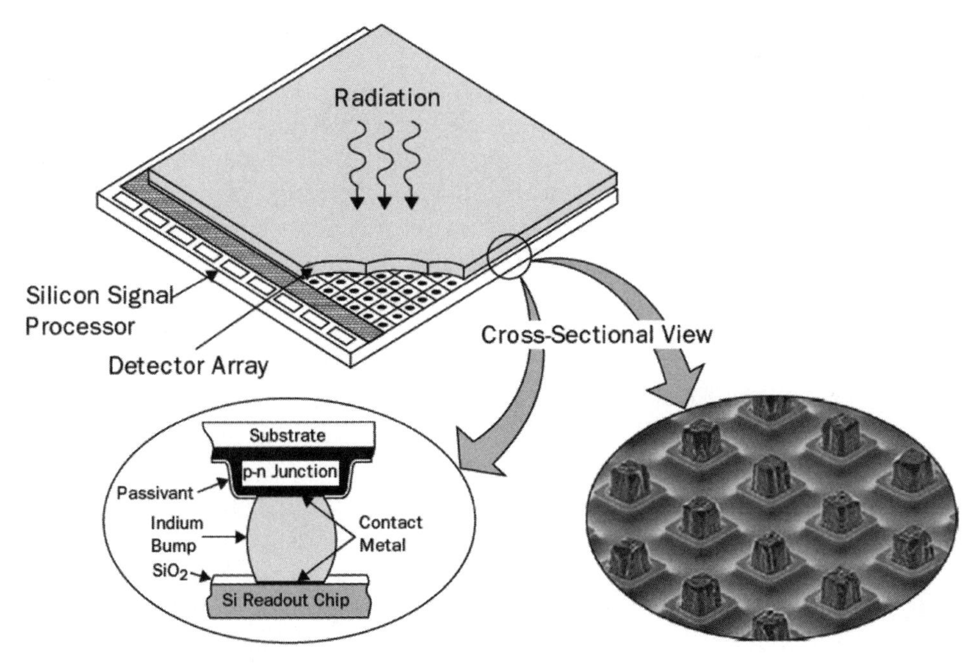


**Figure 7.17** An FPA consists of a detector array and a silicon readout integrated circuit (ROIC). [Reprinted from A. Rogalski, "HgCd Te infrared detectors: historical prospect," *Proc. SPIE* **4999**, pp. 431–442 (2003).]

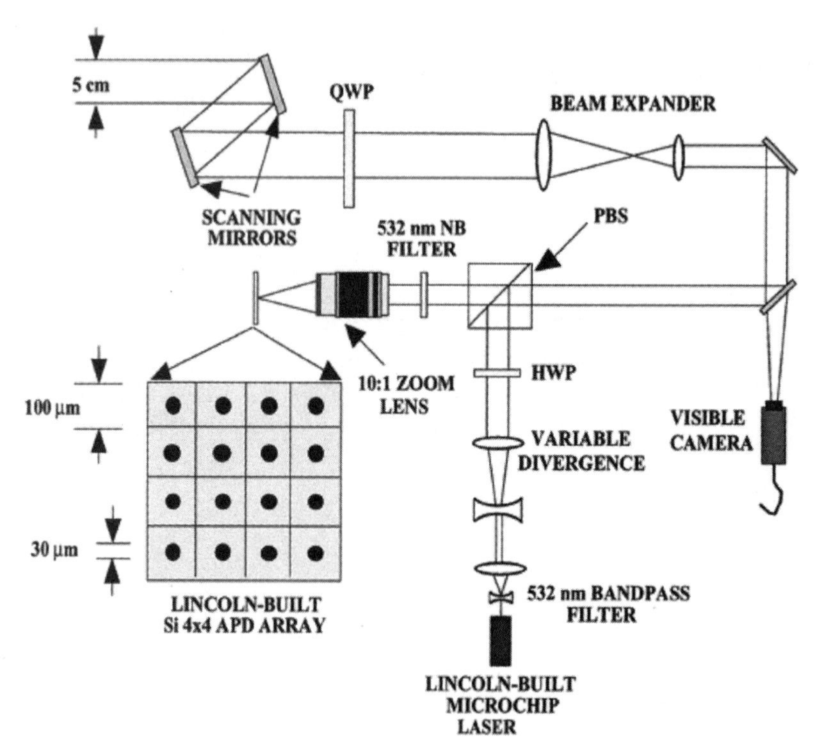


**Figure 7.18** The use of a 4 × 4 GM-APD FPA to collect light reflected from a target is illustrated in a laser radar system. [Reprinted with permission from M. A. Albota, R. M. Heinrichs, D. G. Kocher, et al., *Applied Optics* **41**(36), 7671–7678 (2002).]

hybrid InGaAs FPAs.[24] GM-APD arrays are used in laser radar systems to determine the distance to a target on each pixel (Fig. 7.18), with possible applications to autonomous, self-driving vehicles.[25] Laser spot tracking using direct illumination of FPAs is also possible.[26] The range of performance of commercial FPAs varies from few-photon sensitivity to conventional power measurements of a few milliwatts on each pixel.

What's common to all FPAs is the integration of a large number of individual detectors onto the same photonic chip, thereby allowing digital imaging of a scene. This trend has accelerated over the last 20 years with the development of large-format arrays that feature more pixels (to cover bigger FOVs) and smaller pixels (to obtain better resolution), yielding smaller, lighter systems. Pixel counts for laser-system FPAs are typically limited by the available laser power, with a 256 × 256 pixel arrangement (format) being at the upper end of the range for "flash" (full-FOV illumination) laser radar systems, and 1K × 1K FPAs common for characterization tasks such as Shack–Hartmann wavefront sensors or beam quality measurements. Larger formats require more laser power or better (smaller) detector sensitivity; the laser beam can also be scanned to collect larger images, as is common in biomedical instruments.

In this section, we first take a look at the most important property of FPA imaging, namely, spatial sampling and image resolution (Section 7.4.1). We then review the advantages and disadvantages of the available FPA technologies (Section 7.4.2), as well as FPA specifications unique to laser systems (Section 7.4.3).

### 7.4.1 Sampling

Digital imaging with FPAs presents unique engineering challenges. The most important is that the image is not a point-to-point reproduction of the scene; instead, the pixels "sample" the scene in small IFOV units based on the pixel pitch $x_p$ (Fig. 7.19). This sampling can control the image resolution, particularly if the scene contains periodic patterns that cannot be resolved by the pixel spacing. This is a huge topic applicable to both laser and optical systems, and this subsection only provides a brief summary; more details can be found in Refs. 5 and 27.

The pixel pitch $x_p$—i.e., the distance between pixels—determines the resolution of the FPA. A smaller pitch thus has better spatial resolution for the effective focal length (EFL) of the imaging optics, given that the IFOV ≈ $x_p$/EFL.

While the pixel pitch determines the detector resolution, it is image contrast (or modulation) that determines the FPA's usefulness in discerning these details. This distinction is illustrated in Fig. 7.20, where a series of bright and dark lines (aka line pairs) have been imaged by the lens in Fig. 7.19 onto an FPA. The pixel spacing $x_p$ is too large to distinguish between bright and dark, and each pixel measures a line pair's average as a gray signal; the contrast between pixels is thus zero, or is "cut off" at a line-pair spatial frequency $f_d = 1/x_p$. Note that the pitch is expressed in millimeters, giving units of line pairs per millimeter (lp/mm) for the FPA cutoff frequency.

Different spatial frequencies have different contrast; a plot of how the image modulation (or contrast) varies with spatial frequency is known as a modulation transfer function (MTF)—a common metric for image quality, where a value less than 0.15 or so indicates difficulty in resolving spatial features.[28] Not surprisingly, the MTF for an FPA depends on the pitch:

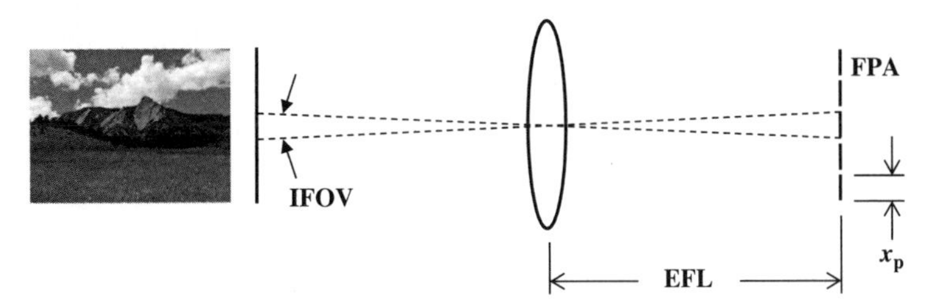


**Figure 7.19** An FPA samples a scene with a pixel-by-pixel instantaneous FOV (IFOV). (Photo credit: Mr. Brian Marotta, Boulder, Colorado.)

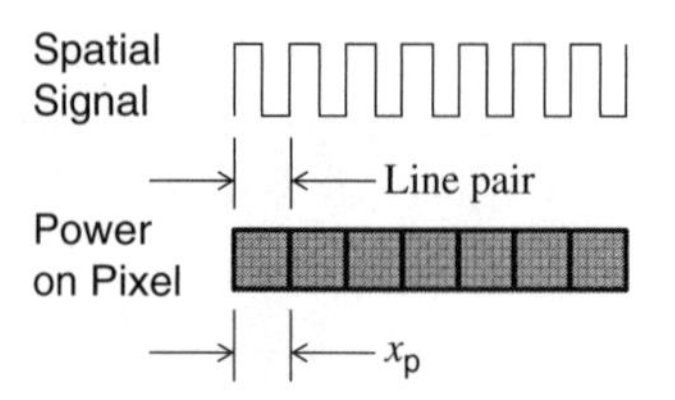


**Figure 7.20** When one line pair is imaged onto one pixel, the pixel-to-pixel contrast is zero, and the FPA cutoff frequency of the line pairs is $f_d = 1/x_p$.

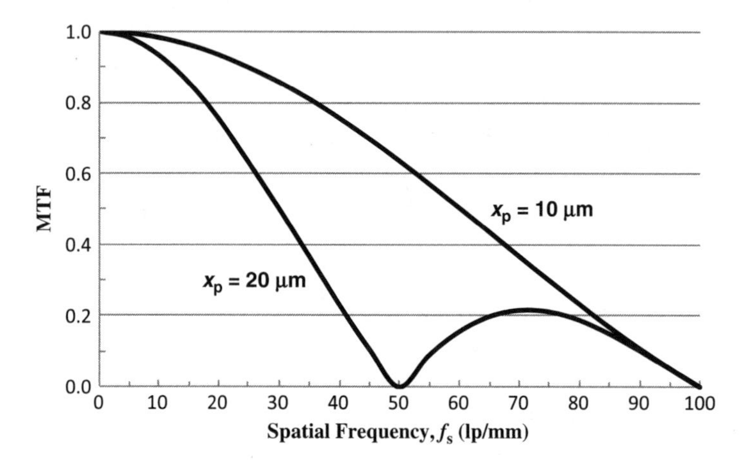


**Figure 7.21** Plot of Eq. (7.8) for $x_p = 10$ μm and $x_p = 20$ μm. The smaller pitch has a higher cutoff frequency (i.e., the first $f_s$ where MTF = 0), potentially allowing better image resolution.

$$MTF_{det} = \left| \frac{\sin(\pi f_s x_p)}{\pi f_s x_p} \right| \tag{7.8}$$

where the spatial frequency $f_s$ is any spatial frequency that may be in the *image*. A plot of $MTF_{det}$ versus $f_s$ is shown in Fig. 7.21 for a pixel pitch $x_p = 10$ μm and 20 μm. Note how the smaller pitch has twice the cutoff frequency, potentially resulting in better image resolution at higher spatial frequencies.

The FPA is only one part of a laser system, however, and a second component that also affects the image resolution is the optical subsystem. The optical subsystem adds diffraction and aberration blur to the system MTF, such that a combination of the optical MTF and detector MTF determines the spatial resolution, not just the detector MTF by itself. Quantitatively,

$$MTF_{sys} = MTF_{opt} \times MTF_{det} \tag{7.9}$$

which is plotted in Fig. 7.22 for $x_p = 20$ μm and an optical system with $\lambda = 0.5$ μm and $f/\# = 20$, with the details of calculating $MTF_{opt}$ given in Ref. 5.

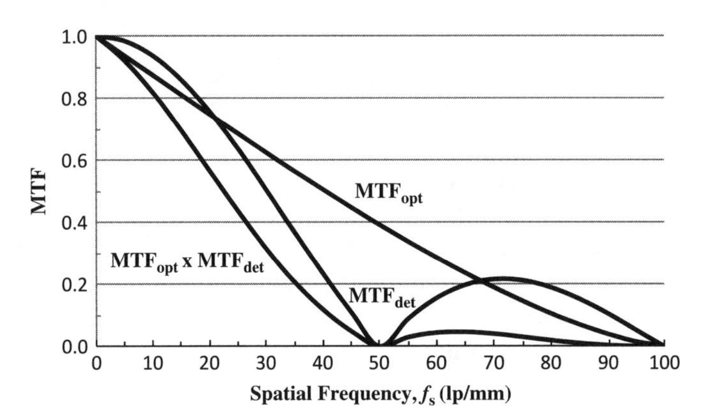


**Figure 7.22** Plot of $MTF_{sys}$ for $x_p = 20$ μm, $\lambda = 0.5$ μm, and $f/\# = 20$. The detector MTF dominates the first spatial frequency at which the MTF = 0, resulting in a detector-limited MTF.

For the particular parameters used in Fig. 7.22, the first zero of the system MTF also occurs at $f_s = f_d = 50$ lp/mm, illustrating a detector-limited system. That is, for a pixel size that is approximately the same size as the diffraction-limited optical blur $B = 2.44\lambda \times f/\#$ for imaging laser illumination scattered from a scene, target, or biomedical sample, the pixel pitch dominates the system cutoff frequency. Other FPAs with smaller pixels will have a system MTF dominated by the size of the optical blur, while others with an intermediate pixel pitch will balance the detector and optical MTF contributions, with neither dominating—a preferred design option resulting in an optical blur $B \approx 2.44 x_p$ in the absence of additional MTF terms such as jitter.[5]

An additional system-design consideration for FPA sampling is radiometric. The power collected by a pixel is proportional to $[d_p/(f/\#)]^2$, where a smaller pixel size $d_p$—limited by, and often equal to, the pitch $x_p$—collects less power than a large pixel if the $f/\#$ of the optics is the same.[5] A faster optical system (smaller $f/\#$) is of course possible to compensate for the "slower" (smaller) pixel, although this reaches the cost-effective limits of lens design at around $f/1.4$ or so for VIS wavelengths, and $f/1$ for LWIR wavelengths. While the large detection area of a PMT is thus good for power collection, it is sometimes unacceptable for spatial resolution.

In evaluating FPA technologies, then, an important consideration will be the available pixel pitch and size. Sections 7.4.2 and 7.4.3 review these and other FPA properties unique to laser systems.

### 7.4.2 FPA technologies

There are a number of different architectures and methods for fabricating FPAs—i.e., FPA technologies. For photon detectors, four primary types are available: charge-coupled devices (CCDs), electron-multiplying CCDs

(EM-CCDs), scientific-grade complementary metal-oxide semiconductor (sCMOS), and hybrid arrays—each with advantages and disadvantages that must be traded off against each other to accommodate multiple laser-system requirements.

The differences between these FPA technologies result in variations in sensitivity, speed, cost, size, weight, and so on. Many of these technologies are made using silicon fabrication processes (CCDs, EM-CCDs, and sCMOS), thus restricting their wavelength response to VIS and NIR; longer wavelengths such as SWIR require InGaAs or MCT FPAs based on a technology reviewed in this subsection known as "hybrid." There are also a couple of miscellaneous technologies—intensified CCDs and electron-bombarded CCDs—which will be briefly summarized.

**Charge-Coupled Devices (CCDs).** CCDs are used for high-performance VIS- and NIR-wavelength applications (scientific, biomedical, etc.) that require low noise and high responsivity. As shown in Fig. 7.23, each pixel in a CCD has an absorbing semiconductor (a silicon *p-n* junction) to convert photons to electrons (charge), a metal-oxide-semiconductor (MOS) capacitor to store this charge, and a clever electrode scheme to couple the charge between pixels for transfer to the end of a row, where it is read out and processed by

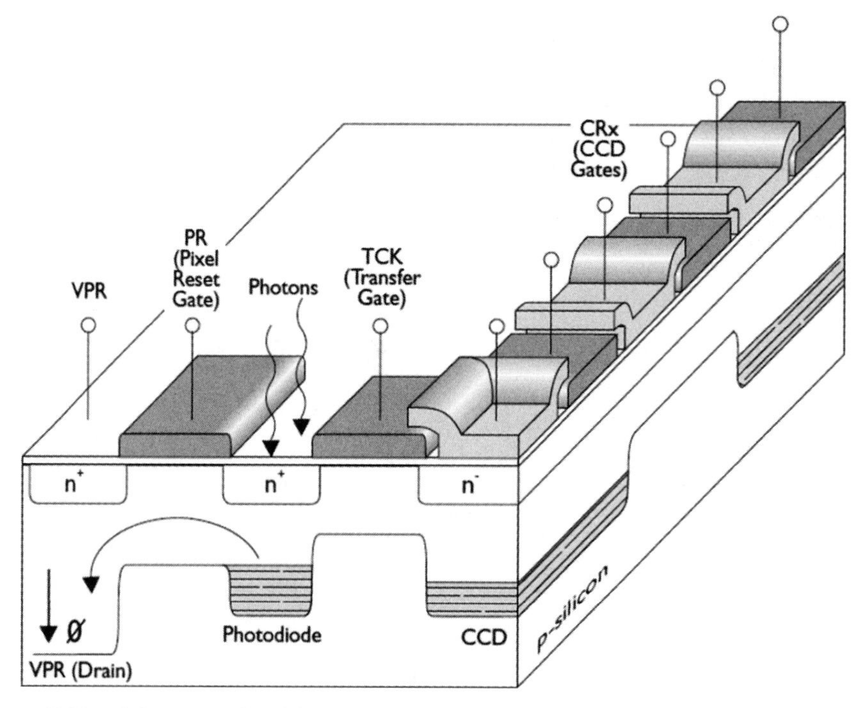


**Figure 7.23** Schematic of a CCD pixel illustrating a *p-n* junction photodiode and charge-transfer gate circuitry. (Credit: Teledyne DALSA Inc.[30])

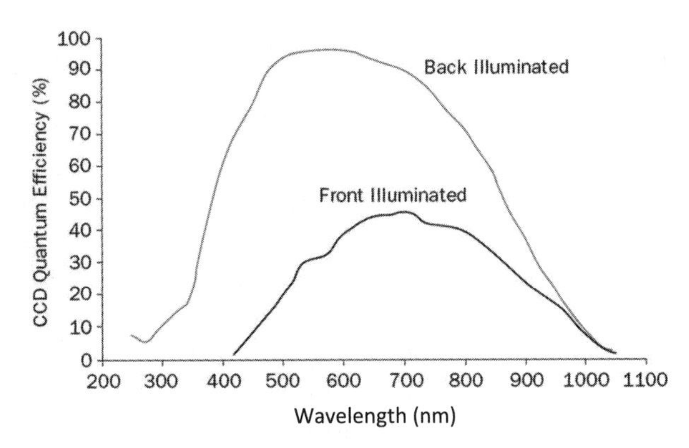


**Figure 7.24** Back-illuminated silicon CCDs have reduced blockage and absorption losses, and therefore have higher quantum efficiency than front-illuminated silicon CCDs. (Courtesy of Princeton Instruments; reprinted with permission.)

electrical circuitry. This transfer is not perfect, and charge-transfer efficiencies (CTEs) of 0.999995 are required (and available) to reduce charge loss for large-format arrays with many pixels along a row.[29]

Figure 7.23 shows that the charge-transfer circuitry blocks photons from reaching the *p-n* junction. The QE for front-illuminated CCDs is thus lower in proportion to the fraction of pixel area covered by the circuitry. It is possible to illuminate pixels from the back of the FPA, but in that case the wafer is relatively thick; hence, it must be thinned to prevent too much absorption by the substrate and not enough absorption by the *p-n* junction's depletion region. The result of this back-illumination technique is an approximate doubling of the average QE as well as an associated increase in UV response (Fig. 7.24).

One disadvantage of the CCD is the relatively long time it takes to transfer the charge to the edge of the FPA for readout; this and read noise limit the rate at which CCDs can collect data to $\approx$ 1–10 frames per second (fps) for 1K $\times$ 1K arrays.[31] As we will see in detail in Section 7.5.2, CCD sensitivity is affected by the various sources of noise, including signal noise, dark current, and read noise. For low signal levels, dark current and read noise are dominant; cooling the CCD to –20 °C to –80 °C with a TEC reduces the dark current to < 1 $e^-$/sec per pixel, leaving a read noise of 2–10 electrons RMS per pixel per frame as the major source of CCD noise for slow-readout commercial products.

While there are a number of variations for the CCD readout architecture that affect sensitivity—frame transfer, interline, etc.—few-photon sensitivity is not possible; nonetheless, CCDs are considered to be the "gold" standard of FPA technologies for a variety of laser-system applications. As reviewed in the next subsection, however, there is a CCD option that multiplies the number of photoelectrons to obtain single-photon sensitivity.

**Electron-Multiplying CCDs (EM-CCDs).** One way to get around the read noise limit for LLL CCDs is to amplify the number of electrons *before* the signal has been read out. As shown in Fig. 7.25, this is done with an electron-multiplying gain sequence that increases the number of electrons by a factor of 100–1000.[32] The process is similar to APD gain based on impact ionization and has the same effects—an increase in signal such that the number of read electrons is insignificant in comparison with the electron-multiplied signal.

If the EM-CCD is deep-cooled to approximately –100 °C to reduce the dark current—which is also amplified by the electron-multiplying gain—the next significant noise is that resulting from amplification of the signal. In this regard, EM-CCDs have very similar performance to HgCdTe LM-APDs and PMTs, with an excess-noise factor $F(G) \approx 1.4$. This is much lower excess noise than can be obtained with silicon [$F(G) \approx 5$] or InGaAs [$F(G) \approx 10$] APDs, and at much lower cost (for now) than MCT-based APD FPAs.

The EM-CCD can also be run at a higher frame rate than a conventional CCD. In a conventional CCD, amplifier read noise limits the frame rates to 1–10 fps; in an EM-CCD, on the other hand, the larger read noise associated with the higher frame rate—and the larger electrical bandwidth $\Delta f$ collecting more noise power [see Eq. (7.18)]—is still insignificant in comparison with the electron-multiplied signal, allowing video frame rates of 30 fps for a 1K × 1K array with an effective read noise of < 1 electron RMS per pixel per frame.

As with CCDs, EM-CCDs are fabricated using silicon *p-n* junction photodiodes; they are also available with both front- and back-illuminated options, with the back-illuminated design having much higher QE over a broader spectral range and a peak $QE > 90\%$ at $\lambda = 500–700$ nm. In

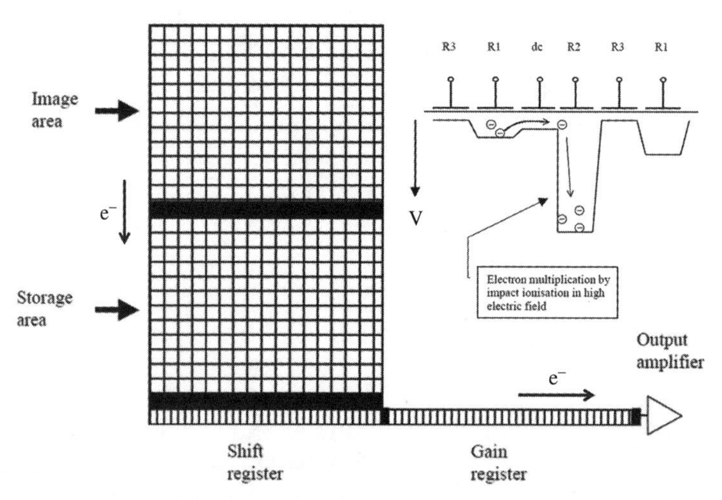


**Figure 7.25** An EM-CCD multiplies the number of photoelectrons from each pixel via impact ionization before the signal is read out at the output amplifier, thus minimizing the relative magnitude of read noise. (Reprinted from Ref. 32.)

combination with low-noise gain and deep cooling to reduce dark current, the large QE contributes to the use of EM-CCDs as high-sensitivity, high-frame-rate FPAs commercially available from camera vendors such as Andor Technology Ltd, e2v, and Princeton Instruments.

**Scientific-Grade CMOS (sCMOS).** Unfortunately, the serial-readout frame rates of EM-CCDs are still too slow for applications such as super-resolution microscopy requiring large arrays of high-resolution (small pixel) detectors.[33] In addition, neither CCD nor EM-CCD fabrication is compatible with high-volume, low-cost production. The CMOS process, on the other hand—initially developed as a set of design rules for silicon-based computer and memory chips—has recently been adapted to consumer "electronics" such as miniaturized ("camera on a chip"), low-power-consumption, low-price FPAs, a typical application being cell-phone cameras where high performance is not critical.

To reduce the size of the FPA's circuit board, readout and processing circuitry are incorporated on each pixel [creating an active-pixel sensor (APS)]. Not surprisingly, reducing this circuitry onto the small size of a CMOS pixel results in design compromises, most notably that CMOS noise is higher than that of a CCD at the frame rates found in consumer cameras. The APS circuitry also takes up some of the pixel area, significantly reducing the fill factor (see Section 7.4.3) and effective responsivity for CMOS FPAs with small pixels ($\leq$ 10 μm).

Because each pixel has readout circuitry associated with it, the collected charge does not have to be transferred down a row. Hence, individual pixels in CMOS FPAs can be read out in parallel, with correspondingly high frame rates of 100 fps for 5.5 Mpixel arrays;[34] additional benefits over CCDs are (1) little electrical power is expended; (2) the readout amplifier for each pixel has extremely low electrical bandwidth $\Delta f$—and thus low noise (see Section 7.5.1)—in comparison with the high-speed amplifier required for the serial readout of 512 or 1024 pixels (e.g.) in a row of CCD data; and (3) no electrons are lost to charge-transfer inefficiencies as they are in a CCD.

Despite the benefits of low cost, low read noise at high frame rates, and low power consumption, laser-system applications of CMOS FPAs were initially lacking due to the disadvantages of the technology: low QE and high noise in comparison with CCDs. As a result, sCMOS FPAs were developed to address these issues.

As with the initial CCD designs, the low CMOS QE was due to on-pixel circuitry blocking photons from reaching the *p-n* junction. By using a microlens array to focus light only on the photosensitive area of each pixel,[5] however, a peak QE as large as 55% at $\lambda = 550$ nm is available with commercial sCMOS products.[34] An alternative approach with higher cost but even better QE and compatibility with low-*f*/# optics is back-thinned illumination, with a QE of 70% at $\lambda = 600$ nm.

With extremely low read noise ( < 1.5 $e^-$ RMS per pixel per read), the dominant noise in conventional CMOS FPAs is due to (1) high dark current associated with the CMOS architecture, and (2) small pixel-to-pixel and column-to-column statistical variations (non-uniformities) in both QE and the charge-to-voltage (units of $\mu V/e^-$) conversion amplifiers, producing a background fixed-pattern noise (FPN) that increases in proportion to the incident power (Section 7.5.1).

Both conventional and scientific CMOS arrays reduce their dark current via cooling, but sCMOS FPAs also use low-dark-current, buried-channel photodiodes similar in design to those developed for CCDs.[35] In addition, the fixed-pattern noise (FPN)—which has been the largest source of noise in conventional CMOS arrays—has been significantly reduced with a signal-processing technique known as correlated double sampling (CDS) to reduce the FPN.[35] In addition to lower dark current and FPN, sCMOS FPAs have also been designed with lower read noise,[34] with a median read noise of < 1.5 electrons RMS per pixel per frame at frame rates of 100 fps.[36]

The bottom line from these improvements is a sCMOS FPA with higher QE, lower dark current, lower FPN, and lower read noise in comparison with the basic CMOS architecture. This combination of high QE and low noise also results in an FPA technology that has equal or better performance compared to EM-CCDs under moderate-to-high light levels.

For low light levels, it is difficult to improve on the benefits of the low-noise, 1000× gain available from EM-CCDs. At higher light levels, however, the excess noise associated with this gain is a disadvantage, and sCMOS—which has no amplification and thus no excess noise—can be the better option. This is illustrated in Fig. 7.26, where the performance of sCMOS

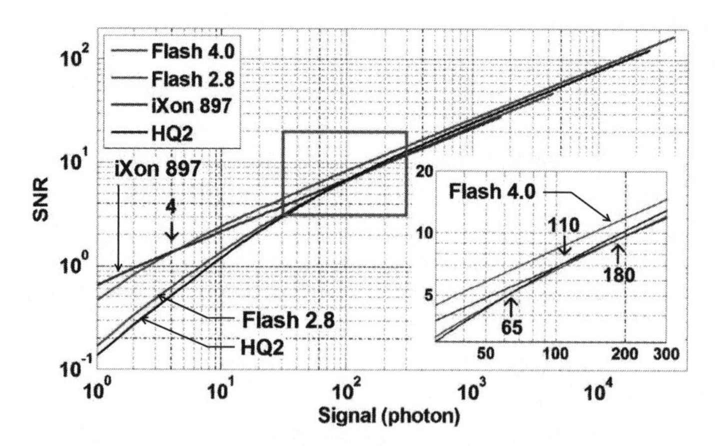


**Figure 7.26** A high-performance sCMOS array (Flash 4.0) has a better SNR than other FPA technologies for a signal photon number greater than 4. [Adapted with permission from F. Long, S. Zeng, and Z.-L. Huang, "Localization-based super-resolution microscopy with an sCMOS camera Part II: Experimental methodology for comparing sCMOS with EMCCD cameras," *Optics Express* **20**(16), 17741 (2012).] (See color plate.)

(Flash 4.0 and Flash 2.8), EM-CCD (iXon 897), and CCD (HQ2) FPAs is compared over a range of incident signal photons. The metric used for the comparison is the signal-to-noise ratio (SNR), where lower FPA noise increases the ratio; details on how to estimate the SNR for a given signal level will be reviewed in Section 7.5.1.

Figure 7.26 shows that the EM-CCD—with the lowest read noise and a higher QE than sCMOS—has the best SNR at signal photon levels up to 4. Beyond that, the high-performance sCMOS array (Flash 4.0) has a better (larger) SNR than the EM-CCD, a result of lack of excess noise for sCMOS. In addition, the Flash 4.0 sCMOS FPA has a better SNR than even the CCD array (HQ2) at high photon numbers. While these trends will vary with pixel size, *f*/# of the optics, exposure time, frame rate, operating temperature, etc., sCMOS can be better than CCDs in some LLL applications, with a photon number $\geq 50$ being the range where sCMOS arrays may be the best FPA technology based on SNR.[33]

**Hybrid FPAs.** Hybrid FPAs address a major weakness of CCD and sCMOS arrays, namely, their reliance on silicon as the same material for both detection and electronics. Both CCD and sCMOS arrays thus take advantage of the fabrication infrastructure that supports the integrated-circuit industry; the problem is that a different semiconductor is required for detecting wavelengths outside the visible and NIR bands (400–1000 nm) to which silicon is mostly sensitive.

The approach taken with hybrid arrays is shown in Fig. 7.17, where one chip is stacked on top of another. The top chip (substrate) is the detector array, which is made of the material (HgCdTe, InGaAs, etc.) appropriate for the wavelengths of interest. The bottom chip is a readout integrated circuit (ROIC), an electronic array typically made out of silicon to leverage the CMOS technology base and capabilities of silicon foundry processes. The two chips are bonded together (hybridized), usually with indium balls (or "bumps") that are small enough to connect each detector pixel electrically to each unit cell in the ROIC, allowing parallel readout.

The detector in a hybrid FPA is usually a PIN or APD; the peak QE from both the thick absorption layer and the absence of circuitry on the photosensitive surface is therefore extremely high, exceeding 95% in some cases. The benefit of parallel readout of photoelectrons that we have seen with sCMOS FPAs also applies to the parallel readout of hybrid arrays, thus producing very low read noise even at high frame rates.

The primary disadvantage of hybrid FPAs is their high cost. That is, rather than processing and packaging of a single CCD or sCMOS silicon chip, the fabrication of hybrid arrays requires processing of two chips—one of which is made of a material that is much more expensive than silicon—and their subsequent bump bonding. This last step is particularly costly, as it is labor ("touch") intensive and can result in low yield if the two chips are not aligned properly in rotation or tilt angle before they are bonded together with the pressure-sensitive indium bumps.

Another disadvantage of hybrid FPAs is that there are technological limitations on minimum pixel size such as the indium bump-bonding process for hybrid arrays. Pixels on the order of 2–10 μm are typical for silicon-based arrays that do not require bump bonding, whereas pixel sizes of about 10 μm are currently the minimum for InGaAs, MCT, and InSb FPAs that do.

Because of their high cost, applications of hybrid FPAs are mostly in aerospace and defense. For example, laser-illumination (active) imaging for night-time viewing has been developed using hybrid InGaAs FPAs. In one demonstration of capabilities, the FPA was sufficiently sensitive to the eye-safe laser wavelength (1570 nm) and pulse energy (8 mJ) to produce good imagery of objects as far away as 1.1 km with an *f*/5 telescope, using a high-speed ROIC to measure 5-nsec laser pulse widths for illumination.[24] While InGaAs FPAs using PIN or APD arrays are also applicable to laser radar systems,[18] hybrid HgCdTe FPAs have been developed to take advantage of the near-noiseless gain of MCT-based LM-APDs.[13,14]

**Miscellaneous.** In addition to CCD, sCMOS, and hybrid arrays, a number of unique FPA technologies have been developed for applications with specialized requirements. In this subsection, we briefly review two of these: intensified CCDs (ICCDs) using MCPs, and electron-bombarded CCDs (EB-CCDs).

An ICCD is useful for applications such as time-resolved fluorescence microscopy requiring high-speed gating and single-photon sensitivity over the fluorescence-emission time. This FPA technology is based on micro-channel plates, i.e., the MCP arrays mentioned at the end of Section 7.3 that do not, by themselves, create an image. They only amplify photons and need an FPA such as a CCD to collect light from the MCP for image capture (Fig. 7.27).

In specifying ICCDs, there are two speeds that must be distinguished. The first is the gating time; the second is the frame readout time. The ICCD has a high-speed on-off gate for collecting data on the order of nanoseconds (via MCP gating), and a typical frame rate of $\approx 30$ fps. With single-photon sensitivity, the ICCD competes with the EM-CCD at these ultra-low light levels; the difference between them is that the EM-CCD is not capable of time-resolved gating. In addition, it is sometimes argued that the higher excess-noise factor of the ICCD—with $F(G) = 2$–$4$ versus $F(G) = 1.4$ for the EM-CCD—is a disadvantage of the ICCD, but this applies only at higher photon levels where excess noise dominates, not at the single- or few-photon level where the ICCD is being compared.

An alternative to the ICCD is the electron-bombarded CCD (EB-CCD); an electron-bombarded CMOS (EB-CMOS) FPA is also available. What is

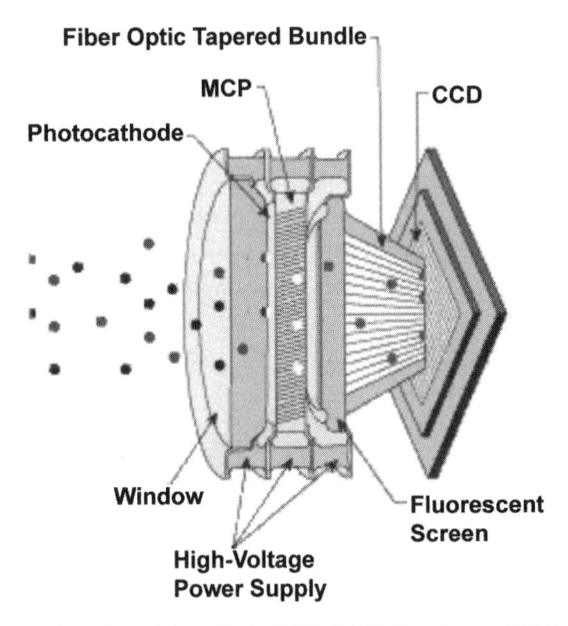


**Figure 7.27** Schematic of an intensified CCD (ICCD) using a MCP and a fluorescent phosphor screen to obtain an intensified image on a CCD. (Courtesy of Princeton Instruments; reprinted with permission.)

common between them is the use of a high-velocity electron beam—by accelerating electrons emitted by a photocathode—to bombard a CCD array, creating additional electrons (gain) via impact ionization with very little excess noise. The photocathode thus determines the wavelength to which the EB FPA is sensitive; the silicon CCD or CMOS array only serves as a low-noise gain-and-measurement device with pixel-scale resolution on the order of 12 μm.

These FPAs have been developed for LLL cameras requiring portability. This comes about because there is no need to cool the FPA, as it is the photocathode temperature that dominates the dark current. Nominal photocathode temperatures of 20–35 °C are common, though this still results in a relatively high dark current; deeper cooling is possible to reduce the dark current, at the expense of reducing the portability. Other disadvantages of the EB technology include the complexity of the electron "optics" required to accelerate electrons, the damage (and resulting increase in FPA dark current) caused by electron impacts to the FPA that shorten its lifetime, and the high cost—all making EB a rarely used FPA technology.

**Summary.** We have reviewed in this section a number of different FPA technologies for creating images, including CCDs, EM-CCDs, sCMOS, hybrids, ICCDs, and EB-CCDs. Many of these are silicon-based *p-n* junction detectors with peak sensitivities in the VIS wavelengths; hybrid arrays extend the peak wavelengths to NIR and SWIR using InGaAs and

MCT. All of the FPA technologies require a ROIC of some sort, either integral to the array or bump bonded as in hybrid FPAs. Single-photon sensitivities are possible with EM-CCDs and ICCDs, where ICCDs also have on-off gating capabilities for time-resolved measurements; sCMOS may have the best overall performance for 50+ photons, although this will depend on the specifics of the laser-system design.

While it is clear, then, that there are a wide variety of FPA technologies, what is not yet clear is that there are a number of commonalities in how FPAs are specified; we review these common specifications in the next section.

### 7.4.3 FPA specifications

In addition to pixel pitch and sampling, there are a number of unique features controlling the use of an FPA in a laser system, including the dependence of the photon detection efficiency on the fill factor, optical crosstalk between pixels, integration time during which signal and noise are collected as charge, low-noise ROICs to read out the charge, and pixel-to-pixel non-uniformities of PIN- and APD-based arrays. The FPA vendor specs for each of these may need to be compared against component-level performance or system-level requirements.

Not covered in this section are topics not specific to FPAs, including linearity, dynamic range, saturation, and others; see Ref. 5 for more details. There are also noise terms that are unique to FPAs, and these will be looked at in Section 7.5.1.

**Photon Detection Efficiency (PDE).** As we have seen in Section 7.1.3, the photon quantum efficiency $\eta_{QE}$ plays a direct role in determining responsivity [Eq. (7.3)] and thus sensitivity for at least one type of limiting noise [Eq. (7.5)]. For single-pixel *p-n* junction, PIN, LM-APD, and PMT detectors, the photon detection efficiency (PDE) is simply the QE; for GM-APDs, the PDE has an additional component based on the probability $\eta_{GM}$ of sustaining a Geiger avalanche, i.e., the $PDE = \eta_{QE} \times \eta_{GM}$.

For FPAs, the fill factor also affects the measured responsivity and QE. As illustrated in Fig. 7.28, fill factor (FF) is the ratio of photosensitive pixel area to pitch area, giving $FF = (d_p/x_p)^2$ for square pixels. This ratio

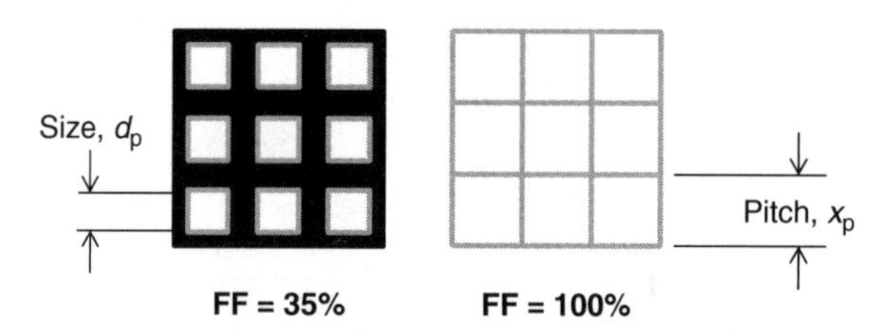


**Figure 7.28** The pixel pitch $x_p$ is the distance between pixels; the pixel size $d_p$ (shown as white squares)—which may be different from the pitch—determines the radiometric collection area.

approaches unity (i.e., 100%) for closely packed *p-n* junction and PIN photodiode arrays but can be much less for high-speed or low-noise pixels requiring a small size. A fill factor of 80%, for example, signifies a ratio of pixel area to pitch area of 0.8; this, in turn, implies that the pixel size is $(0.8)^{1/2} \approx 0.89\times$ the pitch, leaving "dark" gaps between pixels that cannot detect 20% of the incident photons.

This is sometimes specified as an *effective QE* (and responsivity) that is 80% (e.g.) of the inherent material responsivity of a single pixel. For example, a material QE of 80% and fill factor of 95% results in an effective QE $= 0.8 \times 0.95 = 0.76$ for *p-n* junction or PIN photodiodes; this may be listed in some manufacturer's spec sheets as QE × FF, as the FF is difficult to measure directly. In addition, there is also an additional factor of *G* for the effective QE of LM-APDs.

For GM-APD FPAs, the PDE $= \eta_{QE} \times \eta_{GM}$ (without the FF term); the FF for these arrays can be quite small if a microlens array is not used, as a relatively small detector size may be needed to reduce the dark current (Section 7.5.1), and a large pixel pitch (50–100 μm) may be required (as in Fig. 7.18) to reduce the pixel-to-pixel crosstalk.

**Optical Crosstalk.** The close proximity of pixels on an FPA can result in a diffusion of photoelectrons to neighboring pixels; this crosstalk "bleed-over" causes an error in a pixel's output current, smearing the image and reducing the MTF for high-brightness signals.

Crosstalk is not typically a serious problem in *p-n* junction and PIN photodiodes; where it becomes of concern in laser systems is when using APDs, particularly GM-APDs. Remembering that APD gain is due to high-energy electron ionization, additional *photons* are also emitted during avalanche.[37] Such optical crosstalk (OXT) is illustrated in Fig. 7.29, with two crosstalk paths for these additional photons to "contaminate" neighboring pixels.

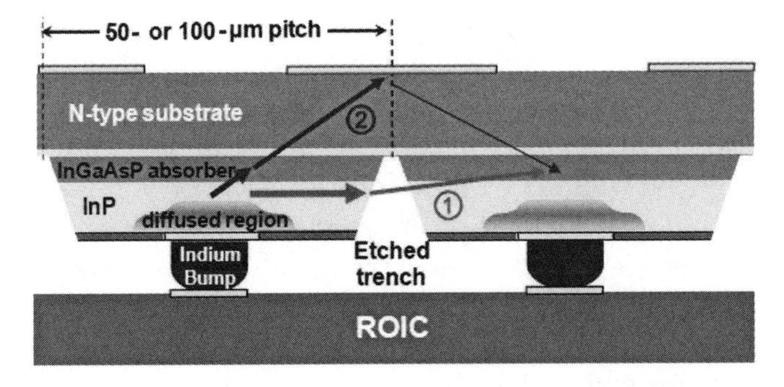


**Figure 7.29** Pixel-to-pixel optical crosstalk in an FPA can occur via direct transfer (path 1) or reflection (path 2). [Reprinted from M. A. Itzler, M. Entwistle, M. Owens, et al., "Comparison of 32 × 128 and 32 × 32 Geiger-mode APD FPAs for single photon 3D LADAR imaging," *Proc. SPIE* **8033**, 80330G (2011).]

These OXT photons are identical to dark counts in that they can trigger an avalanche in the absence of incident photons, and they require afterpulsing dead-time before the pixel can be re-armed for the next event. OXT probabilities are on the order of 35% for commercial InGaAs GM-APD arrays with a peak responsivity at $\lambda = 1550$ nm;[38] quantifying the consequences of false OXT events can be found in Ref. 37. Minimizing OXT requires a large pixel pitch (50–100 μm)—a major design restriction for high-resolution laser systems, requiring a long effective focal length to obtain a small IFOV.

**Integration Time and Frame Rate.** We saw in Section 7.4.1 that the drop in power collected by a smaller pixel—the pixel's radiometric collection area $A_p = d_p^2$—can be compensated with the use of a smaller *f*/# for the collection optics. If this has reached its lens-design limits (of ≈ *f*/1.4 for VIS wavelengths, e.g.), another option for collecting more photons with an FPA is to increase the integration (or shutter, dwell, or exposure) time. This is a unique feature of using FPAs, as they allow the measurement of integrated current (i.e., charge), rather than the current itself.

This design option also has its limitations, as the integration time may instead be limited by the pulse width or similar dynamics (fluorescence emission, e.g.,) of what's being measured. FPAs thus require a range of possible integration times, ranging from nanoseconds for range-gated laser radar systems using hybrid FPAs, to microseconds for laser fluorescence microscopy using sCMOS arrays, to minutes for DNA sequencers requiring an ultralow-dark-current interline CCD to collect very weak signals over a long integration time.

If the signal on a pixel is constant over the integration time $t_{int}$, the number of signal electrons $n_s$ accumulated by the pixel circuitry is given by

$$n_s = i_s \cdot t_{int}/q \qquad [e^-] \tag{7.10}$$

for a signal current $i_s$ (units of C/sec) and an electron charge $q = 1.602 \times 10^{-19}$ C/e$^-$. For example, a Nd:YAG laser directly illuminating an InGaAs pixel with a rectangular pulse width $\Delta t_p = 10$ nsec and a peak power $P_{peak} = 100$ kW generates a peak signal current $i_s = R_o P_{peak} \approx 0.6$ A/W × 100 kW = 60 kA for a pixel responsivity $R_o \approx 0.6$ A/W at $\lambda = 1064$ nm (see Fig. 7.2). From Eq. (7.10), this creates $n_s = i_s t_{int}/q = 60$ kA × 10 nsec/(1.602 × 10$^{-19}$ C/e$^-$) = 3.75 × 10$^{15}$ electrons, vastly exceeding the capacity of the pixel to accumulate charge (see Readout Integrated Circuits below). As we have seen in Chapter 6, however, scattered or fluorescing light results in much lower peak powers, thus allowing the use of FPAs for indirect laser-illuminated imaging.

The integration time applies to the individual pixels of an FPA, yet there is also a time associated with reading out the charge that's been collected by each pixel. This time can be very short even for large-format FPAs with the millions of pixels that constitute a frame, and the total speed at which data can be collected and read out is known as the *frame rate*. A 1K × 1 K array, for example, may have a frame rate FR = 30 fps for the $10^6$ pixels on the array, giving a frame time $t_{fr} = 1/\mathrm{FR} = 33.3$ msec before a new image can be acquired.

If necessary, the integration time can nearly equal the frame time, but is typically much shorter, with limits ranging from $t_{int} \approx 0.25$ μsec → $t_{fr}$. The frame time (or rate) is not always specified on vendor sheets, and pixel readout rate (PRR) is used instead (e.g., 1–20 MHz for CCDs); this is easy enough to convert to frame rate using the expression PRR (Hz) = FR (fps) × $n_{pix}$ (number of pixels per frame). This expression can also be used to first-order estimate the higher frame rate for a selected region-of-interest (ROI) consisting of a smaller number of pixels.

**Readout Integrated Circuits (ROICs).** Controlling the integration time, frame rate, and charge collection in an FPA is the ROIC (pronounced "row-ic"). As shown in Fig. 7.30 for a bump-bonded hybrid FPA, the ROIC can be thought of as a separate silicon component, even if it is integrated on the same chip as the detector array, as it is with CCD and sCMOS FPAs.

The ROIC in Fig. 7.30 consists of individual pre-amplifiers for each pixel (unit cell) known as a capacitive transimpedance amplifier (CTIA). The capacitor (or "well") of the CTIA is what integrates the detector current $i_d = i_s + i_b + i_{dc}$, consisting of signal and background current $i_b$ generated by

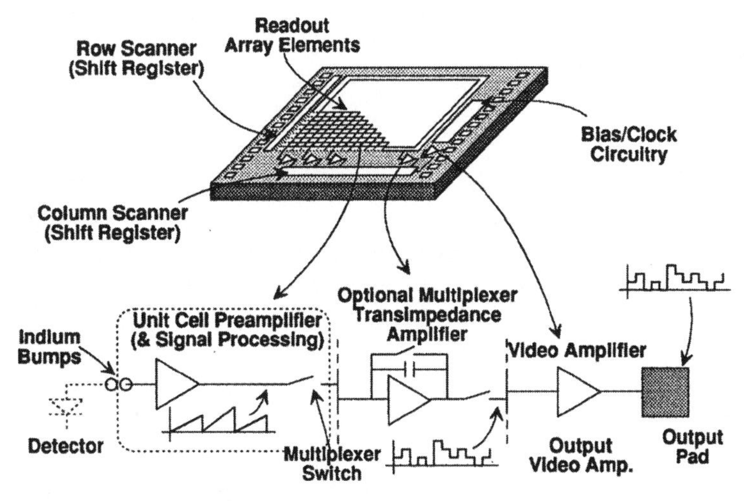


**Figure 7.30** A silicon ROIC consists of pre-amplifiers for each pixel unit cell, a multiplexer to combine the signals in time, and output amplifiers. [Reprinted from J. L. Vampola, "Readout Electronics for Infrared Sensors," in *The Infrared & Electro-Optical Systems Handbook*, Vol. 3, W. D. Rogatto, Ed., ERIM, Ann Arbor, Michigan and SPIE Press, Bellingham, Washington, Chapter 5 (1993).]

the photodiode in response to photon energy $E_p$, as well as detector dark current $i_{dc}$.

The voltage $\Delta V_{out}$ created across the capacitor in such transimpedance (current-to-voltage) amplifiers while accumulating charge during the integration time is approximately given by

$$\Delta V_{out} \approx \frac{i_d \cdot t_{int}}{C_{well}} \quad [\mathrm{V}] \tag{7.11}$$

illustrating that a smaller capacitance $C_{well}$ requires a shorter integration time if the output voltage is fixed—as it must be (at 3.3 V, e.g.) for certain design rules such as silicon CMOS.

The well capacitance expressed in units of electrons is known as the *well depth* $n_w$, with the CTIA preferred for $n_w \approx$ 1–10 Me$^-$ and a ROIC known as a direct-injection (DI) pre-amp having 2–4× larger well capacities—but also higher read noise—for large-photon applications; typical well depths range from 500–1000 e$^-$ per μm$^2$ of CCD or sCMOS pixel area. The well depth (and pixel size $d_p$) thus limits the integration time for a given detector current, as the number of detected electrons generated cannot exceed the depth, i.e., $n_d < n_w$ [see Eq. (7.10)].

Unit-cell pre-amplifiers are also what allow the low-speed and low-read-noise amplifier for a sCMOS or hybrid array—as distinct from a CCD FPA, which has only 1–4 amplifiers for the entire array, thus requiring higher-speed serial readout and a wider electrical bandwidth $\Delta f$.

Specialized ROICs are also used to provide time-of-flight (ToF) and gating capabilities for laser radar systems. The ToF data is determined by the requirement to measure the range $R$, with $2R = c \times t_f$ information on every pixel giving 3D (angle-angle-range) data on the target location.

As we have also seen in Chapter 6, an on-off range-gate time for a detector's reverse bias can prevent backscattered laser light from saturating the detector before a laser radar signal arrives; this requires both a gating start time and a gate width, both functions of which are provided by a ROIC. Resolution on the start time is ≈ 20–100 psec, while gate widths of 10–500 nsec are common. Gating is also used for active illumination; see Ref. 24 for details.

**Uniformity.** Every parameter in an FPA will vary from pixel to pixel to some degree—responsivity, read noise, DCR, bias voltage, optical crosstalk, ToF data, and so on. If we also consider APD-based FPAs, then such non-uniformities will also include the breakdown voltage, APD gain, and PDE.

Of particular interest for assessing image quality is the photo-response non-uniformity (PRNU), a result of any variations that result in pixel-to-pixel or column-to-column differences in output voltage (Fig. 7.31). This may

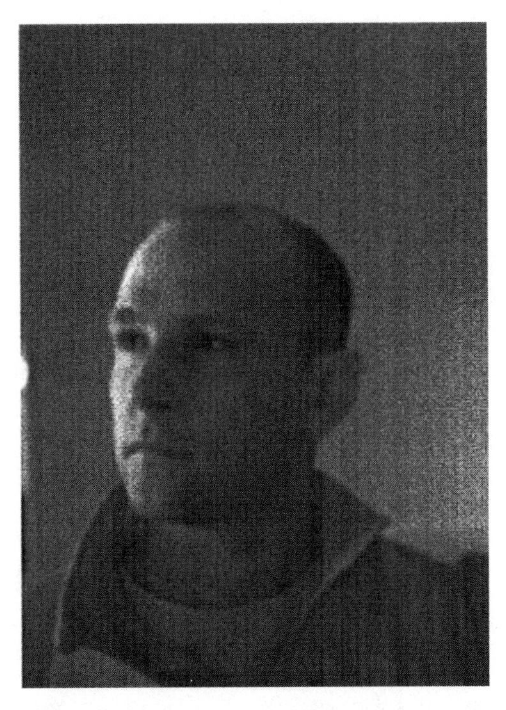

**Figure 7.31** Photoresponse non-uniformities (PRNUs) for each pixel in an FPA are observed as spatial noise in the image. [Reprinted from T. Bakker, D. Turner, and J. Battaglia, "Development of a miniature InGaAs camera for wide operating temperature range using a temperature-parameterized uniformity correction," *Proc. SPIE* **6940**, 69400K (2008).]

include each pixel's responsivity, fill factor, and pre-amplifier gain (as measured by the $\mu V/e^-$ output of the CTIA).

The variations seen in Fig. 7.31 are clearly noise that interferes with our assessment of image quality, and this has in fact been a dominant noise source in CMOS FPAs. Fortunately, this type of FPA fixed-pattern noise (FPN) can be corrected to a large degree, such that the spatial variations are largely unnoticeable by the eye when looking at cell-phone images. Nonetheless, the FPN may still be sufficiently large to interfere with scientific assessments of laser-system image quality—specifically, the SNR. A CCD, for example, may have a PRNU of as much as 1% before non-uniformity correction (NUC), and the resulting noise depends on both the PRNU and the power incident on the pixels (see Section 7.5.1). As a result, correlated double sampling (CDS) and NUC algorithms are commonly used in sCMOS image processing, and a PRNU of less than 0.1% is possible.

Since the SNR depends on the noise, another FPA parameter commonly measured for non-uniformity is the dark current. This is shown in Fig. 7.32, where the number of pixels with a particular DCR is plotted in a histogram, giving both a mean and a variance. These can then be compared against a

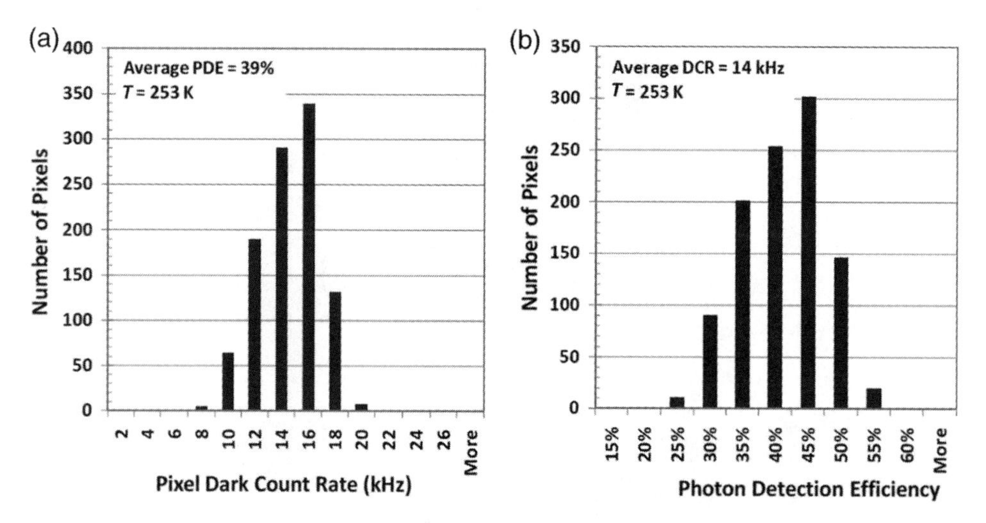


**Figure 7.32** APD dark count rate (DCR) and photon detection efficiency (PDE) are commonly measured for non-uniformity across an FPA. [Reprinted from M. A. Itzler, M. Entwistle, M. Owens, et al., "Comparison of 32 × 128 and 32 × 32 Geiger-mode APD FPAs for single photon 3D LADAR imaging," *Proc. SPIE* **8033**, 80330G (2011).]

system-level requirement such as "Pixel dark count rate must be less than 20 kHz," resulting in some number of pixels not meeting this spec and therefore being "inoperable."[5] High-dark-count ("hot") pixels can be dealt with using a different set of algorithms than FPN—nearest-neighbor averaging, e.g.—but are also a common part of an FPA vendor's specs.

## 7.5 Noise, Sensitivity, and Selection

Summarizing the chapter to this point, we have looked at the concept of a photon detector and its various types, including *p-n* junction, PIN, APD, and PMT. With the exception of PMTs, these detectors can also be integrated into FPAs, leading to a review of the different FPA technologies—CCD, EM-CCD, sCMOS, and hybrid—and their specifications.

Some of the discussion on the advantages and disadvantages of detector types and technologies has been qualitative. For example, we have looked at the effects of APD gain on the collected signal, but have not yet quantified the effects on detected noise. Another example is the effect of amplifier bandwidth on read noise and thus sensitivity at low signal levels—again illustrating the importance of both signal and noise.

Signals and noise can both be measured by the detector subsystem. By themselves these measurements are meaningless numbers; they become useful only when compared with each other by dividing the signal *S* by the noise *N*. This defines the idea of the signal-to-noise ratio (SNR), a key metric for evaluating many laser systems; we will review this metric in Section 7.5.1.

The idea of SNR can be looked at from another perspective that results in the concept of sensitivity (i.e., the smallest signal that the detector subsystem can measure, given the noise). There are a number of variations on this theme, many of which are looked at in Section 7.5.2.

Finally, we review approaches to detector selection in Section 7.5.3, within the context of how detectors influence overall laser-system architectures and design trades.

### 7.5.1 Signal-to-noise ratio

The comparison of the signal and noise on a detector is one of the most important measures of laser system performance. In an imaging application, for example, the SNR affects image fidelity even when the MTF has been optimized (Fig. 7.33); laser tracking systems are similarly affected in that low SNR makes it more difficult to follow an object as its image "dances" around the FPA. Biomedical imaging systems are particularly dependent on SNR, as the probability of correctly detecting an important feature in the image (a tumor, e.g.) is highly sensitive to SNR, as is the minimum SNR necessary to

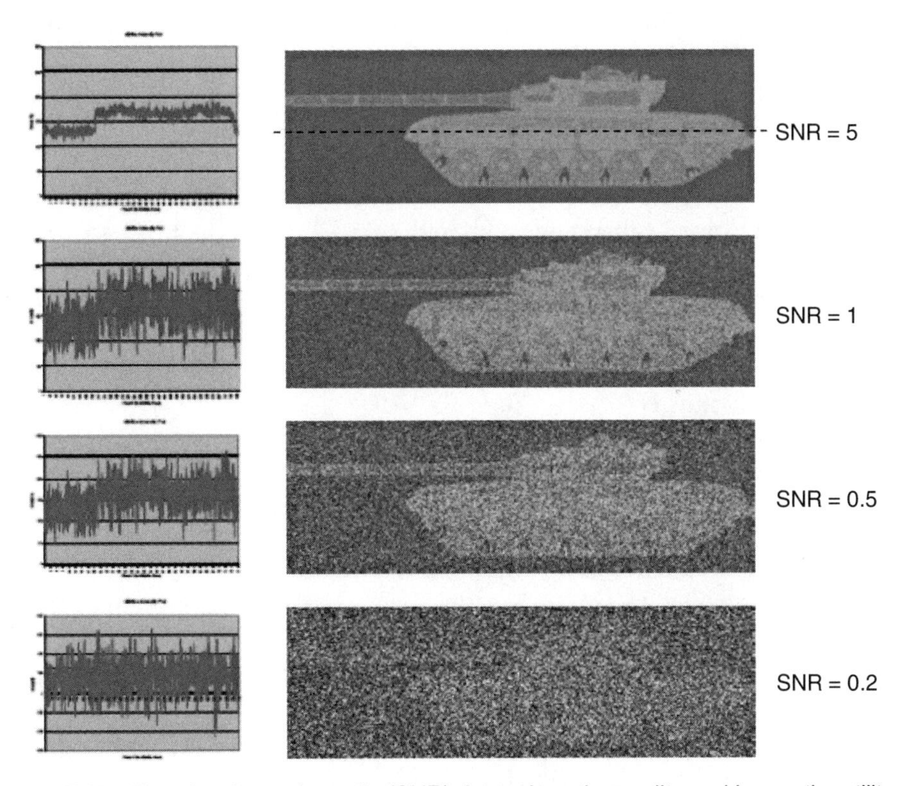


**Figure 7.33** The signal-to-noise ratio (SNR) determines the quality and hence the utility of a signal. (Reprinted with permission from David Schmieder, Instructor, Georgia Tech "Infrared Technology & Applications" Short Course DEF3001P.)

not mistakenly "measure" a tumor when there isn't one (i.e., the probability of a false alarm $P_{fa}$). In all cases, system requirements push the SNR to an optimum range of $\approx$ 5–6; performance drops markedly below this range, and designing an instrument with a higher SNR may involve extraordinary technical, cost, and schedule difficulties.

The SNR for independent noise sources is given by the ratio of detector signal $S = i_s G$ to the standard deviation $\sigma_n$ of the noise current:

$$SNR = \frac{i_s G}{\sigma_n} = \frac{i_s G}{\sqrt{\sigma_s^2 + \sigma_{RIN}^2 + \sigma_b^2 + \sigma_{dc}^2 + \sigma_{amp}^2 + \sigma_{read}^2 + \sigma_{FPN}^2 + \sigma_{sp}^2}} \quad (7.12)$$

where the individual noise terms ($\sigma_s$, $\sigma_b$, etc.) will be defined in the subsections below. Because the noises from different sources are (usually) independent of each other (i.e., they are uncorrelated or *orthogonal*), they can be added in Eq. (7.12) as a root-sum-of-squares [or RSS, shorthand for the "(square) root of the sum of the squares"] of the individual standard deviations to produce a net noise current $\sigma_n$.

Also note that because detectors produce current in response to optical power, the SNR formulation of Eq. (7.12) is the convention used in optical engineering.[2] Electrical engineers use electrical power ($\propto i_s^2$) to define SNR; their SNR is thus the square of that used by optical engineers, giving SNR (electrical) = $SNR^2$ (optical). The SNR will also be expressed in units of number of electrons in Section 7.5.2 when we look at photon counting.

The signal current can be estimated from the power $\Phi$ collected by the optics-plus-detector subsystems, giving $\Phi = TLA_{EP}\Omega_{FOV}$ for an optical subsystem with an entrance-pupil area $A_{EP}$ and a detector subsystem with a collection solid angle $\Omega_{FOV}$ [see Eq. (6.10)]. The average signal current is then given by $i_s = R_o \Phi$ for a *p-n* junction or PIN photodiode, and $i_s$ must be multiplied by any gain to obtain the signal $S = i_s G$ for an LM-APD, PMT, or EM-CCD with gain $G$.

As shown in Eq. (7.12), a number of noise terms are needed to estimate the SNR; these are quantified in the following subsections under the noise categories of signal $\sigma_s$, background $\sigma_b$, dark current $\sigma_{dc}$, amplifier $\sigma_{amp}$, read $\sigma_{read}$, spatial $\sigma_{FPN}$, and speckle $\sigma_{sp}$.

**Signal Noise.** The most basic source of noise is the signal itself. That is, despite the best design intentions and execution, output power from any laser changes over time in response to the quantum-mechanical processes that produce photons. As we have seen in Section 2.1.8, there is also an additional noise—relative intensity noise (RIN)—due to gain-medium or cavity dynamics.

When detecting sources that produce a relatively large number of photons—either directly from the laser or indirectly via scattering—the photodiode current follows Gaussian statistics as a large-photon ($n_p \geq 10$)

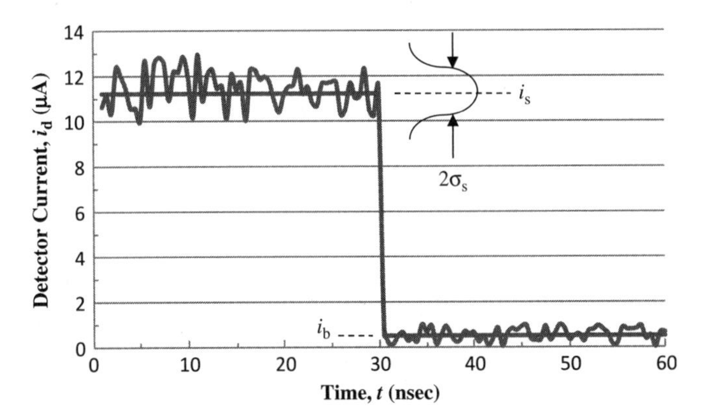


**Figure 7.34** Signal shot noise is assumed to have a white-noise frequency dependence and a standard deviation $\sigma_s$ that increases with mean signal current $i_s$.

approximation to Poisson statistics;[39,40] the attendant quantum-mechanical noise is called *shot noise* because the energy can be associated with the random arrival time of individual photons or "shots." One consequence is that the output fluctuates randomly with a variance $\sigma_s^2$ that grows as the signal current increases (Fig. 7.34).

The standard deviation $\sigma_s$ [root-mean-square (RMS) value] of the signal shot current measured by a photon detector is given by[2]

$$\sigma_s = \sqrt{2qi_s\Delta f \cdot G^2F(G)} \qquad [\text{A}] \tag{7.13}$$

where the $2qi_s\Delta f$ term is due to the signal shot noise for the random photon arrival times as measured with a *p-n* junction or PIN detector, and the $G^2F(G)$ term applies to any detector with gain $G > 1$, such as LM-APDs, PMTs, or EM-CCDs.

The electrical bandwidth $\Delta f$ in Eq. (7.13) assumes that shot noise occurs as white noise—i.e., the noise is equally distributed over a broad range of frequencies. As a result, the more frequencies that are included in the electrical measurement, the more noise that's collected by the detection process. This pushes the system design to as low a bandwidth as possible while maintaining the requirement that the detector be able to measure changes in the signal. The white-noise assumption breaks down when the noise is frequency dependent (typically at very low frequencies where $1/f$ noise is dominant), but it is commonly used nonetheless in system-level calculations.

When the signal's own shot noise is much larger than the other noises in the system—i.e., $\sigma_s \gg \sigma_b$, $\sigma_{dc}$, etc.—then the system is called *signal limited.* Combining Eqs. (7.12) and (7.13), we see in this case that the SNR $\approx [i_s\Delta t/qF(G)]^{1/2}$ for a measurement bandwidth $\Delta f = 1/2\Delta t$. This typically occurs for large signal levels, such as those shown in Fig. 7.26 for $n_p \geq 100$ photons or so.

An important feature of signal-limited detection is that LM-APD, PMT, or EM-CCD gain does not increase the SNR and can only make it worse for an excess-noise factor $F(G) > 1$, a topic we take a closer look at below in "Excess Noise."

Also note that the expression for SNR directly depends on the pulse energy $Q_p$ for applications using pulsed sources such as laser radar. To see why, we note that the signal current $i_s$ depends on the peak power $P_{peak}$ (after reflection loss and scattering), which in turn depends on the pulse energy and pulse width [Eq. (2.3)]. Algebraically, $i_s = R_o\Phi \sim R_o \times Q_p/\Delta t$, giving $i_s\Delta t \sim R_o \times Q_p$. It is for this reason that some laser designers spend much of their time on the development of high-pulse-energy lasers.

As described in Section 2.1.8, the laser RIN is also a source of signal noise and may be large due to inherent laser dynamics such as relaxation oscillations or technical noise due to vibration-induced changes in the length of the laser cavity. Remembering that RIN is defined using the square of the power fluctuations $[\Delta P(f)]^2$, Eq. (2.7) shows that $[\Delta P(f)]^2 = \text{RIN} \cdot \Delta f \cdot P^2$, from which we obtain $\Delta i = R_o\Delta P \equiv \sigma_{RIN}$:

$$\sigma_{RIN} = R_o P \sqrt{RIN \cdot \Delta f \cdot G^2 F(G)} \qquad [\text{A}] \qquad (7.14)$$

where the RIN · $\Delta f$ term is the RIN component for *p-n* junction or PIN detectors, and the $G^2F(G)$ term again applies to any non-Geiger detector with gain $G > 1$. Note that Eq. (7.14) is the RIN for an emitted laser output power $P$; the detected RIN must use the collected power $\Phi$ based on the radiometric methods covered in Chapter 6.

---

**Example 7.3**

It is sometimes mentioned in laser manufacturer's literature that at frequencies above 10 MHz, the noise of the laser is below the shot noise limit of most practical photodiodes. In addition, when comparing photodiodes as in Fig. 7.26, the laser RIN is never included, given the assumption that the RIN is not a significant contributor to detected noise. In this example, we take a look at when this is or is not a valid assumption.

The comparison of RIN with signal shot noise can be found by taking the ratio of Eq. (7.14) to Eq. (7.13), for which the RIN becomes dominant when the ratio $\gg 1$:

$$\frac{\sigma_{RIN}}{\sigma_s} = \sqrt{\frac{R_o P \cdot RIN}{2q}} \gg 1 \qquad (7.15)$$

If the RIN does not depend on the laser output power $P$,[41,42] we can use Eq. (7.15) to estimate the power at which the RIN is much larger than the shot noise:

$$P \gg \frac{2q}{R_o \cdot RIN} \tag{7.16}$$

showing that a noisier laser (larger RIN) has a lower power at which the RIN dominates. To illustrate using a frequency-doubled Nd:YAG laser emitting at $\lambda = 532$ nm, the selected detector is silicon with $\eta_{QE} \approx 0.9$ (Fig. 7.24), from which we find from Eq. (7.3) that the responsivity $R_o = \eta_{QE}\lambda/1.24 = 0.9 \times 0.532$ μm/(1.24 eV-μm) = 0.39 A/W.

The laser RIN for this example is obtained using the low-frequency data in Fig. 2.12, with a value of –135 dB/Hz for a noise frequency $f < 10$ kHz; converting the units of decibels (dB) to real numbers gives us RIN $\approx 10^{-13.5}$/Hz = $3.16 \times 10^{-14}$/Hz. Substituting in Eq. (7.16), we find that $P \gg 2 \times 1.602 \times 10^{-19}/(0.39\ \text{A/W} \times 3.16 \times 10^{-14}/\text{Hz}) = 26$ μW. This is not a huge amount of power, indicating that laser RIN can easily become a dominant noise source at these low frequencies.

RIN can be reduced using electrical noise-reduction techniques.[43] However, Fig. 2.12 also shows a RIN value of approximately –175 dB/Hz at a noise frequency $f > 10$ MHz, with RIN = $3.16 \times 10^{-18}$/Hz smaller by four orders of magnitude than the low-frequency RIN. If the system requirements allow this higher frequency, the power for RIN to dominate over laser shot noise also increases by four orders of magnitude to $P \gg 0.26$ W.

Many systems will require a frequency bandwidth that encompasses the peak RIN shown in Fig. 2.12, and in this case the integrated RIN must be used.[42] Nonetheless, the back-of-the-envelope analysis in this example shows that laser manufacturers' literature is correct in specifying a frequency at which the noise of the laser is below the shot noise limit. We also see that Fig. 7.26 is correct in assuming a "noiseless" laser for which RIN is insignificant at 1–100 photon-level signals. Whether or not shot noise or RIN are small compared with the other detector noises—useful for the design of laser system architectures or the measurement of laser noise itself—depends on the magnitude of these noises, as reviewed in the next subsections.

---

**Background Noise**. With integration times no shorter than 0.25 μsec or so allowed by a ROIC, and signal pulse widths as small as 1 nsec (e.g.), we see that there may be a time period over which an FPA may be collecting photons but not collecting signal. These background photons are also a source of noise, although with appropriate radiometric design and laser selection, the background can be much smaller than the laser signal, as shown in Fig. 7.34 for $t > 30$ nsec.

The detector, of course, does not "know" whether the photons it is measuring come from the signal or the background, and the distinction is arbitrary from the perspective of measured noise. As a result, the equation for background shot noise $\sigma_b$ is identical in form to Eq. (7.13); namely, $\sigma_b = [2qi_b\Delta f \cdot G^2F(G)]^{1/2}$, where the average background current $i_b$ is used instead of the average signal current.

In some situations—for example, trying to identify laser radar pulses reflected from a solar-illuminated scene consisting of cars and pedestrians—the entire background may be considered noise. Techniques such as spatial and spectral filtering can be used to reduce the background level,[5] but despite these efforts, the remaining background current may still be large in comparison with the signal. In such cases, backgrounds can be averaged and subtracted from the measurement, and any remaining current fluctuations are due to noise in the background.

Temporal filtering may also be used to reduce the background noise, and this is the reason for using high-speed ICCDs with nanosecond gating times during which background current is integrated. Using Eq. (7.10), the number of background noise electrons $n_b = \sigma_b(t_{int} - \Delta t_p)/q$, showing that a reduction in integration time $t_{int}$—by using a shorter gate time—directly reduces the background electrons accumulated by a pixel's charge well; the SNR then increases if the gate time is long enough to include the signal's pulse width ($t_{int} > \Delta t_p$). Due to the environmental restrictions of using ICCDs (lifetime and overload), this technique is most useful in biomedical microscopy—e.g., single-molecule fluorescence requiring extremely low backgrounds.

**Dark-Current Noise**. We have seen that there is a random, Poisson-distributed number of photons emitted by a laser in a given time interval; even in the absence of photons, however, there is also a random generation of electrons in photon detectors. This detector "dark current" and its associated shot noise—also known as dark counts for photon-counting measurements—is not due to photons creating conduction electrons; rather, it is the temperature of the detector that gives bound electrons enough thermal energy to conduct even in the absence of photons.

Like the photon noise generated by signal or background light, these dark-current electrons are also randomly generated with a Gaussian amplitude distribution and an assumed white-noise frequency spectrum. Therefore, dark-current shot noise $\sigma_{dc}$ has the same mathematical form as the signal and background shot noises:[2]

$$\sigma_{dc} = \sqrt{2qi_{dc}\Delta f \cdot G^2F(G)} \quad [A] \tag{7.17}$$

where the $2qi_{dc}\Delta f$ term is due to the average bulk dark current $i_{dc}$ (ignoring surface dark currents that are not increased by $G$), and the usual $G^2F(G)$ term applies to LM-APDs, PMTs, and EM-CCDs whenever the number of electrons is multiplied, independent of the gain mechanism.

Dark current creates false indications (false positives) of the presence of light and can be a significant driver in laser system design. If the detector is dark-current limited, then the signal is extremely small or the dark current is excessively large. Inversely, the use of scientific-grade PMTs is commonly used to increase the SNR in low-light situations because the gain $G$ may be greater than $10^6$, while the PMT dark current is extremely low.

Dark current is the consequence of the thermal excitation of electrons to higher-energy conductive states. Because this excitation depends on an Arrhenius relationship, it is exponentially sensitive to temperature. The most commonly used method for reducing dark current is thus reducing the temperature of the detector. For example, we have seen in Section 7.4.2 that EM-CCDs are deep-cooled to approximately –100 °C to reduce the dark current to below the amplification noise. Typical dark-current values for commercial sCMOS cameras are 25 $e^-$/sec per pixel at +20 °C,[34] decreasing to 0.06 $e^-$/sec per pixel at –10 °C,[35] and illustrating the extreme dependence of dark current on detector temperature.

The degree of cooling required will also depend on the detector material. Silicon, for example, is a relatively "quiet" material due to its larger bandgap energy $E_g$, which gives fewer electrons enough energy to conduct at a given temperature. An InGaAs detector, on the other hand, is relatively noisy because of its smaller bandgap energy.

Dark current is affected not only by temperature and material but also by detector reverse bias; this is due to the reduction of the cross-junction energy barrier with reverse bias, giving more low-thermal-energy electrons enough energy to have a high probability of overcoming the barrier and conduct.

Dark current also depends on detector surface area—it is sometimes specified by vendors in terms of nA/cm$^2$—so another method for reducing dark current is to use smaller detectors. A smaller detector has fewer atoms to emit dark current, approximately in proportion to the detector area. Smaller detectors and FPA pixels also have the advantage of enabling a shorter focal length for the same IFOV, which results in smaller, lighter systems. However, due to the smaller etendue $A_d\Omega_{f/\#}$ for a detector area $A_d$ and a solid angle $\Omega_{f/\#}$ associated with the *f*/# of the focusing optics,[5] the disadvantage of smaller detectors is that fewer photons are collected—unless the *f*/# of the optics is also decreased to compensate—and this is one possible trade to be explored if dark-current noise is persistent.

Dark current also depends strongly on the quality of the material growth and etching in the fabrication process. As a result, dark count rates can be much higher ($> 100\times$) for FPA pixels of the same material at the same temperature than for single-pixel detectors fabricated with many fewer processing steps that expose micro-roughness surface area resulting in mobile electrons. In extreme cases—after cooling and pixel size have already been tried—it may be necessary to avoid an FPA and use scanned single-pixel detectors to reduce the dark current.

Finally, just as gating or integration time can be used to reduce background current, it can similarly be used to reduce dark current. In all cases, the use of the dark-current variance in Eq. (7.17) requires the use of dark-current averaging and subtraction for each pixel, as it is $\sigma_{dc}$ that is used in the SNR equation [Eq. (7.12)], not the dark current $i_{dc}$ itself. This data may be obtained, for example, during uniformity measurements as in Fig. 7.32.

**Excess Noise**. We have seen that detector gain adds noise through a $G^2F(G)$ term that increases noise based on *any* current flow—signal, background, or dark current—in a detector with gain $G$, with the excess-noise factor $F(G)$ usually given by Eq. (7.6). This additional noise term is inherent in any detector that multiplies electrons, whether the gain mechanism is a result of avalanching (LM-APDs and PMTs) or electron multiplying (EM-CCDs).

For a signal-limited detector, we have seen that the SNR $\approx [i_s \Delta t / qF(G)]^{1/2}$, illustrating that gain is not necessarily useful in increasing the SNR, and will always be a detriment for signal-limited detection given that $F(G) > 1$ for any detector with gain. Low-noise avalanche materials such as MCT or low-noise gain processes such as PMTs or electron multiplication have $F(G) \approx 1.2$–$1.4$, and this is currently the technological lower limit on $F(G)$. The large noise factors for common detector materials such as silicon [$F(G) \approx 5$ for $G = 150$] and InGaAs [$F(G) \approx 5$ for $G = 10$] limit their use to situations where other noises besides the signal itself limit the SNR. Amplifier noise is one example, and this is seen in detail below in "Amplifier Noise."

The effects of excess noise are shown in Fig. 7.26, where the SNR for the EM-CCD FPA (iXon 897) is lower than that for the high-performance sCMOS FPA (Flash 4.0) for signal-limited detection ($n_p > 100$ photons). This is because the sCMOS does not have gain—giving it a gain $G = 1$ and an excess-noise factor $F(G) = 1$—while the EM-CCD does, resulting in a reduction of the signal-limited SNR for the EM-CCD by a factor of $[F(G)]^{1/2} > 1$. The sCMOS FPA thus provides the best-possible performance known as "shot-noise limited" for noiseless signal-limited detection.

**Amplifier Noise**. Looking next at a noise term associated with the electrical signal, the benefit of parallel readout of accumulated photoelectrons in sCMOS and hybrid FPAs is that the electrical pre-amplifier only needs to work fast enough for 1 pixel, while the amplifier in the serial CCD readout must be fast enough for $10^6$ pixels of data (for a large-format 1K × 1K array, e.g.). As the amplifier noise increases with the bandwidth $\Delta f$ [see Eq. (7.18)], and the noise of a high-bandwidth amplifier is inherently larger than a low-noise amplifier (due to additional $i^2R$ electrical power dissipation at the higher rates), there is a factor of at least 1000 improvement in sCMOS and hybrid amplifier noise in comparison with a large-format CCD. CCDs are thus amplifier limited to either a low bandwidth (and resulting frame rate) or poor sensitivity due to high read noise at higher bandwidths.

To first order, the noise current for an amplifier whose noise spectral density (NSD, units of A/Hz$^{1/2}$) is constant over the bandwidth $\Delta f$ is given by

$$\sigma_{\text{amp}} \approx \text{NSD}\sqrt{\Delta f} \qquad [\text{A}] \tag{7.18}$$

where $\sigma_{\text{amp}}$ starts to dominate over the signal noise at high bandwidths—such as those found in laser communications systems where data rates exceed 10 GHz, e.g.—and typical values of the NSD for a transimpedance amplifier (TIA) are given in Fig. 7.35. The horizontal axis of the figure shows, for example, high-speed (bipolar) TIAs with $\sigma_{\text{amp}}/\Delta f^{1/2} \approx 1$–10 pA/Hz$^{1/2}$ at room temperature. Low-bandwidth field-effect-transistor (FET)-based TIAs are much quieter, with values of $\sigma_{\text{TIA}}/\Delta f^{1/2}$ as low as 0.001–0.01 pA/Hz$^{1/2}$.

Because of the dependence of the NSD on $\Delta f$, Eq. (7.18) cannot be scaled based solely on NSD. For example, an amplifier with a bandwidth of 100 MHz may have an NSD of 0.4 pA/Hz$^{1/2}$ [with a total noise current $\sigma_{\text{amp}} = 0.4$ pA/Hz$^{1/2} \times (10^8$ Hz$)^{1/2} = 4$ nA], whereas a 1-GHz bandwidth amplifier may have an NSD of 4 pA/Hz$^{1/2}$ [and total noise current $\sigma_{\text{amp}} = 4$ pA/Hz$^{1/2} \times (10^9$ Hz$)^{1/2} = 126$ nA]. The wider-bandwidth amplifier thus has significantly more noise current, which is due not only to the wider bandwidth but also to the increase in the intrinsic noise of the higher-speed device. This availability of high-speed amplifiers with sufficiently low noise is one of the practical difficulties in obtaining linear-mode SPADs for the room-temperature detection of single-photon, 10-nsec pulses ($\Delta f = 50$ MHz) for laser radar systems.

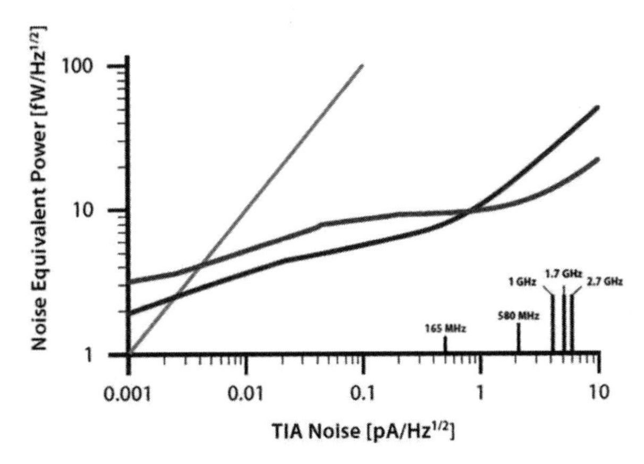


**Figure 7.35** Low-speed (megahertz) transimpedance amplifiers (TIAs) have a much lower noise spectral density (pA/Hz$^{1/2}$) than high-speed (gigahertz) amplifiers. (Data courtesy of Voxtel, Inc.)

In situations where amplifier noise is relatively high, using a linear-mode APD may nonetheless increase the SNR. As shown in Example 7.4, this depends on the relative magnitudes of the amplifier and APD excess noise.

---

**Example 7.4**

A common application for InGaAs LM-APDs is in high-speed laser communications systems operating at speeds of 10 GHz and higher, where amplifier bandwidth and noise are high. Unlike the signal-limited case where the APD's excess-noise factor reduces the SNR, this example illustrates an improvement in SNR up to an optimum APD (or PMT or EM-CCD) gain that depends on the value of the excess-noise factor.

To see why, the SNR equation can be written with only the amplifier and APD signal noises dominant, giving

$$SNR \approx \frac{i_s G}{\sqrt{\sigma_{APD}^2 + \sigma_{amp}^2}} \tag{7.19}$$

where $\sigma_s \equiv \sigma_{APD} = [2qi_s\Delta f \cdot G^2 F(G)]^{1/2}$ from Eq. (7.13), and $\sigma_{amp}$ is given by Eq. (7.18).

When the amplifier noise is much larger than the other noises in the system—i.e., $\sigma_{amp} \gg \sigma_{APD}$ because $\Delta f$ is large, e.g.—then we find that

$$SNR \approx \frac{i_s G}{\sigma_{amp}} = \frac{i_s G}{NSD\sqrt{\Delta f}} \tag{7.20}$$

showing the proportional improvement in the SNR with gain $G$, and the drop in SNR for a noisier amplifier (larger NSD) and wider bandwidth.

As the gain increases, the APD noise in Eq. (7.19) becomes much larger than the other noises in the system—i.e., $\sigma_{APD} \gg \sigma_{amp}$ for large gain—and now we find that

$$SNR \approx \frac{i_s G}{\sqrt{2qi_s\Delta f \cdot G^2 F(G)}} = \sqrt{\frac{i_s \Delta t}{qF(G)}} \tag{7.21}$$

showing that the SNR has become signal limited. That is, the gain has increased the signal strength to beyond the amplifier noise; in doing so, however, it has also increased the APD noise at a faster rate, leading to a decrease in SNR that depends on the value of $F(G)$.

Somewhere between these two extremes, then, is an optimum that depends on the gain. This is illustrated in Fig. 7.36, where the SNR versus gain from Eq. (7.19) shows a peak SNR that depends on $F(G)$ via the ionization ratio $k$. More importantly, Fig. 7.36 shows the peak SNR

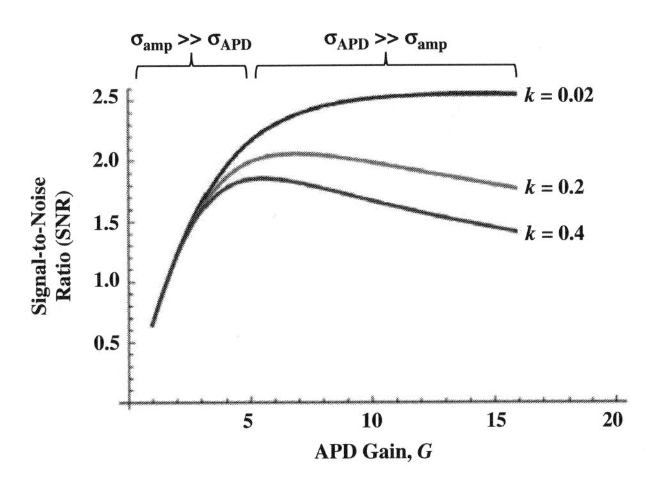


**Figure 7.36** The SNR first increases with APD gain when the amplifier noise is dominant and then decreases with gain as the APD excess noise dominates. (Data courtesy of Voxtel, Inc.)

increasing as the excess noise is lowered ($k = 0.02$), and this is the key reason for the continued development of low-excess-noise APDs with $F(G) \approx 1$ over a range of gain values.[13,14]

---

**Read Noise.** Detector gain is also useful for increasing the SNR in ultralow-light-level measurements such as that shown in Fig. 7.26 for a photon number $n_p \leq 10$. In this case, the gain overcomes a phenomenon known as read noise, significantly improving the ability of a detector to measure a small numbers of photons; at this point in time, the EM-CCD is thus the better detector in this situation, not the sCMOS.

Read noise occurs when the electrons accumulated in the charge-well capacitor for a pixel are transferred from a pre-amplifier for combining (multiplexing) with the electrons from the other pixels before final amplification (Fig. 7.30). In practice, read noise has three components: (1) pre-amplifier noise, (2) thermal variations in the number of electrons accumulated on the capacitor (aka kTC noise), and (3) small variations in the number of electrons remaining on the capacitor after it has been reset by a switching transistor.[44] Combining these effects, manufacturers supply read noise values with their product specs; typical numbers for $\sigma_{read}$ are $\approx$ 1–20 $e^-$ RMS per pixel per read.

These typical numbers depend on the detector temperature and read frequency. Temperature affects the kTC and reset components of read noise; a larger effect is the read frequency, where the pre-amplifier component quickly increases with read bandwidth $\Delta f$ (Fig. 7.37), just as we have seen previously in Eq. (7.18). The parallel-readout pre-amplifiers of sCMOS pixels thus ensure a lower read noise for this FPA technology than the serial readout of CCDs with 1- to 20-MHz pixel readout rates.

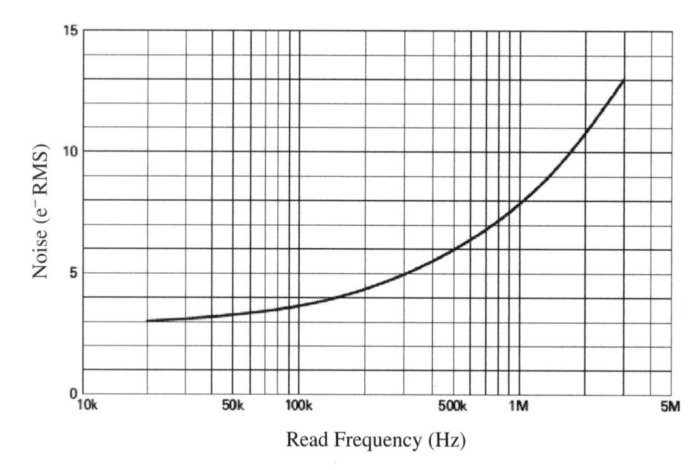


**Figure 7.37** Due to the larger pre-amplifier bandwidth, an increase in read frequency quickly increases the read noise. (Reprinted with permission from e2v Technologies; see Ref 45.)

In contrast with other situations we have looked at, detector gain in this case actually reduces the noise—specifically, the effective read noise by a factor of $G^2$. Physically, this is because the read noise occurs *after* the gain mechanism has already amplified the number of electrons, and is thus a small fraction of the total. Mathematically, we can see this by looking at an approximate SNR equation that includes only APD (or PMT or EM-CCD) shot-noise and read-noise terms:

$$SNR \approx \frac{i_s G}{\sqrt{\sigma_{\text{APD}}^2 + \sigma_{\text{read}}^2}} = \frac{i_s}{\sqrt{2qi_s\Delta f \cdot F(G) + (\sigma_{\text{read}}/G)^2}} \tag{7.22}$$

where we have divided the numerator and denominator of the first expression for SNR by the gain $G$ to obtain the second expression.

For sufficiently large gain, the effective read-noise term [equal to $(\sigma_{\text{read}}/G)^2$] for the APD, PMT, or EM-CCD is small in comparison with $G = 1$ detectors, thus obtaining better SNR than sCMOS FPAs at low photon levels if the responsivity is the same and the excess-noise factor is not large [$F(G) \leq 1.5$ or so]. Alternatively, the increase in read noise at higher read rates can be compensated by an increase in gain, thus allowing higher frame rates. These conclusions depend on the sCMOS values for read noise; the current level of technology is such that detectors with gain and low excess-noise factor—i.e., MCT LM-APDs, PMTs, and EM-CCDs—have better sensitivity, although this could change if the read-noise levels of sCMOS FPAs can be further reduced.

**Spatial Noise.** As we have seen in Section 7.4.3, two major contributors to FPA non-uniformities are pixel-to-pixel differences in responsivity and amplifier gain—differences that result from fabrication variations in the detector array and the ROIC, respectively. These photo-response non-uniformities (PRNUs) can be removed to a large degree,[5] and the remaining pattern of spatial noise is characterized as a percentage of the detector output.

The difference between pixels produces a pixel-to-pixel (or column-to-column) difference in output current (Fig. 7.31), even though the optical source producing the signal or background photons may be perfectly uniform. This phenomenon can limit the detector's sensitivity because the residual fixed-pattern noise (FPN) is directly proportional to the incident power. For an FPA image of a laser-illuminated scene, the standard deviation $\sigma_{FPN}$ of the spatial FPN is

$$\sigma_{FPN} = PRNU \cdot i_d G = PRNU \cdot R_g \Phi \tag{7.23}$$

where $R_g \equiv R_o G$, and the detector current $i_d$ could be due to either the background current $i_b$ or the signal current $i_s$, depending on which is larger.

Note that a larger flux $\Phi$ collected from the source produces a proportional increase in FPN (aka spatial noise). This is distinct from signal and background shot noise, which increase only with the square root of the photon flux [see Eq. (7.13)]. The greater sensitivity to optical flux burdens the laser system designer with reducing the PRNU to low values ($\sim$ 0.1% or lower). The design may thus be pushed to a specific detector material, some of which (e.g., silicon) have a less-variable fabrication process and inherently better uniformity than others (e.g., HgCdTe).

We will see in Example 7.5 that the requirement on PRNU will depend on the magnitudes of the other types of noise present, but non-uniform spatial noise can easily be a limiting factor in FPA selection, especially at high light levels or for long integration times where spatial noise can dominate. The sCMOS FPAs in particular have been designed with a sufficiently low PRNU to successfully compete against CCDs by reducing spatial noise to acceptable levels.[34]

**Speckle Noise.** A type of noise unique to laser systems—and which most people are familiar with—is known as speckle noise. As shown in Fig. 7.38 for an active-imaging application, speckle noise occurs when a laser beam is scattered from a rough surface, as all surfaces are to some degree. For surfaces that are irregular on a scale of at least one-quarter of a wavelength ($\lambda$/4)—this excludes polished mirror surfaces with a 50-Å RMS surface finish, e.g.—the reflected wavefronts can interfere constructively (bright) or destructively (dark), giving the mesmerizing, high-contrast bright-and-dark patterns of a laser-beam scattered from a diffuse surface such as a painted wall.

The random irregularities across most scattering surfaces assure a random speckle pattern. We can see this random pattern with our eyes, and under the right conditions it can also be measured by a detector. For an FPA image of a

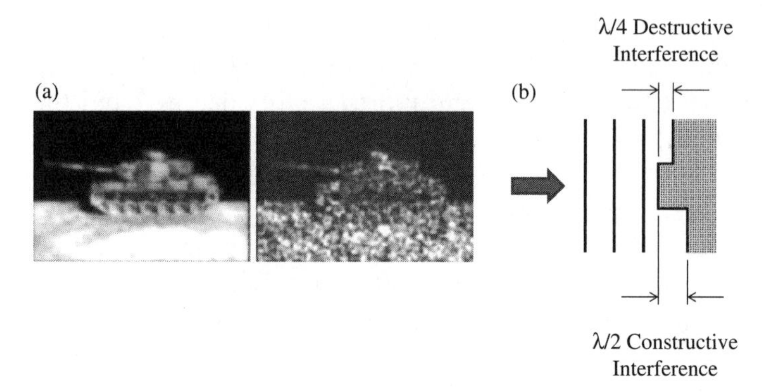


**Figure 7.38** Speckle noise [right photo in (a)] is shown in (b) as a result of the constructive and destructive interference of a reflected wavefront off different heights of the surface. [Photos reprinted from R. G. Driggers, R. H. Vollmerhausen, N. Devitt, C. Halford, and K. J. Barnard, "Impact of speckle on laser range-gated shortwave infrared imaging system target identification performance," *Optical Engineering* **42**(3), pp. 738–746 (2003).]

laser-illuminated scene, the standard deviation $\sigma_{sp}$ of the speckle noise can be approximated by[46]

$$\sigma_{sp} \approx \frac{i_d G}{\sqrt{DoF}} \quad [A] \tag{7.24}$$

where the average detector current $i_d$ can be due to either signal or background flux, and the number of detected electrons $n_d = i_d t_{int}/q \gg DoF$ for this approximation to be valid.

The number of independent degrees of freedom (DoF) can be difficult to quantify, but depends on the spatial and temporal coherence of the laser; an ideal laser that is spatially (single spatial mode) and temporally (single longitudinal mode) coherent has $DoF = 1$. In this case, the speckle noise $\sigma_{sp}$ equals $i_d G$, giving a worst-case speckle contrast $C_{sp} = 1/(DoF)^{1/2} = 1$. A broadband, spatially incoherent source with $DoF \to \infty$ is thus preferred for reducing speckle noise, and this is why it is difficult to see speckle when a rough surface is illuminated with sunlight or other incoherent sources.

Because of their many other advantages—low directionality, high spectral brightness, ultrashort pulses, etc.—lasers are the preferred source of photons for many applications, and the approach taken for systems such as laser projectors[47] or active illumination[48] where speckle noise can be an issue is to increase the number of independent sources of speckle (i.e., the DoF). A number of methods are available to do this, including reducing the temporal and spatial coherence, temporal averaging, angular multiplexing, and polarization diversity.

Since speckle is a result of wavefront interference, the degree of speckle will depend on maintaining the wavefront relationships between the reflected waves. Using Fig. 7.38, for example, the wavefront reflected from the center feature will be one-half of a wavelength out of phase from the wavefront reflected from the "$\lambda/4$ destructive interference" feature. If the wavefronts do not maintain their phase relationship—i.e., their temporal coherence—over the $2 \times \lambda/4$ difference in reflected distance, then the degree of interference is low, as is the speckle contrast. Mathematically, if the coherence length $d_c < 2\delta_{RMS}$ for an RMS surface finish $\delta_{RMS}$ (as in Fig. 4.30), then we can expect low speckle.[49] A reasonably good mirror polish of 10 Å RMS would then require a laser coherence length $d_c < 20$ Å or so to avoid speckle.

It is not difficult to avoid speckle from mirrors with most lasers, but rough, unpolished surfaces can easily have a surface finish on the order of 100 μm or more. One approach to speckle reduction from most surfaces, then, is to decrease the laser's coherence length $d_c = \lambda^2/2\Delta\lambda$. We know that this is possible by increasing the linewidth $\Delta\lambda$ or $\Delta\nu$, i.e., decreasing the temporal coherence [see Eq. (1.3)]. For example, we can see with our eyes that a red HeNe laser reflecting off of a wall with $\Delta\nu_{MLM} = 1$ GHz has a significant degree of speckle, while a supercontinuum laser with $\Delta\lambda = 300$ nm over the VIS band does not.

A narrow-linewidth laser is therefore a disadvantage in laser systems requiring low speckle noise. However, as a supercontinuum laser does not have enough spectral brightness at specific wavelengths such as red-green-blue (RGB) primaries, one method for otherwise increasing linewidth includes direct modulation of a semiconductor-laser's output power, as semiconductor lasers have large amplitude-phase coupling. Alternatively, using multiple lasers with sufficiently separated central wavelengths (wavelength diversity)—approximately 2 nm for each laser to be considered an independent DoF for laser projection systems[50]—is an option that has been used for projection systems using semiconductor lasers.

In addition to decreasing the temporal coherence, another approach to speckle reduction is reducing the spatial coherence with a multimode beam profile. That is, if a spatial beam profile can be decomposed into four modes (for example) *with the same power*, then the speckle noise is reduced by a factor of two. This is not a huge improvement and, as we have seen in Chapters 3 and 4, comes with the disadvantages of an increase in propagation angle and focused spot size.

The degree to which speckle noise reduces the SNR also depends on the speckle size and how it is sampled by the FPA. That is, the speckle size depends on the focusing of each individual coherent wavefront, with an optical resolution thus proportional to $\lambda/D$ for an imaging lens or mirror with aperture $D$.[49] At the same time, the speckles are sampled by the FPA, and small speckles in comparison with the pixel size results in an averaging of the speckle patterns, in that multiple speckles will be superimposed on one pixel and measured as current.

Additional methods for reducing speckle noise include polarization diversity, angular multiplexing, and temporal averaging over the integration time of the detector; details for each of these are reviewed in Ref. 49. As laser systems engineers, we know that these efforts will reach a point of diminishing returns, and our efforts at reducing speckle noise will eventually lead to another noise in the system being dominant. Example 7.5 looks at the specific comparison of speckle noise with FPA spatial noise.

---

**Example 7.5**

A typical active-imaging application to collect FPA snapshots using laser illumination has two possible sources of spatially varying noise: (1) speckle noise and (2) FPA fixed-pattern noise (FPN) due to photoresponse non-uniformities. Both noises are directly proportional to the signal current; as a laser systems engineer, where should you prioritize your efforts at reducing either of these noises?

The SNR equation for a *p-n* junction or PIN FPA that includes these noises is given by

$$\mathrm{SNR} \approx \frac{i_s}{\sqrt{\sigma_{\mathrm{FPN}}^2 + \sigma_{\mathrm{sp}}^2}} = \frac{i_s}{\sqrt{(PRNU \cdot i_s)^2 + i_s^2/DoF}} \tag{7.25}$$

where the spatial noise $\sigma_{\mathrm{FPN}}$ is given by Eq. (7.23), and the speckle noise $\sigma_{\mathrm{sp}}$ by Eq. (7.24). Note that we could include LM-APDs or EM-CCDs as FPA options, but given that the signal and noises are directly proportional to the gain, the gain $G$ cancels in numerator and denominator, also giving Eq. (7.25) for the SNR.

For the situation where the spatial noise is much larger than the speckle noise ($\sigma_{\mathrm{FPN}} \gg \sigma_{\mathrm{sp}}$), the SNR equation is

$$SNR \approx \frac{i_s}{\sqrt{\sigma_{\mathrm{FPN}}^2}} = \frac{i_s}{PRNU \cdot i_s} = \frac{1}{PRNU} \tag{7.26}$$

illustrating the importance of non-uniformity correction (NUC) to reduce the PRNU noise.

When the speckle noise is much larger than the spatial noise ($\sigma_{\mathrm{sp}} \gg \sigma_{\mathrm{FPN}}$), the SNR equation becomes

$$SNR \approx \frac{i_s}{\sqrt{\sigma_{\mathrm{sp}}^2}} = \frac{i_s}{i_s/\sqrt{DoF}} = \sqrt{DoF} \tag{7.27}$$

where the increase in the number of independent sources of speckle quantified by the DoF improves the SNR at a slow rate in comparison with the reduction in PRNU.

Comparing Eqs. (7.26) and (7.27) with $(DoF)^{1/2} \ll 1/PRNU = 1/0.001 = 1000$ (e.g.), speckle noise from a laser clearly places a lower limit on the SNR in Eq. (7.25) when the photoresponse non-uniformities have been reduced to a reasonably low PRNU. In practice, the direct proportionality with detector current ensures that, unless specific measures are taken to reduce it, speckle noise will also dominate over other sources of noise—signal, background, and dark current—that vary only with $i^{1/2}$.

---

**Summary.** While reducing speckle noise will be a key driver for laser-based imaging with FPAs, we have seen in this section that a number of other noise sources can dominate single-pixel detectors under specific situations such as high bandwidth (amplifier noise), high temperature (dark current), ultralow signal (read noise), or large signal (signal, spatial, and speckle noise).

We have also seen how detector gain $G$ for an LM-APD, PMT, or EM-CCD is not useful in all situations, specifically when the noise increases with $G$ at the same rate as the signal, as with signal noise [Eq. (7.13)], RIN [Eq. (7.14)], background noise, dark-current noise [Eq. (7.17)], spatial noise [Eq. (7.23)], and speckle noise [Eq. (7.24)]. In the cases of signal, RIN, background, and dark-current noise, the gain actually reduces the SNR due to the excess-noise factor $F(G)$. That being said, detector gain is useful when the noise does not increase with gain, such as increasing the SNR when amplifier noise dominates (Example 7.4) or even reducing the effective read noise for EM-CCDs to sub-electron levels [Eq. (7.22)].

These dependencies for each type of noise are summarized in Table 7.2. A noisier detector is one that is not as sensitive, and the table lists various design options for improving sensitivity; how to quantify the degree of sensitivity for a given noise is reviewed in Section 7.5.2.

**Table 7.2** Direct and indirect dependencies of the various types of detection noise found in a laser system.

| Noise | Dependencies | Equation |
|---|---|---|
| Signal | Signal current $i_s$; bandwidth $\Delta f$; RIN; gain $G$ | $\sigma_s = [2qi_s\Delta f \cdot G^2F(G)]^{1/2}$ |
| Background | Background current $i_b$; bandwidth $\Delta f$; gain $G$ | $\sigma_b = [2qi_b\Delta f \cdot G^2F(G)]^{1/2}$ |
| Dark | Temperature $T$; detector size; integration time; gain $G$ | $\sigma_{dc} = [2qi_{dc}\Delta f \cdot G^2F(G)]^{1/2}$ |
| Excess | Gain $G$; excess-noise factor $F(G)$ | $G^2F(G)$ |
| Amplifier | Amplifier NSD; bandwidth $\Delta f$ | $\sigma_{amp} = NSD \cdot (\Delta f)^{1/2}$ |
| Read | Read bandwidth $\Delta f$; temperature $T$; gain $G$ | Vendor spec ($e^-$/read) |
| Spatial | Detector current $i_d$; PRNU; gain $G$ | $\sigma_{FPN} = PRNU \cdot i_d G$ |
| Speckle | Detector current $i_d$; DoF; gain $G$ | $\sigma_{sp} \approx i_d G/(DoF)^{1/2}$ |

### 7.5.2 Detector sensitivity

Detector sensitivity—i.e., the smallest detectable power—can range from a single photon to many orders of magnitude more. One determinant of a detector's sensitivity is the noise, and in this section we take a deeper look at the connection between these two parameters.

The most basic measure of sensitivity is the noise-equivalent power (NEP). This is the optical power required to produce a signal $S = i_s G$ equal to the noise $N = \sigma_n$, i.e., SNR = 1. As has been mentioned, an SNR ≈ 5–6 is required for a high probability of detection and a low probability of false positives,[5] but using SNR = 1 establishes a standard for comparing detectors, even if the number must be scaled up to be useful for design.

As an example of how to estimate the NEP, we first look at a signal-limited detector whose SNR is given by the RHS of Eq. (7.21). Setting this expression to equal 1, and using the fact that $i_s = R_o \Phi_s$, we find that the signal flux $\Phi_s$ required for $SNR = 1$ is given by

$$\Phi_s \equiv NEP_s = \frac{2q\Delta f \cdot F(G)}{R_o} \qquad [\mathrm{W}] \qquad (7.28)$$

where the variable $\Phi_s$ is re-named the signal-limited $\mathrm{NEP_s}$, and we have brought the bandwidth $\Delta f = 1/2\Delta t$ back into the equation because NEP is sometimes defined as $NEP/\Delta f$ [$\mathrm{W/Hz^{1/2}}$].

Physically, Eq. (7.28) tells us that a larger bandwidth or excess-noise factor increases the optical power required for the signal to equal the noise; as both $\Delta f$ and $F(G)$ increase the signal noise $\sigma_s$ [see Eq. (7.13)], we would expect the NEP to increase. In addition, a larger responsivity $R_o$ in converting signal power into current decreases the NEP—i.e., makes the detector more sensitive—as the signal increases more than its own noise with a larger $R_o$. Also note that the responsivity is related to the QE at a particular wavelength using Eq. (7.3), illustrating why a higher QE results in a more-sensitive detector.

This method for finding an equation for the NEP can also be applied to other limiting noises—background, dark-current, amplifier, and so on—and different physical trends are found. For example, using Eq. (7.20) for the SNR for a detector with amplifier-limited noise, we find that we obtain a form of Eq. (7.5) modified for detector gain, giving $NEP_{amp} = NSD(\Delta f)^{1/2}/R_o G$. A quieter amplifier (smaller NSD) thus decreases (improves) the NEP, as does a larger LM-APD, PMT, or EM-CCD gain—illustrating yet again the benefits of gain in amplifier-limited measurements. Also note that the bandwidth increases the NEP, so it is often removed from the detector comparison by dividing both sides of the equation for $\mathrm{NEP_{amp}}$ by $(\Delta f)^{1/2}$, giving the units of $\mathrm{fW/Hz^{1/2}}$ seen in the vertical axis of Fig. 7.35 for the NEP of TIAs.

There are, of course, many situations where it is not possible to identify one specific noise such as signal or amplifier as being dominant, and in that case the full SNR expression given by Eq. (7.12) must be used; numerical and graphical solutions for the NEP in that case are straightforward.

There are a number of variations on the NEP theme. The most common in laser systems is the number of noise-equivalent photons (NEPh), obtained by multiplying the NEP by the integration or rectangular pulse time over which photons are collected, giving the noise-equivalent energy; this result is then divided by the energy per photon $E_p = hc/\lambda$:

$$NEPh \approx \frac{NEP \cdot t_{\text{int}}}{E_p} \tag{7.29}$$

The NEPh is a common metric for laser systems only because of the need for some systems—single-molecule fluorescence microscopy[11] or long-range laser radar,[14] e.g.—for single-photon sensitivity. Unfortunately, single-photon sensitivity is not the same as single-photon measurement (or counting), and there are practical difficulties with both of these concepts.

Looking at the practicality of single-photon sensitivity, we can re-write the SNR equation in terms of the number of signal and noise electrons:

$$SNR = \frac{n_s G}{\sqrt{n_{\sigma s}^2 + n_{\sigma \text{RIN}}^2 + n_{\sigma b}^2 + n_{\sigma \text{dc}}^2 + n_{\sigma \text{amp}}^2 + n_{\sigma \text{read}}^2 + n_{\sigma \text{FPN}}^2 + n_{\sigma \text{sp}}^2}} \tag{7.30}$$

which looks similar to Eq. (7.12) for the standard deviation $n_{\sigma s}$ of the signal-noise electrons, the standard deviation $n_{\sigma \text{RIN}}$ of the RIN-noise electrons, and so on. The fun starts when we look at the individual expressions for each of these noise terms. For example, using Eq. (7.10) to convert Eq. (7.13) from signal-noise current to signal-noise electrons, we obtain

$$n_{\sigma s} = \sqrt{n_s \cdot G^2 F(G)} \qquad [\text{e}^-] \tag{7.31}$$

which does not depend explicitly on bandwidth $\Delta f$. It is implied, however, as the number of signal electrons $n_s$ is proportional to the integration time or pulse width, which in turn determines the measurement bandwidth.

We can now combine Eqs. (7.30) and (7.31) to determine the feasibility of single-photon sensitivity when the signal noise is dominant. As in Eq. (7.22), this may be possible with a high-gain EM-CCD with low read noise. In this case, the SNR is given by

$$SNR_{\text{sig}} \approx \frac{n_s G}{\sqrt{n_{\sigma s}^2}} = \sqrt{\frac{n_s}{F(G)}} \tag{7.32}$$

which is already showing us that the EM-CCD excess noise reduces the SNR, as expected when the signal and noise both increase by $G$. Going down this trail one more step leads us to an estimate of the signal-limited noise-equivalent photons ($NEPh_{sig}$), obtained by setting $SNR_{sig} = 1$ in Eq. (7.32) and solving for the mean number of photons $n_p \equiv NEPh$:

$$NEPh = \frac{F(G)}{\eta_{QE}} \qquad [\text{\# of photons}] \tag{7.33}$$

where we have used the detector QE to connect the mean number of signal electrons to the mean number of photons $n_p = \eta_{QE} \times n_s$.

This fascinating result clearly shows us the difficulty in obtaining single-photon sensitivity: *Eq. (7.33) is always greater than one*. For example, for an EM-CCD with $F(G) = 1.4$ and $\eta_{QE} = 0.8$, we find that the best-possible detector sensitivity $NEPh_s = 1.4/0.8 = 1.75 \approx 2$ photons (as shown in Fig. 7.26 for the iXon 897 EM-CCD). Even if a perfectly noiseless detector with $F(G) = 1$ were available—they are in the form of sCMOS and CCD FPAs, but these do not have the gain required to reduce the effective read noise to below the signal shot noise, thus invalidating Eq. (7.33)—we still find that $NEPh_s = 1/0.8 > 1$, but also illustrating why vendors continue to develop detectors such as MCT LM-APDs with low excess noise and high QE.

So how do we obtain single-photon sensitivity? Another situation we have looked at where detector gain is useful is when the amplifier noise dominates (Example 7.4). In this case, the SNR equation becomes

$$SNR_{amp} = \frac{n_s G}{n_{\sigma amp}} = \frac{n_s G}{(\Delta t/q) \cdot NSD\sqrt{\Delta f}} = \frac{2qn_s G\sqrt{\Delta f}}{NSD} \tag{7.34}$$

where we have used Eq. (7.10) to convert $\sigma_{amp}$ in Eq. (7.18) to $n_{\sigma amp}$ and Eq. (7.4) to relate amplifier bandwidth $\Delta f = 1/2\Delta t$. The gain $G$ thus directly improves the SNR; is it good enough to get to single-photon sensitivity?

The amplifier-limited noise-equivalent photons ($NEPh_{amp}$) is obtained by setting $SNR_{amp} = 1$ in Eq. (7.34) and solving for the mean number of photons $n_p \equiv NEPh_{amp}$:

$$NEPh_{amp} = \frac{1}{\eta_{QE} G} \cdot \frac{NSD}{2q\sqrt{\Delta f}} \qquad [\text{\# of photons}] \tag{7.35}$$

which does not give us much physical insight, but does allow us to quantify the conditions under which $NEPh_{amp} \leq 1$ for single-photon (or better) sensitivity.

Specifically, we note that in this case $NEPh_{amp}$ gets smaller with gain $G$. So let's look at how much gain is needed for the detector to be sensitive to one photon or less:

$$NEPh_{\mathrm{amp}} \leq 1 \Rightarrow G \geq \frac{1}{\eta_{\mathrm{QE}}} \cdot \frac{NSD}{2q\sqrt{\Delta f}} \tag{7.36}$$

which requires amplifier data to see if single-photon sensitivity is possible with state-of-the-art technology. Using the data from Fig. 7.35, we find that the $NSD = 6$ pA/Hz$^{1/2}$ at $\Delta f = 2.7$ GHz for a commercial, low-noise TIA. Substituting in Eq. (7.36) with $\eta_{\mathrm{QE}} = 0.8$, we find that we need a gain $G \geq 450$ for single-photon sensitivity. This gain is easily obtainable with HgCdTe LM-APDs (see Fig. 7.11), GM-APDs (SPADs or FPAs), PMTs, and EM-CCDs—though not necessarily with the low level of amplifier noise needed to obtain single-photon sensitivity.

While Eq. (7.36) does not include any excess noise associated with the gain, in practice it is still important to reduce $F(G)$ to $\leq 1.5$ or so. That is, there is rarely a pure situation of amplifier-dominated noise—particularly at high gain—and the signal noise will contribute to the total noise as the gain increases, as seen in Eq. (7.31) and Fig. 7.36 of Example 7.4. As a result, the excess-noise factor $F(G)$ does play a role, but only after the gain has increased the signal to the point where the signal noise is comparable to the amplifier noise.

Also note that the low QE of PMTs (see Fig. 7.16) can be compensated by the extremely high gain ($10^6$ or higher) to obtain single-photon sensitivity with this type of detector. Another trade to be considered for all detector types with $G > 1$ is the use of lower-speed (and therefore lower-noise) amplifiers. This reduces the gain required for single-photon sensitivity given the assumption of amplifier-limited noise; a lower speed, however, may also imply a longer integration time over which dark counts are collected, possibly pushing Eq. (7.36) outside the bounds of its amplifier-limited validity.

### 7.5.3 Detector selection

There are, then, a number of trades between different detectors—trades that depend on the system requirements. In light of the wide range of details that must be considered in specifying detectors—that is, responsivity, bandwidth, pixel size, linearity, power range, saturation, uniformity, operability, and so on—it is no surprise that detector selection is one of the most challenging aspects of laser systems engineering.

Detector selection requires a power (or photon) budget to determine system sensitivity, a noise budget to calculate SNR, and a comparison of detector specs from different vendors—none of whom has exactly what's needed. The process may require an iteration (or three) if the detector has too much noise, or isn't available in a material that matches the source wavelengths, or if the system requirements are such that it's not possible to lower the bandwidth to reduce some of the noise components, and so on.

In this section, we look at detector selection from two perspectives. The first is a comparison of the different detectors we have reviewed in this book, categorized as PIN (and *p-n* junction), APDs, and PMTs. We then finish the book with a discussion of how detector options influence the overall system architecture, including design trades between the laser, optical, scanning, and detector subsystems.

**Detector Trades.** It sometimes happens that detectors are selected based on a single criterion such as sensitivity or bandwidth; while this is occasionally necessary, this is in general not a good systems-engineering strategy. The trades between detector materials, types, geometries, and FPA technologies reveal a number of important differences, and these trades—in addition to the system-level trades discussed below—will drive detector selection.

Detector selection starts, then, with a comparison of the different detector types based on four or five of the most critical specifications. These are usually wavelength coverage, detector geometry, sensitivity (which includes dominant noise terms), cooling requirements, and total cost (including cooler); other known specs could also be included in the comparison. Table 7.3 summarizes some of the most important properties for each detector type.

Focusing on critical differences between detectors such as those listed in Table 7.3 allows us to reduce the number of options to a few promising candidates. The specs for the ideal candidate often must be changed and

**Table 7.3** Key properties of detector types reviewed in this book. PIN photodiodes also includes *p-n* junction detectors; SWaP = size, weight, and electrical power consumption.

| Detector Type | Key Properties |
|---|---|
| PIN Photodiodes | • UV to LWIR wavelengths (0.3–12 μm)<br>• Few-photon sensitivity (EM-CCDs)<br>• Available in large-format FPAs (1K × 1K)<br>• Low cost (single pixel or CMOS FPA) |
| APDs | • VIS to SWIR wavelengths (0.4–2 μm)<br>• Single-photon sensitivity (GM or MCT LM)<br>• High speed ($\Delta f$ > 1 GHz)<br>• Available in moderate-format FPAs |
| PMTs | • Restricted wavelength range (UV to NIR)<br>• Single-photon sensitivity; low excess noise<br>• High speed ($\Delta f$ > 1 GHz)<br>• Higher SWaP and voltage |

design compromises (trades) made. Even without a trade study, having data such as Fig. 7.26 can help us make design decisions, even if we don't understand the details as to why the curves look the way they do, or what is limiting them.

Unfortunately, Fig. 7.26 is incomplete in that it only provides data on one aspect of comparing sCMOS with EM-CCD cameras, namely, SNR. There are, however, a number of other criteria that must be used for detector selection. For example, deep cooling may be required to reduce the sCMOS dark current and read noise to a level where they are competitive with EM-CCDs; the cooling, however, increases the size, weight, power consumption, and cost—and these disadvantages must be balanced against the improvement in sCMOS noise.

A trade study, then, compares an improvement in one aspect of detector performance against disadvantages in others. This can lead to an optimization (as in Example 7.4) or at least a better understanding of which detector specs are critical. We have seen a number of these trades throughout this book; looking in more detail at the sCMOS (Hamamatsu Flash 4.0) versus EM-CCD (Andor iXon 897) comparison for Fig. 7.26, we can summarize the key trades as follows:

- Wavelength: Both are silicon detectors, with a back-illuminated QE > 90% (iXon 897) versus QE > 70% (Flash 4.0) in the VIS band for super-resolution imaging of biomedical samples.
- Detector Geometry: Both are FPAs used for imaging, with the EM-CCD format having 512 × 512 pixels and the sCMOS having 2048 × 2048. With a resolution of 16-μm square pixels, the EM-CCD covers a FOV of 512 pixels × 16 μm/pixel = 8,192 μm projected onto the sample; with 6.5-μm pixels, the sCMOS covers a FOV of 13,312 μm—1.62× larger FOV in each dimension, and $(1.62)^2 \approx$ 2.6× more area coverage in a sCMOS frame.
- Sensitivity: As shown in Fig. 7.26, the EM-CCD—with its lower read noise, higher QE, and larger pixels—is better at detecting ultralow-light levels on the order of a few photons. At higher levels, however, the EM-CCD excess noise reduces the SNR in comparison with zero-excess-noise sCMOS FPAs.
- Frame Rate: Even though the sCMOS has 16× more pixels than the EM-CCD, both are used at a nominal full-frame rate of 30 fps, restricted by CCD serial-amplifier read-noise bandwidth.
- Cooling: With dark current that is multiplied by a factor of 500–1000, deep thermoelectric cooling down to –85 °C or lower is required for the EM-CCD FPA. This significantly increases the size, weight, and power consumption (SWaP) in comparison with a lightly cooled sCMOS FPA at –10 °C.

Which of these is preferred depends on the system requirements. For example, is the sensitivity of the EM-CCD important? If so, is it so important that the customer is willing to pay the price for it in terms of cooling and SWaP? For biomedical instruments used in a laboratory this is reasonable; for aerospace customers, maybe not so much. Or perhaps image resolution (smaller IFOV) is also a key driver? Even though the better resolution (smaller pixel) sCMOS does not have the LLL sensitivity of the EM-CCD?

It's also necessary to include in a trade study the programmatic requirements such as total lifecycle cost (including unit, operating, and maintenance costs), reliability, technology readiness level, etc. Equally important are another set of studies that take into account the other subsystems, namely, the system trades.

**System Trades**. Detector selection is not an isolated process, and we must also include the other subsystems to make intelligent design choices. It sometimes happens, for example, that the most sensitive detector is selected for a system even though there may also be trades between the other subsystems that allow use of a less-sensitive (and much less expensive) detector. As we have seen in Table 1.4, these trades are between the laser, optical, and detector subsystems; we now also include the possibility of a scanning subsystem.

To illustrate the trades in detail, the number of signal electrons $n_s$ collected by an integrating detector such as an FPA depends on a number of system parameters:

$$n_s = \frac{i_s t_{int}}{q} = \frac{R_o \Phi_s \cdot t_{int}}{q} = \frac{R_o \cdot T L_s A_p \Omega_{f/\#} \cdot t_{int}}{q} \quad [e^-] \tag{7.37}$$

where we have used Eq. (7.10) for the first equality, and Eq. (6.10) and the conservation of étendue ($A_{EP}\Omega_{IFOV} = A_p\Omega_{f/\#}$) for the expression on the RHS when collecting scattered laser light with either an FPA or a scanned single-pixel detector from an illuminated scene. If we instead directly illuminate the optical aperture with a laser with intensity $I$ (Fig. 6.10), then the $TL_sA_p\Omega_{f/\#}$ term is replaced by $TI\Omega_{EP}$ (as in Section 6.3).

To increase the number of scattered-signal electrons—without worrying about noise electrons for the moment—a detector with a larger responsivity $R_o$ (or QE) could be used, but so could a more powerful laser to increase the scene radiance $L_s$, a larger pixel area $A_p$, a larger solid angle $\Omega_{f/\#}$ for the image *f*-cone, or a longer integration time $t_{int}$. These options may be incompatible with other requirements—a larger pixel trades against better image resolution, e.g., or a longer integration time may not be compatible with object motion, or an increase in responsivity using a detector with gain may also increase the noise—but Eq. (7.37) and Table 7.4 summarize the laser-system trade-space options for signal collection.

**Table 7.4** Subsystem trades and their dependencies that influence the signal $S = n_s G$ in the SNR equation for electrons [Eq. (7.30)].

| Subsystem | Signal Dependencies |
|---|---|
| Laser | Scene radiance $L_s$ via laser output power $P$ and $M^2$ |
| Scanning | Integration time $t_{int}$ |
| Optics | Transmission $T$; solid angle $\Omega_{f/\#}$ |
| Detector | Responsivity $R_o$; area $A_p$; gain $G$; integration time $t_{int}$ |

As we have seen in detail in this chapter, including noise electrons has its own set of dependencies for a given type of noise (Table 7.2). In the following paragraphs, we include both signal and noise electrons to give an overview of the laser system design process by going into more detail on some of these trades.

The first and most fundamental of these are the wavelength trades. The most obvious of these is the matching of the laser wavelengths in Table 2.8 with the detector wavelengths in Table 7.1. The subtlety here, of course, is the degree of "matching" that is required, and this can be determined by a trade between laser power (or pulse energy) and detector sensitivity via responsivity $R_o$.

As a simple example, using a solid-state Nd:YAG laser emitting at $\lambda$ =1064 nm seems to require an expensive InGaAs detector and thus excludes the use of the Nd:YAG as a laser option. It turns out, however, that even though silicon typically has a low responsivity at this wavelength, it can be increased with a thicker intrinsic region, giving it sufficient QE to make the relatively low-cost Nd:YAG laser and an enhanced-silicon detector a reasonable match. The trade in this case is that by increasing the intrinsic-region thickness, the detector is not optimized for speed and may no longer be able to meet the bandwidth requirements of short pulses.

Second, more laser power can be traded off against better sensitivity in scanning systems as well. We have seen this previously in Chapter 6, where we compared the power required for obtaining sufficient signal on a scanned single-pixel detector versus that for a flash FPA. What was found was that spreading the laser power over a large area reduced the scene radiance by the number of pixels illuminated—a factor of 16,384 for a relatively small $128 \times 128$ FPA. This is clearly a huge increase in peak power required for the laser, or an equally huge improvement in the sensitivity for the FPA's pixels. A scanning system—despite the increase in complexity and imaging time—is thus a reasonable system design for some applications where things are not moving or image-collection time is not critical, as in biomedical laser-scanning microscopes.

Third, poor laser power or detector sensitivity can sometimes be compensated for by the use of larger pixels. The PMT, for example, often has an extremely low QE, but a large collection area $A_d$ in comparison with

10- to 100-μm detectors; the product of $R_o \times A_d$ is thus sufficient to generate enough signal electrons for LLL applications.

The disadvantage, of course, is that PMTs are not available in FPA format, and the larger area degrades the image resolution (IFOV) or requires an extremely long effective focal length for a given $IFOV = x_p/EFL \approx d_p/EFL$ for $FF \approx 1$. The longer EFL, in turn, reduces the *f*-cone solid angle $\Omega_{f/\#}$ of the optics, offsetting the advantage of the larger detector area if the IFOV is the same. In terms of optical and detector subsystem variables, it can be shown that the quantity $\pi[d_p/(f/\#)]^2/4$ determines the optical power collection from an area source through the etendue term ($A_{EP}\Omega_{IFOV}$ or $A_p\Omega_{f/\#}$) in Eq. (7.37), giving another set of system trades to consider.

Specifically, a smaller pixel size is required for a smaller IFOV and better image resolution, but the disadvantage of smaller pixels is that fewer photons are collected—unless the detector integration time $t_{int}$ can be increased or the *f*/# of the optics can be decreased to compensate. Even if the integration time or *f*/# is not changed, however, and less power is collected for the signal in the SNR equation, the detector MTF improves with smaller pixels (see Fig. 7.21). So now we see a trade between SNR and MTF, where SNR and MTF are the two most "primal" metrics for evaluating the performance of laser imaging systems, as they both determine image contrast (as in Fig. 7.33)—SNR with respect to detector noise, and MTF with respect to neighboring pixels.

How these trades must balance out, of course, depends on the system requirements. Additional system-level metrics such as size, weight, power consumption, and cost must also be included in the design. For example, it has been said that creating photons is less expensive than detecting them, but that is certainly not true if the laser is already at the high end of its output power, or the detector has a poor NEP. In other applications such as manufacturing-process monitoring, detection may be a secondary consideration, and the laser trades we looked at in Chapter 2 govern the design.

Returning to Eq. (7.37) for one last look before it sets below the horizon, we see that there are ten possible trades between $R_o \times L_s$, $R_o \times A_p$, $A_p \times t_{int}$, etc., if we do not include optical transmission $T$. In addition, there is also the gain $G$ and noise, resulting in a nearly infinite number of system trades—and the ones that we have not included in this book can now hopefully be approached by the reader in a systematic manner.

## 7.6 Problems

**7.1** Using Eqs. (7.1) and (7.2), predict the slope of the responsivity curve given in Fig. 7.2 for $\lambda = 0.7$–$1.4$ μm. What accounts for any discrepancies between your prediction and the data? Hint: What assumption do you have to make as to the number of electrons that are created per photon?

**7.2** The bandgap energy of a HgCdTe detector is approximately 0.25 eV at 77 K. How many joules of energy does this correspond to? Would you expect the bandgap energy to increase or decrease as the temperature is increased?

**7.3** How many photons are in a 1064-nm pulse that is 10-nsec wide and carries 10 mJ of energy? What about a 532-nm pulse of the same energy and pulse width? Is the pulse width relevant?

**7.4** A Nd:YAG laser generates pulses of 10-nsec duration, with a 2-nsec rise time on the leading edge of the pulse. What electrical bandwidth is required to measure the rise time?

**7.5** Why is the gain of an InGaAs APD typically limited to $G \approx 10$, while that of a silicon APD can be increased to $G \approx 100$?

**7.6** In Example 7.1, a pulse width of 10 nsec was used to find the maximum DCR for single-photon detection. What is the DCR if we instead use 5-nsec pulses?

**7.7** If the DCR increases with temperature at an exponential rate, and the DCR for an InGaAs GM-APD is 10 kHz at $T = 250$ K, what is the DCR at $T = 300$ K? What NEP does this imply at room temperature, assuming the same parameters as in Example 7.1?

**7.8** Assuming the same parameters as in Example 7.1, compare silicon with InGaAs for single-photon detection at $\lambda = 1064$ nm. Note that the PDE of silicon is 4% at this wavelength.

**7.9** A PMT has a dark count rate of 100 cps. What is the dark current in amps?

**7.10** What is the gain–bandwidth product ($G \cdot \Delta f$) of a PMT? How does it compare with that of an APD? Does the PMT have a factor limiting this product, as does the APD?

**7.11** In Fig. 7.21, we see that the MTF curve for $x_p = 20$ μm first goes to zero at $f_d = 50$ lp/mm, but then rises up a little and again goes to zero at $f_s = 100$ lp/mm. Physically, why does the curve again go to zero at 100 lp/mm? Hint: See Fig. 7.20.

**7.12** In Fig. 7.22, what is the diffraction-limited optical blur $B$? What is the ratio of the blur size to the pixel pitch? Does this ratio have any significance? Hint: See Ref. 5.

**7.13** For single-photon sensitivity, is it best to use an EM-CCD at a low or a high frame rate?

**7.14** Which produces more signal electrons: a USP laser with a peak power $P_{peak} = 10$ MW over a pulse width $\Delta t_p = 10$ psec, or a Nd:YAG laser with

$P_{peak} = 100$ kW over a pulse width $\Delta t_p = 10$ nsec? Which collects more dark current during the integration time if a silicon sCMOS FPA is used to collect pulse energy? And which has the better ratio of signal to dark current?

**7.15** Combining Eqs. (7.10) and (7.11), what is the well depth of a CMOS preamplifier measured in units of electrons? Assume a square pixel size $d_p = 10$ μm, a maximum $V_{out} = 3.3$ V, and a capacitor thickness $t_C = 0.5$ μm.

**7.16** We can solve Eq. (7.16) for the largest-allowable RIN for the detector noise to be limited by the laser's shot noise. What is this value (in units of real numbers and decibels) for $P = 1$ μW? Assume the same responsivity as in Example 7.3.

**7.17** In Fig. 7.26, will a PMT have better, worse, or the same SNR performance as an EM-CCD for signal-limited detection ($n_p > 100$ photons or so).

**7.18** In Fig. 7.36, the use of the ionization ratio $k$ assumes that the McIntyre model is valid for the APD excess noise. Plot the SNR versus gain for a PMT or EM-CCD with $F(G) = 1.4$ for any value of gain (assume that $NSD = 6$ pA/Hz$^{1/2}$ at $\Delta f = 2.7$ GHz). Is there an optimum SNR?

**7.19** Referring to Example 7.5, how large can the PRNU be for speckle noise to dominate the SNR? Assume that $DoF = 10$.

**7.20** We saw in Section 7.5.2 that a larger QE improves (decreases) the NEP for signal- and amplifier-limited situations. Are there any situations where a larger QE does not improve the NEP?

**7.21** Show that Eq. (7.29) is equivalent to Eq. (7.33).

**7.22** Using the data from Fig. 7.35, how much detector gain $G$ is needed for amplifier-limited single-photon sensitivity for a low-speed TIA with $\Delta f = 165$ MHz?

## Notes and References


1. E. Friedman and J. L. Miller, *Photonics Rules of Thumb*, Second Edition, SPIE Press, Bellingham, Washington (2004).
2. E. L. Dereniak and G. D. Boreman, *Infrared Detectors and Systems*, John Wiley & Sons, Hoboken, New Jersey (1996).
3. In alphabetical order, the materials are: cadmium sulfide (CdS), germanium (Ge), indium antimonide (InSb), indium gallium arsenide (InGaAs), indium gallium nitride (InGaN), lead selenide (PbSe), lead sulfide (PbS), mercury cadmium telluride (HgCdTe or MCT), quantum-well infrared photodetector (QWIP), silicon (Si), silicon carbide (SiC), and silicon doped with arsenic (Si:As).

4. S. B. Alexander, *Optical Communication Receiver Design*, SPIE Press, Bellingham, Washington (1997) [doi: 10.1117/3.219402].

5. K. J. Kasunic, *Optical Systems Engineering*, McGraw-Hill, New York, Chapter 6 (2011).

6. Electron drift across the intrinsic layer also influences modulation speed, and detector designers must balance the decrease in capacitance against the increase in drift time in determining an optimal thickness of the intrinsic layer.

7. J. F. James, *A Student's Guide to Fourier Transforms*, Cambridge University Press, Cambridge (1995).

8. P. R. Norton, "Infrared image sensors," *Optical Engineering* **30**(11), 1649–1663 (1991) [doi: 10.1117/12.56001].

9. R. J. McIntyre, "Multiplication noise in uniform avalanche diodes," *IEEE Transactions on Electron Devices* **ED-13**(1), 164–168 (1966).

10. The impact ionization ratio $k$ is the ratio of hole-to-electron ionization. Holes are typically heavier than electrons and are thus more difficult to ionize, leading to $k < 1$ and the excess-noise factor $F(G) > 2$ at high gain due to statistically independent amplification of holes and electrons. With extremely heavy holes, $k \approx 0$, and only electrons provide avalanche gain, giving $F(G) \approx 2$.

11. R. Lang, Ed., *Biomedical Optical Imaging Technologies*, Springer-Verlag, Berlin-Heidelberg (2013).

12. X. Sun and F. Davidson, "Photon counting with silicon avalanche photodiodes," *Journal of Lightwave Technology* **10**(8), 1023–1032 (1992).

13. J. D. Beck, R. Scritchfield, P. Mitra, W. W. Sullivan, A. D. Gleckler, R. Strittmatter, and R. J. Martin "Linear mode photon counting with the noiseless gain HgCdTe e-avalanche photodiode," *Optical Engineering* **53**(8), 081905 (2014) [doi: 10.1117/1.OE.53.8.081905].

14. M. Jack, G. Chapman, J. Edwards, W. Mc Keag, T. Veeder, J. Wehner, T. Roberts, T. Robinson, J. Neisz, C. Andressen, R. Rinker, D. N. B. Hall, S. M. Jacobson, F. Amzajerdian, and T. D. Cook, "Advances in LADAR components and subsystems at Raytheon," *Proc. SPIE* **8353**, 83532F (2012) [doi: 10.1117/12/923683].

15. G. M. Williams, M. A. Compton, and A. S. Huntington, "High-speed photon counting with linear-mode APD receivers," *Proc. SPIE* **7320**, 732012 (2009) [doi: 10.1117/12.817862].

16. For FPAs, the PDE also includes a third component known as the fill factor; see Section 7.4 for details.

17. J. G. Rarity, T. E. Wall, K. D. Ridley, P. C. M. Owens, and P. R. Tapster, "Single-photon counting for the 1300- to 1600-nm range by use of Peltier-cooled and passively quenched InGaAs avalanche photodiodes," *Applied Optics* **39**(36), 6746–6753 (2000). Note that Eq. (7.7) is also used in frequency-normalized form by dividing both sides of the equation by $(\Delta f)^{1/2}$, giving units of W/Hz$^{1/2}$.

18. K. E. Jensen, P. I. Hopman, E. K. Duerr, E. A. Dauler, J. P. Donnelly, S. H. Groves, L. J. Mahoney, K. A. McIntosh, K. M. Molvar, A. Napoleone, D. C. Oakley, S. Verghese, C. J. Vineis, and R. D. Younger, "Afterpulsing in Geiger-mode avalanche photodiodes for 1.06 μm wavelength," *Applied Physics Letters* **88**, 133503 (2006).

19. C. Jackson, K. O'Neill, L. A. Wall, and B. McGarvey, "High-volume silicon photomultiplier production, performance, and reliability," *Optical Engineering* **53**(8), 081909 (2014) [doi: 10.1117/1.OE.8.081909].

20. X. Sun, M. A. Krainak, J. B. Abshire, J. D. Spinhirne, C. Trottier, M. Davies, H. Dautet, G. R. Allan, A. T. Lukemire, and J. C. Vandivrer, "Space-qualified silicon avalanche-photodiode single-photon-counting modules," *Journal of Modern Optics* **51**(9–10), 1333–1350 (2004).

21. Hamamatsu Photonics, *Photomultiplier Tubes: Basics and Applications*, Third Edition, Chapter 6 (2007).

22. V. Sivaprakasam, A. L. Huston, C. Scotto, and J. D. Eversole "Multiple UV wavelength excitation and fluorescence of bioaerosols," *Optics Express* **12**(19), 4457–4466 (2004).

23. W. Becker and A. Bergmann, "Detectors for high-speed photon counting," Becker & Hickl GmbH, Berlin (2015).

24. T. J. Martin, R. M. Brubaker, V. Burzi, M. H. Ettenberg, K. Forsyth, J. Groppe, M. Line, and T. Sudol, "A 640 × 512 InGaAs camera for range-gated and staring applications," *Proc. SPIE* **6206**, 620609 (2006) [doi: 10.1117/12.666021].

25. M. Juberts and A. Barbera, "Status report on next-generation LADAR for driving unmanned ground vehicles," *Proc. SPIE* **5609**, 1–9 (2004) [doi: 10.1117/12.580235].

26. A. Cordes and A. Davidson, "CMOS cameras allow robust active stabilization of laser beams," *Laser Focus World*, Aug. 2011, pp. 73–76.

27. R. H. Vollmerhausen and Ronald G. Driggers, *Analysis of Sampled Imaging Systems*, SPIE Press, Bellingham, Washington (2000) [doi: 10.1117/3.353257].

28. Image contrast is defined as $C_i = I_{max} - I_{min}$, which is the same as the modulation except that this difference is not divided by twice the average. Image contrast is related to image modulation $m_i$ by $C_i = (1 + m_i)/(1 - m_i)$.

29. J. R. Janesick, *Scientific Charge-Coupled Devices*, SPIE Press, Bellingham, Washington (2001) [doi: 10.1117/3.374903].

30. Teledyne DALSA Inc., "CCD Technology Primer" (2015).

31. Princeton Instruments, "CCD Camera Selection Chart," *Imaging* brochure (2015).

32. D. J. Denvir and E. Conroy, "Electron multiplying CCDs," *Proc. SPIE* **4877**, 55–68 (2003) [doi: 10.1117/12.463677].

33. F. Long, S. Zeng, and Z.-L. Huang, "Localization-based super-resolution microscopy with an sCMOS camera Part II: Experimental methodology for comparing sCMOS with EMCCD cameras," *Optics Express* **20**(16), 17741 (2012).

34. B. Fowler, C. Liu, S. Mims, J. Balicki, H. Do, J. Appelbaum, and P. Vu, "A 5.5 Mpixel 100 frames/sec wide dynamic range low noise CMOS sensor for scientific applications," *Proc. SPIE* **7536**, 753607 (2010) [doi: 10.1117/12.846975].

35. Hamamatsu Corp., "ORCA-Flash 2.8 Technical Note" (2010) and "ORCA-Flash 4.0 V2" data sheet (2014).

36. Andor Corp., "Neo 5.5 sCMOS" data sheet (2015).

37. Q. Chau, X. Jiang, M. A. Itzler, M. Entwistle, B. Piccone, M. Owens, and K. Slomkowski, "Analysis and modeling of optical crosstalk in InP-based Geiger-mode avalanche photodiode FPAs," *Proc. SPIE* **9492**, 949200 (2015) [doi: 10.1117/12.2177082].

38. Princeton Lightwave, Product Summary, Part Number CAM32X32B-GMA-0 (2015).

39. B. R. Frieden, *Probability, Statistical Optics, and Data Testing*, Second Edition, Springer-Verlag, Berlin, Heidelberg (1991).

40. G. R. Osche, *Optical Detection Theory for Laser Applications*, John Wiley & Sons, Hoboken, New Jersey (2002).

41. At a given frequency, RIN typically decreases at higher power; see Ref. 42 for more details.

42. G. P. Agrawal, *Fiber-Optic Communication Systems*, Second Edition, John Wiley & Sons, Hoboken, New Jersey (1997).

43. P. C. D. Hobbs, *Building Electro-Optical Systems*, Second Edition, John Wiley & Sons, Hoboken, New Jersey (2009).

44. See J. L. Vampola, "Readout Electronics for Infrared Sensors," in *The Infrared & Electro-Optical Systems Handbook*, Vol. 3, W. D. Rogatto, Ed., ERIM, Ann Arbor, Michigan and SPIE Press, Bellingham, Washington, Chapter 5 (1993); and J. D. Vincent, S. E. Hodges, J. Vampola, M. Stegall, and G. Pierce, *Fundamentals of Infrared and Visible Detector Operation and Testing*, Second Edition, John Wiley & Sons, Hoboken, New Jersey (2016).

45. See e2v Technologies, "CCD57-10 AIMO Back-Illuminated CCD" data sheet or Hamamatsu Corp., *Opto-Semiconductor Handbook*, "Chapter 05 Image Sensors," Fig. 1–43 (2015).

46. R. D. Richmond and S. C. Cain, *Direct-Detection LADAR Systems*, SPIE Press, Bellingham, Washington, Chapter 1 (2010) [doi: 10.1117/3.836466].

47. J. I. Trisnadi, "Speckle contrast reduction in laser projection displays," *Proc. SPIE* **4657**, 131–137 (2002) [doi: 10.1117/12.463781].

48. R. G. Driggers, R. H. Vollmerhausen, N. M. Devitt, C. E. Halford, and K. J. Barnard, "Impact of speckle on laser range-gated shortwave infrared imaging system target identification performance," *Optical Engineering* **42**(3), 738–746 (2003) [doi: 10.1117/1.1543159].

49. J. W. Goodman, *Speckle Phenomenon in Optics: Theory and Applications*, Ben Roberts & Company, Greenwood Village, Colorado, Chapter 5 (2007). While Goodman does not explicitly state the coherence length condition $d_c < 2\delta_{RMS}$ for low speckle, it can be derived from Eq. (5-43) of this reference.

50. P. Janssens and K. Malfait, "Future prospects of high-end laser projectors," *Proc. SPIE* **7232**, 72320Y (2009) [doi: 10.1117/12.808106].

# Glossary of Symbols and Acronyms

| | |
|---|---|
| $A$ | area ($m^2$); optical absorption |
| $A_b$ | beam area ($mm^2$) |
| $A_d$ | detector area ($mm^2$) |
| $A_{EP}$ | entrance pupil area ($mm^2$) |
| $A_o$ | illuminated object area ($mm^2$) |
| $A_p$ | pixel area ($\mu m^2$) |
| AO | acousto-optic |
| AOI | angle of incidence (rads) |
| APD | avalanche photodiode |
| APS | active-pixel sensor |
| AR | antireflection |
| ASE | amplified spontaneous emission |
| $A\Omega$ | étendue ($m^2$-sr) |
| $B$ | focused blur diameter ($\mu m$); PSD frequency exponent |
| $B_{SA}$ | focused blur diameter due to spherical aberration ($\mu m$) |
| BFD | back focal distance |
| BPF | bandpass filter |
| BPP | beam-parameter product (mm-mrad) |
| BSDF | bidirectional scatter distribution function |
| $c$ | speed of light, $\approx 3 \times 10^8$ m/sec |
| $C$ | wavefront or surface curvature (1/mm) |
| $C_o$ | wavefront curvature incident on lens (1/mm) |
| $C_i$ | wavefront curvature exiting lens (1/mm); image contrast |
| $C_{sp}$ | speckle contrast |
| $C_{well}$ | charge-well capacitance (pF) |
| CA | clear aperture |
| CCD | charge-coupled device |
| CDS | correlated double sampling |
| CMOS | complementary metal-oxide semiconductor |

| | |
|---|---|
| CoO | cost of ownership |
| COTS | commercial off-the-shelf |
| cps | counts per second |
| CRT | cathode-ray tube |
| CTE | charge-transfer efficiency; coefficient of thermal expansion |
| CTIA | capacitive transimpedance amplifier |
| CW | continuous wave |
| | |
| $d$ | distance (m) |
| $d_c$ | coherence length (m) |
| $d_{c,n}$ | coherence length in a medium of index $n$ (m) |
| $d_{FP}$ | Fabry–Pérot cavity thickness (mm) |
| $dn/dT$ | change in index with temperature (1/K) |
| $d_p$ | pixel size (μm) |
| $D$ | lens diameter or aperture size (mm); fiber diameter (μm) |
| $D_{1/e^2}$ | beam diameter ($1/e^2$) incident on or exiting from a lens (mm) |
| $D_b(z)$ | beam diameter (mm) |
| $D_{EP}$ | entrance-pupil diameter (mm) |
| $D_o$ | waist diameter (mm) |
| DBR | distributed Bragg reflector |
| DCR | dark-count rate [$e^-$/sec or counts per sec (cps)] |
| DE | directed energy |
| DFG | difference-frequency generation |
| DI | direct injection |
| DLC | diamond-like carbon |
| DoF | degrees of freedom |
| DOF | depth of focus (μm) |
| dpi | dots per inch |
| DPSS | diode-pumped solid-state |
| DWDM | dense wavelength-division multiplexing |
| | |
| $E$ | irradiance (W/m$^2$); Young's modulus (GPa) |
| $E_g$ | bandgap energy (J or eV) |
| $E_i$ | electron energy for energy level $i$ (J or eV) |
| $E_o$ | Gaussian peak irradiance (W/m$^2$) |
| $E_p$ | photon energy (J or eV) |
| EB-CCD | electron-bombarded CCD |
| EB-CMOS | electron-bombarded CMOS |
| EFL | effective focal length (mm) |
| EM | electromagnetic |
| EM-CCD | electron-multiplying CCD |
| EOL | end of life |

| | |
|---|---|
| EOM | electro-optic modulator |
| ESD | energy spectral density |
| | |
| $f$ | focal length (mm); electrical frequency (Hz) |
| $f_d$ | FPA cutoff frequency (lp/mm) |
| $f_{RO}$ | relaxation-oscillation frequency (Hz) |
| $f_s$ | spatial frequency (lp/mm); mirror scan frequency (Hz) |
| $f/\#$ | relative aperture, $\equiv f/D$ |
| $F$ | fluence (J/m$^2$) |
| $F(G)$ | excess noise factor |
| $F_R$ | cavity finesse based on power reflectivity $R_P$ |
| FBG | fiber Bragg grating |
| FET | field effect transistor |
| FF | FPA fill factor |
| FHG | fourth-harmonic generation |
| FOI | field of illumination (rad) |
| FOR | field of regard (rad) |
| FOV | field of view (rad) |
| FP | Fabry–Pérot |
| FPA | focal plane array |
| FPN | fixed-pattern noise |
| FR | frame rate [Hz or frames per sec (fps)] |
| FSM | fast-steering mirror |
| FSR | free spectral range (Hz) |
| FWHM | full-width at half-maximum |
| | |
| $g$ | laser gain (1/cm) |
| $g_i$ | laser-cavity stability parameter |
| $G$ | detector gain; thermo-optic constant (1/K) |
| GM-APD | Geiger-mode APD |
| GVD | group-velocity dispersion |
| | |
| $h$ | Planck's constant, $= 6.626 \times 10^{-34}$ J-sec; mirror thickness (mm) |
| HFOV | half-FOV (rad) |
| HAZ | heat-affected zone |
| HPD | hybrid photodetector |
| HR | high reflectivity |
| HSF | high spatial frequency |
| HT | high transmission |
| HWP | half-wave plate |
| | |
| $i$ | current (A) |
| $i_b$ | detector background current (A) |

| | |
|---|---|
| $i_d$ | detector current (A) |
| $i_{dc}$ | detector dark current (A) |
| $i_s$ | detector signal current (A) |
| $i_{th}$ | laser threshold current (A) |
| $I$ | intensity (W/sr) |
| IAD | ion-assisted deposition |
| IBS | ion-beam sputtering |
| ICCD | intensified CCD |
| IFOV | instantaneous FOV (μrad) |
| IR | infrared |
| IRCM | IR countermeasure |
| ISO | International Standards Organization |
| $J$ | rotational moment of inertia (kg-m$^2$) |
| $k$ | APD ionization coefficient; thermal conductivity (W/m-K) |
| $K_{SA}$ | blur size factor due to spherical aberration |
| $K_T$ | truncation factor |
| KTP | potassium titanium-oxide phosphate |
| $L$ | length (m); radiance or brightness (W/m$^2$-sr) |
| $L_i$ | image radiance (W/m$^2$-sr) |
| $L_s$ | source radiance (W/m$^2$-sr) |
| $L_\lambda$ | spectral radiance or brightness (W/m$^2$-sr-nm) |
| LAM | laser additive manufacturing |
| LCOS | liquid crystal on silicon |
| LCPG | liquid crystal polarization grating |
| LDT | laser damage threshold (J/cm$^2$ or W/cm$^2$) |
| LED | light-emitting diode |
| LIDT | laser-induced damage threshold |
| LLL | low light level |
| LMA | large mode area |
| LM-APD | linear-mode APD |
| lp | line pair |
| LWIR | longwave IR |
| $m$ | integer, 1, 2, 3...; waist magnification $w_{02}/w_{01}$; mass (kg) |
| $m_i$ | image modulation; image magnification |
| $m_{lens}$ | lens object-image magnification |
| $m_p$ | peak waist magnification $w_{02}/w_{01}$ at $1f$:$1f$ conjugates |
| $M$ | square-root of $M^2$ |
| $M^2$ | beam quality compared with a diffraction-limited TEM$_{00}$ beam |

$M_a$ afocal telescope magnification
MCP micro-channel plate
MCT mercury cadmium telluride
MEMS micro-electromechanical system
MLM multiple longitudinal mode
MMF multimode fiber
MOPA master-oscillator power amplifier
MPE maximum permissible exposure; multiphoton excitation
MPN mode-partition noise
MPPC multipixel photon counter
MRF magneto-rheological finishing
MSF mid-spatial-frequency
MTF modulation transfer function
$MTF_{det}$ detector MTF
$MTF_{opt}$ optical MTF
$MTF_{sys}$ system MTF
MTTF mean time-to-failure
MWIR midwave IR

$n$ refractive index
$n_e$ number of electrons
$n_f$ number of polygon facets
$n_p$ number of photons
$n_s$ number of signal electrons
$n_w$ well depth ($e^-$)
$n_{\sigma amp}$ number of amplifier noise electrons ($e^-$)
$n_{\sigma b}$ number of background noise electrons ($e^-$)
$n_{\sigma dc}$ number of dark-current noise electrons ($e^-$)
$n_{\sigma FPN}$ number of spatial noise electrons ($e^-$)
$n_{\sigma read}$ number of read noise electrons ($e^-$)
$n_{\sigma RIN}$ number of RIN noise electrons ($e^-$)
$n_{\sigma s}$ number of signal noise electrons ($e^-$)
$n_{\sigma sp}$ number of speckle noise electrons ($e^-$)
$N$ number of longitudinal modes; resolvable spots; detector noise (A or $e^-$)
$N_e$ number of electrons per second ($e^-$/sec)
$N_i$ number of electrons per unit volume in energy level $i$ ($1/m^3$)
$N_p$ number of photons per second (#/sec); number of pixels
NBF narrow-band filter
NEP noise-equivalent power (W or $W/Hz^{1/2}$)
$NEP_{amp}$ amplifier-limited NEP (W or $W/Hz^{1/2}$)
$NEP_s$ signal-limited NEP (W or $W/Hz^{1/2}$)

NEPh noise-equivalent photons (# of photons)
NIR near-IR
NPRO nonplanar ring oscillator
NRE nonrecurring engineering
NSD noise spectral density ($A/Hz^{1/2}$)
NUC non-uniformity correction
NUV near UV

OCS optical cross-section ($m^2/sr$)
OCT optical coherence tomography
OPA optical phased array
OPL optical path length (= *nd*, μm or waves)
OPO optical parametric oscillator
OPSL optically pumped semiconductor laser
OXT optical crosstalk

$P$ CW output power (W)
$P_{avg}$ average output power (W)
$P_{elec}$ electrical power (W)
$P_d$ probability of detection
$P_{fa}$ probability of false alarm
$P_h$ horizontally polarized power
$P_{inc}$ optical power incident on a lens or surface (W)
$P_{peak}$ peak output power (W)
$P_r$ optical power reflected by a lens or surface (W)
$P_t$ optical power transmitted by a lens or surface (W)
$P_{th}$ thermal heat load due to lens absorption (W)
$P_v$ vertically polarized power
PBS polarizing beamsplitter
PCF photonic crystal fiber
PDE photon detection efficiency
PDH Pound, Drever, and Hall
PER polarization extinction ratio
PIB power-in-bucket
PIN *p-i-n* photodetector
PM polarization-maintaining
PMT photomultiplier tube
PRF pulse repetition frequency (Hz)
PRNU photo-response non-uniformity
PRR pixel readout rate (Hz)
PSD power spectral density ($nm^2$-m), aka energy spectral density
PV peak to valley; photovoltaic
PZT piezoelectric transducer

| | |
|---|---|
| $q$ | electron charge, $= 1.602 \times 10^{-19}$ C/e$^-$; lens shape factor |
| $Q$ | heat load (W) |
| $Q_c$ | cavity quality |
| $Q_p$ | pulse energy (J) |
| $Q_{store}$ | cavity photon-energy storage (J) |
| QCL | quantum-cascade laser |
| QCW | quasi-continuous wave |
| QE | quantum efficiency |
| QWP | quarter-wave plate |
| | |
| $r$ | radial coordinate (m) |
| $R$ | average power reflectivity; diffraction ripple; range (m) |
| $R(z)$ | Gaussian wavefront radius of curvature (mm) |
| $R_f$ | Fresnel surface reflectivity |
| $R_g$ | responsivity after including detector gain $G$ (A/W) |
| $R_i$ | wavefront radius of curvature exiting lens (mm) |
| $R_o$ | wavefront radius of curvature incident on lens (mm); detector responsivity (A/W) |
| $R_p$ | reflectance of $p$-polarized light |
| $R_{pi}$ | power reflectivity of surface $i$ |
| $R_s$ | reflectance of $s$-polarized light |
| $R_t$ | thermal resistance (K/W) |
| RHS | right-hand side |
| RIN | relative intensity noise (1/Hz or dB/Hz) |
| RMS | root mean square |
| ROI | region-of-interest |
| ROIC | readout integrated circuit |
| RPM | revolutions per minute |
| RSS | root sum square |
| | |
| $s$ | incoherent source size (mm) |
| $s_o$ | object distance (mm) |
| $s_i$ | image distance (mm) |
| sCMOS | scientific-grade CMOS |
| $S$ | Strehl ratio; mirror width (mm); detector signal (A or e$^-$) |
| SA | spherical aberration |
| SAM | saturable-absorber mirror |
| SESAM | semiconductor saturable-absorber mirror |
| SFE | surface figure error (μm or waves) |
| SFG | sum-frequency generation |
| SHG | second-harmonic generation |
| SiPM | silicon photomultiplier |
| SLM | single longitudinal mode |

| | |
|---|---|
| SMF | single-mode fiber |
| SNR | signal-to-noise ratio |
| SPAD | single-photon avalanche detector |
| SPCM | single-photon counting module |
| SPDT | single-point diamond turning |
| SRS | stimulated Raman scattering |
| STED | stimulated emission depletion |
| SWaP | size, weight, and power |
| SWIR | shortwave IR |
| $t$ | time (sec) |
| $t_f$ | time of flight (sec) |
| $t_{int}$ | detector integration time (sec) |
| $t_s$ | scan time (sec) |
| $T$ | truncation ratio; optical transmittance; temperature (K); torque (N-m) |
| $T_{atm}$ | atmospheric transmission |
| $T_{ext}$ | external transmission |
| $T_{int}$ | internal transmission |
| $T_{opt}$ | optical transmission |
| $T_p$ | pulse period (sec) |
| $T_{PIB}$ | transmitted power-in-bucket |
| $T_{trunc}$ | optical transmission after truncation losses |
| TCK | transfer clock |
| TDL | times diffraction limited |
| TEA | transversely excited atmospheric |
| TEC | thermoelectric cooler |
| $TEM_{pq}$ | transverse electro-magnetic mode with integer number of nodes $p$ and $q$ |
| THG | third-harmonic generation |
| TIA | transimpedance amplifier |
| TIR | total internal reflection |
| TIS | total integrated scatter |
| ToF | time of flight (sec) |
| ULE | ultralow expansion |
| USP | ultrashort pulse |
| UV | ultraviolet |
| $v$ | scan velocity (m/sec) |
| $v_g$ | group velocity (m/sec) |
| $V$ | volume ($cm^3$) |
| $V_b$ | bias voltage (V) |

| | |
|---|---|
| $V_{br}$ | breakdown voltage (V) |
| VAC | volts of alternating current |
| VCSEL | vertical-cavity surface-emitting laser |
| VECSEL | vertical-external-cavity surface-emitting laser |
| VIS | visible |
| VPR | pixel reset voltage |
| VUV | vacuum UV |
| $w(z)$ | Gaussian $1/e^2$ beam radius (mm) |
| $w_o$ | Gaussian $1/e^2$ waist radius (mm) |
| $w_{01}$ | Gaussian $1/e^2$ object-waist radius (mm) |
| $w_{02}$ | Gaussian $1/e^2$ image-waist radius (mm) |
| $w_{oM}$ | laser waist radius for an embedded beam with quality $M^2$ (mm) |
| WD | working distance |
| WFE | wavefront error (μm or waves) |
| WP | wall plug |
| $x$ | transverse coordinate (m) |
| $x_p$ | pixel pitch (μm) |
| $y$ | transverse coordinate (m) |
| $y_{MSF}$ | surface error (nm) |
| $z$ | axial (or longitudinal) propagation axis (m) |
| $z_1$ | object waist-to-lens distance (mm) |
| $z_2$ | lens-to-image waist distance (mm) |
| $z_{FF}$ | far-field distance (m) |
| $z_R$ | Rayleigh range (m) |
| $z_{R1}$ | Rayleigh range of the object waist (m) |
| $z_{R2}$ | Rayleigh range of the image waist (m) |
| $\alpha$ | angular acceleration (rad/sec$^2$) |
| $\alpha_{int}$ | internal loss (1/cm) |
| $\alpha_m$ | mirror loss (1/cm) |
| $\alpha_m(\lambda)$ | material attenuation coefficient (1/cm) |
| $\alpha_t$ | coefficient of thermal expansion (1/K) |
| $\beta_{SA}$ | angular blur size due to spherical aberration (μrad) |
| $\delta$ | mirror dynamic deflection (μm) |
| $\delta_{RMS}$ | RMS surface finish (Å or nm) |
| $\delta_T$ | mirror thermal distortion (μm) |

| | |
|---|---|
| $\Delta d$ | surface figure error (SFE) or irregularity (μm or waves) |
| $\Delta f$ | electrical bandwidth (Hz) |
| $\Delta L$ | change in cavity length (μm) |
| $\Delta L_t$ | change in cavity length due to thermal expansion (μm) |
| $\Delta Q$ | gain bandwidth (J) |
| $\Delta R$ | range resolution (m) |
| $\Delta t_p$ | pulse width (sec) |
| $\Delta T$ | temperature change (C or K) |
| $\Delta v$ | velocity variation (m/sec) |
| $\Delta x$ | distance between spatial features (mm) |
| $\Delta y$ | change in beam-pointing location (μm) |
| $\Delta z_{ast}$ | axial astigmatism (μm) |
| $\Delta \phi$ | phase difference (rad) |
| $\Delta \lambda$ | emission linewidth (μm or nm) |
| $\Delta \lambda_g$ | gain bandwidth (μm or nm) |
| $\Delta \nu$ | emission linewidth (Hz) |
| $\Delta \nu_a$ | axial mode spacing (Hz) |
| $\Delta \nu_g$ | gain bandwidth (Hz) |
| $\Delta \nu_L$ | frequency shift or broadening due to change in cavity length (Hz) |
| $\Delta \nu_{MLM}$ | multi-longitudinal-mode emission linewidth (Hz) |
| $\Delta \nu_R$ | laser or etalon cold-cavity transmission bandwidth (Hz) |
| $\Delta \nu_{SLM}$ | single-longitudinal-mode cold-cavity linewidth (Hz) |
| $\Delta \nu_{ST}$ | Schawlow–Townes single-longitudinal-mode emission linewidth (Hz) |
| $\Delta \theta$ | mirror misalignment angle or change in beam pointing angle (μrad) |
| $\Delta \theta_d$ | diffraction angle |
| $\Delta \theta_m$ | change in mirror mechanical pointing angle |
| $\Delta \omega$ | linewidth (rad/sec) |
| $\Delta \omega_a$ | axial mode spacing (rad/sec) |
| | |
| $\varepsilon$ | obscuration ratio |
| | |
| $\Phi$ | optical power collected by an optical system (W) |
| $\Phi_L$ | refractive or reflective power of a lens or mirror (1/m) |
| | |
| $\gamma_{obs}$ | obscuration loss |
| | |
| $\eta$ | polygon geometric efficiency factor |
| $\eta_{GM}$ | Geiger-mode avalanche efficiency |
| $\eta_s$ | slope efficiency (W/A) |
| $\eta_{QE}$ | quantum efficiency – also see QE |
| $\eta_{WP}$ | wall-plug efficiency (%) |

| | |
|---|---|
| $\lambda$ | wavelength (μm or nm) |
| $\lambda_o$ | center wavelength (μm or nm) |
| | |
| $\nu$ | optical frequency (= $c/\lambda$, Hz) |
| $\nu_m$ | axial mode frequency (Hz) |
| $\nu_p$ | pump optical frequency (Hz) |
| $\nu_{pqm}$ | transverse mode frequency (Hz) |
| | |
| $\theta$ | angular coordinate or angular scan range (rad) |
| $\theta_{01}$ | far-field half-divergence angle incident on lens (rad) |
| $\theta_{02}$ | far-field half-divergence angle exiting lens (rad) |
| $\theta_d$ | diffraction angle (rad) |
| $\theta_{DL}$ | diffraction-limited full-divergence angle (rad) |
| $\theta_o$ | far-field half-divergence angle (rad) |
| $\theta_s$ | scatter angle (rad) |
| $\theta_{slow}$ | slow-axis full-divergence angle (rad) |
| $\dot{\theta}$ | angular velocity (rad/sec) |
| $\ddot{\theta}$ | angular acceleration (rad/sec$^2$) |
| | |
| $\rho$ | power reflectivity; mass density (kg/m$^3$) |
| | |
| $\sigma_{amp}$ | amplifier noise (A) |
| $\sigma_{APD}$ | APD-detector signal noise (A) |
| $\sigma_b$ | detector background noise (A) |
| $\sigma_{dc}$ | detector dark-current noise (A) |
| $\sigma_{FPN}$ | detector spatial noise (A) |
| $\sigma_n$ | detector noise current (A) |
| $\sigma_o$ | second-moment beam radius (mm) |
| $\sigma_P$ | standard deviation of output power (W) |
| $\sigma_{read}$ | detector read noise (A) |
| $\sigma_{RIN}$ | detected RIN noise (A) |
| $\sigma_s$ | detector signal noise (A) |
| $\sigma_{sp}$ | detected speckle noise (A) |
| | |
| $\tau_c$ | coherence time (sec) |
| $\tau_p$ | photon lifetime or energy storage time (sec) |
| | |
| $\omega$ | optical frequency (= $2\pi\nu$, rad/sec) |
| $\Omega$ | modulation frequency (rad/sec); solid angle (sr) |
| $\Omega_{f/\#}$ | solid angle of lens focusing cone (sr) |
| $\Omega_{IFOV}$ | solid angle of pixel IFOV (sr) |

# Index

**Keith J. Kasunic** has more than 30 years of experience developing optical, electro-optical, infrared, and laser systems. He holds a Ph.D. in Optical Sciences from the University of Arizona, an M.S. in Mechanical Engineering from Stanford University, and a B.S. in Mechanical Engineering from MIT. He has worked for or been a consultant to a number of organizations, including Lockheed Martin, Ball Aerospace, Sandia National Labs, and Nortel Networks; he is currently the Technical Director of Optical Systems Group, LLC. He is also the author of two textbooks [*Optical Systems Engineering* (McGraw-Hill, 2011) and *Optomechanical Systems Engineering* (John Wiley, 2015)], an Instructor for SPIE, an Affiliate Instructor with Georgia Tech's SENSIAC, and an Instructor for the Optical Engineering Certificate Program at Univ. of California – Irvine.